"We are indebted to Dr. Libster and Sr. Betty Ann McNeil for this well-researched book. Not only will it significantly contribute to our understanding of ~ ~ing and some of its true 19th-century heroines, it gives us a m~~ ~ ~fining nursing at a time when that was unheard ~f ~ nurse, devoted to what was best for the care o learly about how care should be given, no m~ ; just such a nurse. She will be an inspiration llow her example. Even though the technolo; ...~ struggles Sr. Matilda had will resonate with nurses ~ ~joice in her successes."

Sr. Carol Keehan, DC, RN, MS
President/CEO
The Catholic Health Association of the United States

"*Enlightened Charity* is an intriguing, convincing, and groundbreaking history that contributes to our understanding of the consequences of choices made in the past for current nursing practice. This book presents an American history of nursing that claims a much earlier emergence than the traditionally held view that sees American nursing practice beginning in the late 19th century. This portrayal of the life and nursing of Sister Matilda is a work of art that offers valuable insights into the components of effective nursing practice. It is a most delightful read!"

Sylvia Rinker, RN, PhD
President, American Association for the History of Nursing

"*Enlightened Charity* is a book that will enlighten anyone who is concerned with the history and future of nursing. It raises critical issues about the promise and problems of the religious origins of the profession and the continued use of religious metaphors in framing nursing work. Beautifully written, it brings to our attention not only a lost tradition but also the skills and intelligence that nurses master and practice and that are too often concealed in an etherealization of both the nurse and her practice. We understand from this book how nurses lived their history and traditions and what has been their true legacy. I recommend it not only for the way it unearths this invisible tradition but for the analytical issues it raises and that desperately need discussion in the contemporary nursing universe."

Suzanne Gordon,
Co-Author, *Safety in Numbers:*
Nurse-to-Patient Ratios and the Future of Health Care
Co-Editor, *The Culture and Politics of Health Care Work Series,*
Cornell University Press

"*Enlightened Charity* succeeds as a history that recovers lost memory about the indispensable role of nurses in the 19th-century development of professionalized health care as science and as service. It does so through a relatively unknown account by a very unknown early nurse in the United States who also happened to be a Roman Catholic sister belonging to the Daughters of Charity of St. Vincent de Paul: Matilda Coskery. As a member of a community with a long nursing tradition dating back to the 17th century, Matilda Coskery emerges from the shadows as a towering and paradigmatic figure of wisdom, professionalism, and care. The authors of this study have made a wonderful contribution not just to the histories of nursing but also to the present debate about how nursing can evolve to shape the future of health-care delivery.

Rev. Edward Udovic, CM, PhD
Senior Executive for University Mission
DePaul University

"*Enlightened Charity* is a comprehensive historical perspective of the work of the Sisters and Daughters of Charity and their extraordinary contribution to the foundations of holistic concepts in nursing. It is a delightful read that adds a rich dimension to our knowledge of nursing's holistic roots. This wonderful book really brings forth the importance of understanding our infinite and sacred nature and its centrality in healing."

Lucia Thornton, RN, MSN, AHN-BC
President, American Holistic Nurses Association
Founder of the Model of Whole-Person Caring™

"*Enlightened Charity* is an important contribution to the care and treatment of the mentally ill in America, the hitherto neglected relationship between religion and medicine, and the history of nursing. It sharply revises the traditional history of nursing, which dates the beginning of professionalization in the late nineteenth century, by pointing to the role of religious orders such as their Sisters of Charity who founded the Mount Hope Institution in Baltimore in 1840. Focusing on the career of Sister Matilda Coskery and her hitherto ignored *Advices Concerning the Sick*, Martha M. Libster, PhD, and Sister Betty Ann McNeil have produced an enlightening history that deserves a wide audience."

Gerald N. Grob, PhD
Henry E. Sigerist Professor of the History of Medicine, Emeritus
Rutgers University

"Enlightened Charity is a detailed account of a significant piece of nursing history that offers depth to one's identity as a nurse. The fundamentals of nursing are expressed throughout the book as the story of Sister Matilda and the Sisters of Charity unfolds. Examples of initial assessments, continuous monitoring of patient responses, critical thinking, and planning for individualized care are clearly spelled out in Sister Matilda's writings and the authors' account of their practice. The book grounds nursing practice in a long history of care and concern for the sick. I loved it!"

Cathy Bair McLean, RN, MSN, LMFT, MS
Clinical Assistant Professor of Nursing
East Carolina University College of Nursing

"The authors of *Enlightened Charity* open a window into the nineteenth century, a hidden period of American nursing history. In the book, they describe a religious tradition of nursing, which pre-existed the Nightingale model, and continues today. The exemplar of the tradition, Sr. Matilda Coskery, DC (1799–1870), emerges as an advanced-practice nurse who models a mode and style of psychiatric nursing practice that is enviable. As the reader follows the amazing Sr. Matilda, who founded and managed the first nurse-run psychiatric hospital in the United States, one enters an era where knowledge of neurophysiology and evidenced-based treatment of mental illness was primitive. Yet Sr. Matilda and her religious and medical colleagues practiced moral therapy by creating healing environments and providing compassionate care for psychiatric patients. Interestingly, these nineteenth-century practitioners assessed their patients, were conscious of health-care costs, and reported outcome measurements. During their research for the book, the authors made a wonderful discovery, an unpublished text written by Sr. Matilda Coskery. This primer, *Advices Concerning the Sick*, gives insight into the meaning of a religious tradition of care of the sick poor, which was developed by Vincent de Paul and Louise de Marillac in seventeenth-century Paris and was brought to the United States by Elizabeth Ann Seton. It also sheds light on the beliefs and modalities of nursing in the period. You must read this delightful book."

Sr. Rosemary Donley, SC, PhD, APRN
Ordinary Professor of Nursing, The Catholic University of America
and the Designated Laval Professor of Justice for Underserved People,
Duquesne University School of Nursing

Also by Dr. Martha Libster

Herbal Diplomats:
The Contribution of Early American Nurses
(1830–1860) to Nineteenth-Century Health Care
Reform and the Botanical Medical Movement

Demonstrating Care: The Art of Integrative Nursing

The Integrative Herb Guide for Nurses (Book and CD-Rom with videos)

Also by Sister Betty Ann McNeil, DC

15 Days of Prayer With Saint Elizabeth Ann Seton

The Mountain and Valley of Saint Elizabeth Ann Seton

The Vincentian Family Tree:
A Genealogical Study (Vincentian Studies Institute monographs)

Enlightened Charity

The Holistic Nursing Care, Education,
and Advices Concerning the Sick
of Sister Matilda Coskery, 1799-1870

DR. MARTHA MATHEWS LIBSTER, Ph.D., R.N.

SISTER BETTY ANN McNEIL, D.C., M.S.W.

GOLDEN APPLE PUBLICATIONS

All good wishes —
May this history inspire
memories of your own charitable
to our caring community!

Martha

Editor/Indexer: Triple SSS Press Media Development, Inc.
Book design: Mark Gelotte, www.maeric.com

Printed in the United States of America

Library of Congress Catalog Number: 2009920410

Libster, Martha M, 1960-
    Enlightened charity: holistic nursing care, education,
and "advices concerning the sick" of sister Matilda Coskery,
1799-1870 / Martha M. Libster, Ph.D, R.N. , Sister Betty Ann
McNeil, D.C., M.S.W.
    xxii, 506 p.:ill., p. cm.
    Includes bibliographical references and index
    ISBN 9780975501825

1. Nursing–United States–History 2. United States History -
19th Century 3. Religion-Spirituality-Women's 4. Women–
United States–History   I. Title: Enlightened Charity.
II., McNeil, Sister Betty Ann, 1945-

This book is dedicated to

Sister Aloysia Dugan, DC
(1918–2006)

Teacher—Nurse—Nurse-Educator
Provincial Archivist (1979–1995), Daughters of Charity of
Saint Vincent de Paul Province of Emmitsburg, Maryland

for her humble service and professionalism in the
meticulous preservation of historic records of enduring
value and for sharing her wisdom about the significance
of Sister Matilda Coskery's Advices Concerning the Sick
for study, scholarship, and compassionate nursing care
in the tradition of Sts. Louise de Marillac and
Vincent de Paul.

This book is also dedicated to

Sister Matilda Coskery and Dr. William Stokes,

whom we thank for leaving such a clear trail of healing
inspiration. Finally, this book is dedicated to American
nurses, who we hope will discover a connection with
this caring community of nurses whose history waits
for the weaving of new "threads" into the tapestry of
an important nursing tradition. May you find many
treasures in this early history and a path of enlightened
charity that can transform as well as inform.

— Dr. Martha Mathews Libster and Sister Betty Ann McNeil

Table of Contents

LIST OF FIGURES

Acknowledgments

~ ♏ ~

Enlightened Charity would not have been possible without the assistance of many. While the responsibility for the accuracy of the historical work rests solely with us, we would like to thank the following people and institutions for their kindness and enthusiastic support of this work:

Dr. Libster's research was generously supported by an East Carolina University Research and Creative Activity Grant and a Vincentian Studies Institute Research Grant. We thank Vice Chancellor Dierdre Mageean; Vice Chancellor Phyllis Horns; Dean Sylvia Brown; Associate Deans Alta Andrews, Marti Engelke, and Marie Pokorny; Dr. Mary Ann Rose; and the faculty and staff of the College of Nursing at East Carolina University. We thank Rev. Edward Udovic, CM, presiding officer; and Mr. Nathaniel Michaud, executive director of the Vincentian Studies Institute of the United States, DePaul University in Chicago, Illinois, for their support. We thank Sister Elyse Staab, DC; Sister Claire Debes, DC; and their provincial councils, who supported Sister Betty Ann's involvement in this project from its inception. We are especially grateful for the assistance of Vincentian-Louisian scholar Sister Marie Poole, DC, editor-in-chief and translator, *Vincent de Paul Correspondence, Conferences, and Documents,* for sharing her insights, experience, and expertise.

We thank Ms. Bonnie Weatherly, archives manager; Ms. Selin James and Ms. Mary Anne Weatherly, archival assistants at the Daughters of Charity Archives, Province of Emmitsburg, Maryland, for their gracious assistance, patience, and dedication throughout these many years of detailed research and writing. We also thank Sister Mary Jo Stein, DC, for her assistance and insight during the early stages of research on Sister Matilda Coskery.

Thank you to Dr. Ruth Moskop, Ms. Sue Henry, Ms. Melissa Nasea, and the staffs of the William E. Laupus Health Sciences Library and J. Y. Joyner Library, East Carolina University, Greenville, North Carolina; Mr. Richard Behles, Health Sciences and Human Services Library, University of Maryland; Dr. Rob Schoeberlein, Ms. Nancy Bramucci, and Mr. Michael McCormick of the Maryland State Archives, Annapolis, Maryland; Ms. Andrea Bainbridge, American Medical Association; Ms. Lois Martin and the staff at the Mater Dei Provincialate, Daughters of Charity Archives, Evansville, Indiana; Rev. John Schipp and staff at the Old Cathedral Library and Museum in Vincennes, Indiana; Dr. Tricia Pyne, Ms. Allison Foley and the staff of the Associated Archives of the Archdiocese of Baltimore at St. Mary's Seminary & University; Mr. John Diefenderfer, DePaul Provincial House, Albany, New York; Sister Ellen Clifford, Archives of the Sisters of Charity of Nazareth in Bardstown, Kentucky; Ms. Morgen MacIntosh and Ms. Kathryn De Graff, DeAndreis-Rosati Memorial Archives, DePaul University; Sister Ana Maria Olmeda, DC, secretary general, and Sister Christa Bauer, DC, general councillor, Company of the Daughters of Charity of Saint Vincent de Paul, Paris, France; Mr. Ted Delaney and Ms. Jane White of the Old City Cemetery and Museum, Lynchburg, Virginia; Mr. James McColery of Thomson Reuters for his help with Endnote; John Hargett; Ms. Glenda Stewart, administrative assistant to Dr. Libster; Ms. Natasha Worthington, administrative assistant to the ECU Research Faculty; and student research assistants Ms. Allison Morgan, Ms. Carol Ann Rose, and Ms. Gillian Jones.

We appreciate the input of the following reviewers, who provided important perspectives as we finalized the work:

Dr. Sylvia Rinker

Dr. Mary Johnson

Ms. Cathy McLean

On a more personal note, we are eternally grateful for the interest and encouragement of the Daughters of Charity at Mother Seton House in Emmitsburg, Maryland; Harold Libster; and our families and friends, who provided ongoing support to us during this project. We also would like to thank our book designer, Mark Gelotte, and our editors, Eileen Clawson, Josephine Cepeda, and Susan Simpfenderfer, for their attunement to this historical work and their tireless attention to detail.

Finally, we would like to thank St. Vincent, St. Louise, and St. Elizabeth Ann Seton for inspiration that always seemed to manifest as impeccable timing, synergistic interaction, historical discovery, and insight.

— Dr. Martha Mathews Libster and Sister Betty Ann McNeil

Professional Nursing in America before the Nightingale Model

Some years ago I was researching the history of the nineteenth-century botanical health reform movement for a book project on nurses and herbal remedies. Text after historical text revealed nothing. I even spoke to the scholars who had written the histories of the American Botanical Movement as well as other historians of early and mid-nineteenth-century America. They confirmed that I would have a hard time finding evidence of the nurses of the period. By the end of two years of searching, however, I had acquired more data on early and mid-nineteenth-century *professional* nursing, midwifery, and nurse-herbalism than I had dreamed was possible.

It was during that historical quest that I met Sister Betty Ann McNeil, a Daughter of Charity and archivist for the community of religious women, who introduced me to a very special book, *Advices Concerning the Sick*. The Daughters have deduced that *Advices* was written by Sister Matilda Coskery in the mid-nineteenth century as an instruction manual for the novice nurses whom Sister Matilda prepared for caring missions. Neither *Advices* nor the early nursing history of the American Daughters has ever been published.

In fact, very little historical scholarship has been conducted on the subject of American nursing prior to the Civil War. Perhaps this is because many twentieth- and twenty-first-century textbooks and nursing histories state that "professional" nursing in America began in 1873 with the adoption of the Nightingale model of nursing at Bellevue Hospital in New

York. Many American textbooks deem British nurse Florence Nightingale to be the "mother of modern nursing" and her advice book, *Notes on Nursing*, an early treatise on nursing care. I, like many others, have had little reason to question this history; Nightingale was and is an incredibly influential nurse. But then I discovered the histories of American nurses of the early nineteenth century—Shakers, Mormons, and Daughters of Charity—and my interest was piqued. Florence Nightingale's work became prominent after her trip to the Crimea and the publication of her book in 1859. The nurses I found as a result of my research into the history of the American Botanical Movement were working as professional nurses within their religious communities and in some cases serving the larger public decades before 1859. These women, it seemed, had also had a hand in the "mothering" of American nursing!

As my historical research was transformed into the book titled *Herbal Diplomats*,[1] I realized that I could not end my work with the American Botanical Movement. I became increasingly interested in the period leading up to the adoption of the Nightingale model, which represented the introduction of secularization reform of American nursing in the later nineteenth century. The meaning of secularization in nursing at that time specifically meant the distancing of the practice of nursing from its centuries-old religious ties. The reform movement focused on creating opportunities for women to be educated as nurses without having to enter religious life. However, as will be explained in this book, secularization also became equated with professionalism. This ultimately led to the removal of the early contributions of religious nurses such as the Daughters of Charity in American nursing history.

I felt a calling from the early "mothers" of American nursing in religious communities to tell their stories and to examine secularization reform within a broader historical context that included the work of religious nurses. I decided to focus my research specifically on Sister Matilda Coskery's work and the nursing care provided by American Sisters of Charity from Emmitsburg, Maryland, known after 1850 as "Daughters of Charity." My hope was that I would glean a greater understanding of early and mid-nineteenth-century nursing culture through the lens of the Daughters of Charity community. I found the Sisters' history helpful in illuminating the movement from nursing in a religious community to secularization and also very relevant to contemporary nursing practice.

The healing heritage of the American Sisters of Charity was inspired by the seventeenth-century community of the Daughters of Charity, founded by Vincent de Paul and Louise de Marillac in Paris, France. The Vincentian-Louisian tradition[2] of nursing the "sick poor"[3] was carried to America in 1809 by Elizabeth Ann Seton, the foundress of the American Sisters of Charity. Chapters 1 and 2 of this book provide an overview of the underlying French and American history of the Community. While the Community's mission included the education and care of the poor in schools and orphanages, the focus of this history is the Sisters' nursing ministry from hospitals and asylums to the battlefield. Chapters 3 through 6 explore the contributions to the professional nursing of the period by Sister Matilda Coskery, her *Advices* text, and her Sister-Nurse companions. Sister Matilda and the Daughters of Charity were contemporaries of Florence Nightingale. They were influenced by European nursing, but they were American—it is important for American nurses to know the history of nursing spawned on American soil because that is the foundation for their professional identity.

For the past four years, Sister Betty Ann and I have been researching the life, the ministry, and the nursing care of Sister Matilda and the early Sister-Nurses. We bring our backgrounds in writing histories of nursing, religious women living in community, and American healthcare culture to this twenty-first-century mission; to tell a story of a humble yet powerful woman who, with many other devoted Sisters of her community as well as visionary physicians, helped launch a national mission of charity expressed in the Vincentian-Louisian tradition of nursing care of the sick poor and the insane. This is a history of leadership; early American nursing education; and a holistic approach to care that addressed the spiritual, emotional, and psychological as well as the physical needs of all patients. It is a history of the migration of caring knowledge from Europe to America and of the relationship of nurses and physicians who chose to share responsibility for building an enlightened healthcare system.

The history of Sister Matilda moves me as a human being and as a professional psychiatric nurse. Her work compels me to find meaning in the works of nineteenth-century nurses that might also inspire nurses today. British historian Edward Hallett Carr wrote that "learning from history is never a one way process" and that "the function of history is to promote a profounder understanding of both past and present through interrelation between them."[4] I agree. The motivation for writing this history is indeed to promote understanding. Raising awareness of early American nursing through the study of history is important to professional and personal identity; I believe this because my students have shown me that this is so.

Many American nurses and nursing students with whom I have interacted over the years since my first early American research know about Florence Nightingale and *Notes on Nursing*. And yet none seemed to know about the work of the Daughters of Charity. I found myself wondering what would happen if American nurses knew that there were *professional* nurses, formal vocational education, and at least one nursing textbook prior to 1873. In the four years since the completion of the research for *Herbal Diplomats*, I have had the opportunity to introduce many American nurses, educators, and historians as well as undergraduate, graduate, and doctoral students to the work of the early Daughters of Charity *(See Appendix E)*. The response is the same; they say, "I had no idea that there were professional nurses back then" and "how come more people don't know about this part of our history?" They are often astonished to find the professional values they hold, such as evidence-based reflective practice; critical thinking; leadership; professional ethics; and holistic, spiritually guided service described in the history of the early Sisters.

I am not surprised at their wonder because I have searched for early American histories and found there to be a distinct lack of detail on early American nursing and the professional nurse before 1873. Their questions and enthusiasm for understanding the history have served as the primary inspiration for writing this book. I approached Sister Betty Ann and the Daughters of Charity at St. Joseph's Provincial House in Emmitsburg, Maryland, with the stories of my students and colleagues who recognized that their lives had been "changed" professionally and personally and that their sense of the purpose for nursing had been deepened by studying the history of the early Sisters and Daughters of Charity.

This experience was not new to the Daughters! Soon after Sister Betty Ann was appointed archivist for the Emmitsburg Province of the Daughters of Charity, she invited her predecessor, Sister Aloysia Dugan, DC, to walk through the collection and highlight various record groups that contained valuable documents or artifacts that might otherwise be overlooked. As a nurse for over thirty years and chair of the Nursing Department of Saint Joseph College for ten years, Sister Aloysia, who had begun her formation with the Daughters of Charity at the Mount Hope Retreat, delighted in explaining the historic significance of Sister Matilda's *Advices Concerning the Sick* to Sister Betty Ann, a clinical social worker. Sister Aloysia expressed regret at never having the opportunity or time to promote public knowledge of this manuscript or publish it. Thus the seed was planted and germinated as Sister Betty Ann prayed for the opportunity for this document to be the subject of research and publication. A few years later when I met Sister Betty Ann, we decided to write the history, and our mission began.

American nurses of all faiths, races, genders, ethnicities, and cultures have responded similarly to the historical evidence I share with them of the professional nurses of the early nineteenth century. They marvel at the professional roots of the discipline. But while history has a way of offering new and refreshing perspectives, it can also be quite challenging. Historical evidence is not always what we want it to be, just as the outcomes of a clinical trial may not support the initial hopes embedded in the desire of the scientist. The historian is also a scientist whose object is the exploration of the patterns of human behavior as data over time. The study of history, like the study of science, is about putting the "things" and "events" of the universe in order so patterns can be seen, heard, and intuited. As we researched Sister Matilda and the early nursing missions of the Sisters and then Daughters of Charity it became evident that the history, the patterns emerging from the archival records, was not the history we "knew." We have had years during the research process to adapt to the notion that there were professional nurses in the early and mid-nineteenth century and that the history we were constructing would suggest a significant change in the historical literature on the history of American nursing. Some readers of this history may adapt to the change in a matter of pages, but we also understand that for others hearing this new historical piece of the creation story of professional culture in American nursing may be more challenging.

For over a century American nurses have read histories that state that nurses who cared for patients before the adoption of the Nightingale model were not professional. As will be discussed in more detail later in this book, they are often portrayed as uneducated, ill prepared for their work, and merely empirical in their approach. At best, nurses were characterized as disobedient to physicians, a quality that proper training could fix. At worst, nurses were depicted as drunkards and whores who could not be trusted to perform the real work of caring and curing. But nurses at times could be counted on for the custodial care that few in society would agree to do for little if any pay. Hearing this story so many times over the years left me with a sense that there was certainly nothing redeeming in the history of American nursing prior to the adoption of the Nightingale model of training. When I found evidence of early professional American nursing, I was overjoyed, but I did not know why. It took me a while to understand the beauty and importance of *national* heritage and professional identity. Nurses' professional heritage informs our ability to build a strong community of scholars, healers, and educators. Community can be a balm for healing the sense of isolation and loneliness that can occur in the health professions. The history of the Sisters and Daughters of Charity offers nurses the opportunity to engage in historical study as a professional community-building experience.

The Sisters and Daughters of Charity healing tradition was founded in the mission of community. This history is the story of their early service to the sick poor, particularly the insane. Sister Matilda's story of professional practice is significant and extensive enough to fill this book. But she did not work alone. In fact, as you will read here, she is rarely mentioned by name in historical documents. We surmise that in her devotion to her spiritual mission of charity, simplicity, and humility she would not have allowed herself to be mentioned or singled out by name. Her focus would have been the work of the "little company," as the cofounders called the community of women from the time of their inception. There are no personal diaries written by Sister Matilda, but Community history and historical evidence provides support that she authored a journal account of the early history of the Mount Hope Retreat, the asylum she started in the 1840s, and *Advices Concerning the Sick*, the nursing fundamentals textbook for new Sister-Nurses that demonstrates her nursing skill as well as her thoughts and feelings about nursing the sick and insane. The two documents, the journal and *Advices*, became the focus for our construction of this history. We felt that *Advices* most certainly needed to be published for American nurses, as well as those globally who are interested in the history of women, the Sisters and Daughters of Charity, women in religious life, and nursing. Sister Matilda's text exemplifies the level of knowledge, skill, and expertise of an early American nurse who led a group of religious women into a public sphere of male physicians and hospital administrators where they would care for and serve without hesitation the sick poor and the insane, a patient population who were repugnant to society.

The importance of humility and community to Sister Matilda and the early Sisters posed a challenge for this history. It is important to stay true to the data in any research-based project, and therefore a history that focused on Sister Matilda had to stay true to and respect her chosen path of humility and community. While there are biographical sections about Sister Matilda placed chronologically throughout this book that describe her charitable work and service, this history is not a biography of Sister Matilda Coskery per se. The difference is subtle, but as one gets to know Sister Matilda and the Community of early American Sister-Nurses, it becomes clear that the truest characterization of any sister discussed individually should be represented within the context of her role as a vessel for the spirit of community mission.

We hope that this history of the nursing care of the Sisters and Daughters of Charity, which includes Sister Matilda's *Advices,* brings the work of the Vincentian-Louisian nursing tradition into the public eye in a new way and shows that Sister Matilda Coskery and her companion nurses were archetypal professional nurses of the nineteenth century. This period was formative in American nursing and in the development of American hospitals and healthcare culture. We realize that this work of discovery of a lost period in American nursing is just a beginning. More research is needed to produce the fullest account of nursing during a time in American history when the social, religious, and political issues of health reform were the center of public attention.

American nursing history, like the history of American medicine, is connected culturally with the histories of other countries. Early American nurses' history of caring for the sick has its roots in the nursing heritage of France, Ireland, England, West Africa, Mexico, and China. In addition,

American nursing history is rooted in the healing practices of the indigenous people of Turtle Island (United States and Canada). There are many early histories needed to mend the gap in knowledge about early American nursing history. This book will provide one perspective, that of the migration of the French Vincentian-Louisian nursing tradition to America in the work of the Sisters and Daughters of Charity.

This book is a history of Catholic-American women nurses. It is an exploration of the nature of early and mid-nineteenth-century American nursing, most particularly nursing education and clinical skills, the relationship between nurses and physicians, and nurse autonomy as a measure of professionalism. The details of Sister Matilda's instruction manual for nurses, *Advices Concerning the Sick,* are examined for keys to understanding the thoughts, beliefs, and motivations of nurses of the period who, like Sister Matilda, were called spiritually to the practice of nursing. Physicians, writers, and some among the public said that it was the Sisters' "enlightened charity" that made them stand out as professionals from among the larger society of caring women. This is the story of that "something different" they were said to have possessed.

Dr. Martha M. Libster
Farmville, North Carolina

Sister Betty Ann McNeil
Emmitsburg, Maryland

That Something Different

Upon his retirement in the year 1887, William Hughes Stokes (1812–1893), had been a physician for fifty-three years. He received his medical degree at the University of Maryland in 1834 and gained his early clinical experience "reading medicine" with Drs. Donaldson and Stewart of Baltimore before interning at the Baltimore Infirmary.[1] At the infirmary Stokes worked alongside the Sisters of Charity Nurses who had assumed the "whole direction and management of the institution"[2] in 1823 at the request of Dr. Granville Sharp Pattison (1791–1851) and the professors of the College of Medicine of Maryland at the University of Maryland. After receiving his degree, Stokes accepted a position as resident physician for the Maryland Hospital for the Insane,[3] a state hospital. During his time at both institutions as he worked with the Sisters of Charity of St. Joseph's (SC), Stokes developed a love for the care of the insane, who were some of the most marginalized and misunderstood of early nineteenth-century society. He wrote in 1843 that "in the whole catalogue of human maladies there is no one calculated to enlist so profoundly the sympathies of the physician, and to animate him to a diligent endeavor to possess himself of the means ascertained to be most available for relieving it, than insanity."[4]

Stokes's quest for the most compassionate care of insane patients forced him to leave the Maryland Hospital for the Insane. After only one year Stokes moved to Georgia in 1835, where he held a general practice for five years. He would later write that the "whole system of treatment" of the insane at the Maryland Hospital had been "radically wrong."[5] In 1841 he visited the Hanwell Asylum in England to study the implementation of Dr. John Conolly's new system of nonrestraint used in the care of persons suffering from insanity. Upon his return Stokes joined SC Nurse Matilda Coskery, with whom he had worked at the Maryland Hospital, to open the Mount Saint Vincent's Hospital,[6] referred to after 1844 as the Mount

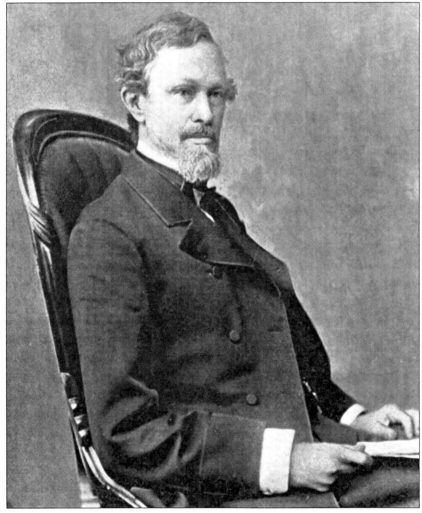

Fig. I-1   *Dr. William Hughes Stokes*

Hope Institution or Retreat, the first Catholic hospital for the insane in the United States. Sister Matilda and the other SC left the Maryland Hospital in 1839 because they also were unable to influence administration to make changes the Sisters felt were necessary. Sister Matilda was the Sister Servant or head nurse of the new hospital. Stokes served only as consulting physician to the SC Nurses who owned and administered all activities at the hospital, an unusual achievement for women of the period.

By establishing his role as "consulting" physician rather than "resident" physician, Stokes and the Sisters of Charity challenged the emerging medical dominance in American healthcare. In the early years of the Mount Hope mission, Dr. Stokes defended not only his right to serve Mount Hope as a consultant but also the right of the Sisters to hold administrative and clinical control within their facility. He also supported their right to lead the mission of reinventing the care of the institutionalized insane, at least those entrusted to their care. Dr. Stokes wrote in an institutional report:

> We have endeavored . . . not only to keep pace with the advancing science in the treatment of the insane, but have earnestly labored to raise it to a higher and broader plane of service; and thus fulfill its great mission of benevolence and charity, with a rigor, which would increase, rather than diminish, with age.[7]

By 1852 the work of Dr. Stokes, Sister Matilda, and the SC Nurses (now the Daughters of Charity) was acknowledged nationally. Just twelve years into their mission, Dorothea Dix, the renowned American reformer of mental health institutions, reported (despite being notably anti-Catholic) that Mount Hope was one of two successful facilities for the treatment of persons with mental illness in the state of Maryland.[8] The Stokes-SC model of care for persons who were insane was based upon a "law of humanity and kindness," for which Stokes determined the SC were "peculiarly qualified."[9] The Sisters who were educated for their service following the healing tradition of seventeenth-century French founders Vincent de Paul (1581–1660) and Louise de Marillac (1591–1660) were known for possessing something different in the way they cared for persons who were sick and insane. The American Sisters and their French counterparts, the Daughters of Charity, held an international reputation for benevolence, charity, and excellence in nursing care. Stokes stated in his third annual report that the SC Nurses practiced an "enlightened and universal charity."[10]

Enlightened charity was a virtue venerated by early nineteenth-century Europeans and Americans alike. For example, woman's rights activist Catherine Barmby of England wrote in 1839 that enlightened charity was a "lovely attribute of humanity" for which she prayed that she and her "fellow creatures might in all our future words and deeds be under its controul.[sic]"[11] She cited the following example:

> True it is, that for all the evils man has committed, for all the sufferings woman has endured, and great they are, and have been, — there is none among the living or the dead that justly we should censure or condemn. Charity, enlightened charity, gives us the key to this fact.[12]

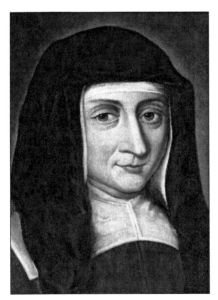
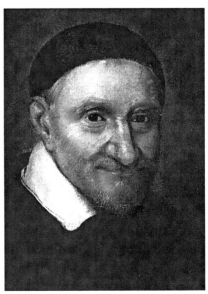

Fig. I-2   *Louise de Marillac and Vincent de Paul*

Courtesy, Daughters of Charity Archives, Emmitsburg, Maryland

4

During the eighteenth and into the early nineteenth century, Americans and Europeans engaged in a period often referred to historically as the Enlightenment, a time when the exploration of reason was prevalent in society, particularly among the elite. Practically all key Enlightenment thinkers were men, such as Voltaire, who argued that true knowledge was gleaned through experience and experiment rather than the a priori reasoning of seventeenth-century thinkers.[13] Reason and science, "Enlightened" thinkers believed, would lead potentially to a more satisfied and humane existence but separated from experience and sensitivity could lead to error. By the nineteenth century Victorians were often dismissing the Enlightenment movement as mechanical, bereft of deep thought, and in some instances immoral. Some scholars have argued that those with authority and power in society who exercised their "reason" did so to "increase their power and enhance their authority, in ways which often penalized the poor, weak, and inarticulate."[14]

Stokes, a learned and well-traveled man, often emphasized in his written reports the importance of utilizing a rational approach in the medical care of the insane. The practice of the enlightened physician of the period was to be based on "experience guided by reason."[15] While Stokes's rational treatments included the "careful deliberation" and "cautious investigation of the peculiarities of each case,"[16] he assigned the "enlightened charity" of the SC Nurses to a different origin more in keeping with nineteenth-century Romantic thought, the soul. In 1845 Stokes stated that the virtues of kindness and benevolence demonstrated by the SC Nurses at Mount Hope in the care of the insane were the "direct emanations and blessed fruits of that enlightened and universal charity which they so beautifully illustrate by their lives, and which has its imperishable root in the Christian religion."[17] The "roots" of the charitable works of the Sisters' enlightened care lay in a healing tradition to uplift and heal the sick poor by serving the insane patient with a love that the SC Nurse would extend to Jesus Christ himself.

This healing, nursing tradition was established by Vincent de Paul and Louise de Marillac in the original confraternity[18] of sisters in France in 1633, soon named by the people the Daughters of Charity (DC). The nursing tradition observed as "enlightened and universal charity" by Stokes was witnessed by many others in Europe and America. In both domestic and public circles the Vincentian-Louisian nursing tradition was considered different from the care of the sick observed in other nurses, attendants, and community women healers of the time.

By the mid-nineteenth century the reputation of the American SC Nurses was well established in the minds of the public and its healthcare providers. Popular nineteenth-century domestic-advice writers Catharine Beecher and Harriet Beecher Stowe told of an exchange concerning the Sisters' reputation that Beecher had with a woman at the time of the American Civil War:

> "Are the Sisters of Charity really better nurses than most other women?" I asked an intelligent lady who had seen much of our military hospitals. "Yes they are," was her reply. "Why should it be so?" "I think it is because with them it is a work of self-abnegation, and of duty to God, and they are so quiet and self-forgetful in its exercise that they do it better, while many other women show such self-consciousness and are so fussy![19]

Catholic and Protestant women sought to "emulate" the Sisters of Charity of St. Vincent de Paul in "number and usefulness."[20] The authors of a popular book on sickroom management wrote, "A Society has been formed in London for the instruction of sick nurses. Those sent out go by the name of the Protestant Sisters of Charity, and are taught to perform all the offices of charity for which the Roman Catholic Sisters of Charity have been so long distinguished."[21]

Physicians too sang the praises of the DC and SC. In 1825 Dr. Robert Gooch, a renowned British medical authority of the nineteenth century, suggested that "all real Christians join and found an order of women like the Sisters of Charity in Catholic countries" such as France and Belgium.[22] And in 1869 a report of the American Medical Association's Committee on the Training of Nurses specifically recognized the works of the SC:

> The Committee cannot permit this opportunity to pass without paying a feeble tribute of respect and admiration to the Sisters of Charity, on account of the noble work

in which, for upwards of two centuries, they have been steadily engaged, in carrying out the objects for which their order and the various branches growing out of it were originally instituted. A more honest, upright, and devoted, self-sacrificing body of women never existed. The Catholic Church, under whose direction and auspices they have so long and so faithfully labored, has set an example worthy of the imitation of all denominations of Protestants, who it cannot be denied, have too long stood aloof from this great work which reflects so much credit upon their Catholic brethren. No one can witness the disinterested sacrifices of the Sisters of Charity—their unceasing devotion to the sick and the dying, their unflinching courage in times of epidemics, their daily toils, and their midnight vigils for the benefit of suffering human beings—without the most profound admiration for their character, and a deep sense of gratitude to Almighty God for permitting such beings to dwell among men.[23]

The American Catholic community was well aware of the achievements of their nursing sisterhoods. News of the success of the SC quickly pervaded Catholic social networks. In 1834 the Rev. Frederick Rese, Bishop of Detroit, wrote the following in a letter to the SC leadership in Maryland: "Your Sisters have been successful by a particular blessing and Providence in gaining the fond wishes of the good citizens nearly all over the United States, and are therefore very well calculated to further the interests of the Kingdom of God here on earth."[24] By midcentury, at the time of the opening of the St. John's Infirmary in Milwaukee, the *Catholic Almanac* reported that "the very title and profession of a Daughter of St. Vincent de Paul are sufficient guaranties to the public that there will be no departure from the strictest order, the greatest cleanliness and the most unremitting attention."[25]

The enlightened charity of the early and mid-nineteenth century SC Nurses detailed in subsequent chapters was a result of the successful cultural migration, transmission, and integration of a two-hundred-year-old Vincentian-Louisian healing heritage from France to the United States.

The humility, simplicity, and charity of the Community of American SC Nurses was translated into a holistic nursing practice and educational preparation for nurses that conveyed the deeply devout intentions of the Sisters for their healing missions to serve both the corporal and spiritual needs of the sick poor. The following chapters provide definition and context for the enlightened charity demonstrated by American SC in the early and mid-nineteenth century. The SC's contributions to the development of an American healthcare system, its health policies regarding the care of the mentally ill, nursing education, and the doctor-nurse relationship are also explored. For decades Dr. Stokes, a devout Episcopalian, in collaboration with the SC, reevaluated, researched, and ultimately reconstructed the treatment of the insane into a holistic model that encompassed the care of body, mind, and spirit. His writings and his long tenure with the SC demonstrate that he had realized a dream with the SC nurses: to implement what he thought to be the most innovative care representative of an ethic of charity and kindness that both Stokes and the Sisters believed had the greatest potential to fully heal the insane, some of the most marginalized people in nineteenth-century American society.

The women of the Vincentian-Louisian nursing tradition valued and continued to hold their spirit of community in highest regard. As will be demonstrated throughout this account of one small but significant part of their history, individual SC did not and do not, for the sake of the mission, set themselves apart from their sisters in community. For this reason, it was uncharacteristic (although not forbidden) for any SC to keep a personal diary or journal other than a spiritual journal for personal reflection and devotion. However, the Sisters did keep Community and mission records, many of which have been used to construct this historical account of early nursing missions. The most lengthy and detailed of early Sisters' nursing-mission records are two accounts attributed to Sister Matilda Coskery: *Cradle of Mount Hope: Historical Account of Mt. St. Vincent Hospital/Mount Hope Retreat*[26] and an instruction book for nurses entitled *Advices Concerning the Sick.*[27] These two manuscripts provide extraordinary insight into the lives and works of professional nurses in the early and mid-nineteenth century. They also explain the unique perspectives and practices that served as foundation for the enlightened charity of Sister Matilda and other SC Nurse pioneers.

This book draws extensively from both of the documents attributed to Sister Matilda. Matilda's history would be incomplete, however, without the specific context for those documents. The chapters that follow describe the spiritual tradition that formed and enlightened her, the community life that prepared and nurtured her, and the nursing service that sustained her. Some of Sister Matilda's biographical history is included throughout the chapters, but the focus of this work is her mission and ministry. The nursing missions of the SC and Sister Matilda in particular serve as the contextual center for this book. While we are by necessity singling out Sister Matilda and her missions in order to tell a story, we want to state clearly that we have made every attempt to honor the spirit of the Vincentian-Louisian tradition and the memory of Sister Matilda by writing a history that elucidates her lived experience within an apostolic[28] community of religious women. It is in the Community of the Sisters of Charity of St. Joseph's in Emmitsburg, Maryland, that this story begins for Sister Matilda Coskery.

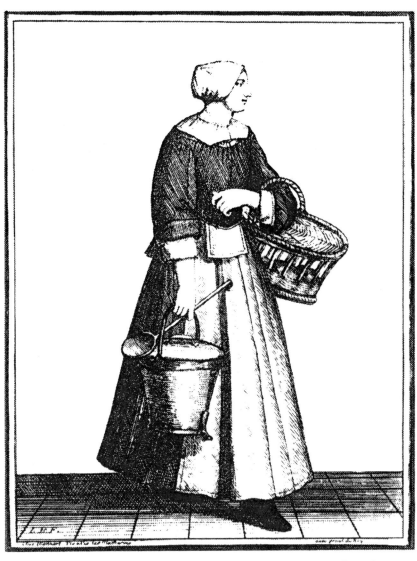

Fig. 1-1   *17th Century Daughter of Charity of St. Vincent de Paul in France*

CHAPTER I

A Healing Heritage of
Holistic Nursing Care

The care of the sick poor and the insane has historically been a challenge for society. The American Sisters and Dr. Stokes embarked upon a very difficult mission in 1840 that was not without precedent. The French Daughters of Charity, predecessors of and models for the American SC, had been working with the sick poor and the insane for nearly two centuries when the American Community began. On November 29, 1633, a French priest named Vincent de Paul and a widow from an aristocratic family, Louise de Marillac,[1] founded the Company of the Daughters of Charity (DC), Servants of the Sick Poor, at Paris. Three years earlier Vincent had entrusted Louise with the formation and training of the young women who were volunteering to devote themselves to the work of parish-based Confraternities of Charity. Vincent had been directing Confraternities of Charity throughout the countryside of France since the movement's inception at Châtillon-les-Dombes (l'Ain)[2] in France, August 23, 1617. The first Confraternity of Charity in Paris was established in the parish of Saint-Sauveur in 1629. The next year Marguerite Naseau (1594–1633) of Suresnes offered her services to Vincent to nurse the sick. Vincent sent Marguerite and others who followed her example to Louise for training in nursing and ministry. For Marguerite and the DC throughout the years and to the present day, the mission is the same:

> The charity of Jesus Christ crucified, which animates and
> sets afire the heart of the Daughter of Charity, urges her

to hasten to the relief of every type of human misery.[3]

Louise and Vincent held "conferences" regularly after 1641 to form the confraternity of sisters to serve with gentleness, courtesy, and deep respect the sick poor who were in need.[4] Documents from these conferences provide a running commentary on the way of life of the DC. Initially, the sisters, called "servants of the poor," provided nursing care as well as education and ministry to poor people in the towns and villages surrounding Paris. Over time, as the need arose, Louise and Vincent sent the DC Nurses to care for the sick in hospitals, orphanages, prisons, the battlefield, and insane asylums throughout the country. Within a twenty-year period (1640–1660), the early sisters managed nursing care in eight general hospitals throughout France. The cofounders devised innovative ways to avoid the conventions of their day that confined religious women to the cloister. One of these was the development of a nomenclature unique to the DC and their mission. For example, the sisters lived in houses, not convents; their religious formation was in seminaries, not novitiates; and their vows were made annually in private instead of perpetual profession in public. The Protestant Reformation had suppressed noncloistered religious life for women, and the Tridentine decrees of the Catholic Reformation in 1563 demanded that all nuns live within convent walls. By the early seventeenth century, there were no Protestant communities of nurses remaining, and Catholic leadership had also denied the requests of their religious women to practice nursing.

Francis de Sales (1576–1622) and Jane Frances de Chantal (1572–1641) cofounded the Visitation of Holy Mary, a community of religious women in Annecy in 1610. After the death of de Sales, who had established a Visitation Monastery in Paris in 1621, Vincent de Paul became the ecclesiastical superior of the nuns. Vincent and Louise both had become acquainted with Francis de Sales and knew him well. Francis de Sales's writings, in particular his *Introduction to the Devout Life*, were part of Vincent's, Louise's, and their followers' spiritual readings.[5] The spiritual foundation for the nursing ministry of the Visitadines (Visitation nuns) and the Vincentian-Louisian DC (apostolic Community) was influenced by the teachings of Francis de Sales and Jane de Chantal. For these two leaders, friendship was a unique form of love that served as a "medium for which the love and knowledge of the loving God was cultivated."[6] They held the beliefs that the individual heart of all devout persons, who came from every walk of life, could be transformed to the heart of Jesus and that it was through the transformation of the heart in friendships between people that societies were transformed.[7]

The nursing tradition of Vincent and Louise was cofounded upon this heartfelt friendship and mutuality in ministry. Louise and Vincent collaborated in governing and instructing the growing Community through visits, advices, correspondence, and Community documents. They negotiated business arrangements together and developed education for the DC Nurses in the spiritual and corporal care of the sick. To prepare the women for their work, Vincent and Louise instructed the sisters in Community life and nursing skills, which included the spiritual values essential for service to the poor. The teachings of the founders shaped the DC tradition of service, influenced their ministries, and over time enabled them to maintain a clear focus on their mission to serve "Our Lord in the person of His poor people," believing that Jesus Christ "recognizes as done to Himself the service they render to the sick poor."[8]

Initially, the DC provided pastoral care but not nursing care in hospitals. Louise was concerned about the poor sanitation in the facilities and also the state of physician care. Vincent de Paul noted public sentiment about physicians in a letter to Louise, saying, "After all, people think that doctors kill more patients than they cure."[9] Louise had expressed her "anxiety" for the health of her son, an only child, who was under the care of a physician. Even after the DC began managing large hospitals, Vincent de Paul admonished Louise to be submissive to physicians' recommendations.[10] Louise was also concerned that hospital service would distract the DC from their primary vocation of serving the sick poor in their homes. She was concerned that the sick poor would have to leave their homes to obtain care from the DC in the hospitals and that the affluent in society who had fallen on hard times would not come to a public institution such as a hospital for care.[11] Impelled by the Charity of Jesus Christ, which drove the DC in their mission of serving their "Lords and Masters the Poor" despite penal attitudes and societal regulations of the Great Confinement of persons in abject poverty, the sisters, just seven years after being founded, entered into hospital nursing in addition to their home care of the sick in the parishes.[12] Louise de Marillac signed the contract for their first hospital mission February 1, 1640, at the Hôtel-Dieu in Angers.[13] The vision and mission of the DC at Angers was "to honor Our Lord, Father of the Poor, and His Holy Mother, in order to assist, corporally and spiritually, the sick poor of the Hôtel-Dieu of the town: corporally, by serving them and giving them food and medicine; spiritually, by instructing the patients in things necessary for salvation.[14] The Angers mission laid the foundation for the DC's holistic nursing tradition.

∼ The Spirit of the Company ∼

Vincent de Paul and Louise de Marillac, by referring to their Community as a "Company" or "Confraternity of Charity" and not as a religious order, were able to successfully petition the Archbishop of Paris for approval of the women's ministry as a Confraternity in 1655. The DC ultimately received approval from Pope Clement IX in 1668. The nursing care of the sick poor in their homes was a clear demonstration of the divergence from the work and social position of other religious women, and yet their work was founded upon deep spiritual roots. The following is a poetic description of the DC's simple lifestyle of service:

> They [the Daughters of Charity] shall keep in mind that they [have] for monastery only the houses of the sick; for cell a rented room; for cloister the streets of the city; for enclosure obedience going only to the homes of the sick and to places necessary for their service; for grill fear of God; for veil holy modesty; and making no other profession to ensure their vocation than their constant trust in Divine Providence and the offering they make to God of all that they are and of their service in the person of the poor.[15]

Francis de Sales had referred to women who participated in the ministry as "women apostles."[16] The DC were not established as "nuns" but as "apostolic women." The difference was very meaningful at the time because the new company entered the homes of the sick poor. They were not cloistered as were the nuns of the period but were women who would "come and go like seculars"[17] as they fulfilled their missions. Vincent preferred the vocabulary of "mission"[18] to refer to the DC's service to God, which in the Vincentian-Louisian tradition meant serving the poor. Louise encouraged the DC to work together for the sake of mission and to be particularly mindful of interpersonal relationships—the "support of one another, graciousness and submission, and perfect harmony."[19] It was the imitation of Jesus Christ in their apostolic ministry or mission of the DC Nurses that led them to strive for humility, simplicity, and charity in their ministry and service.

Holy Practices— Humility, Simplicity, and Charity ⌒

The DC sought involvement in God's charitable work. They were urged by their founders to be the instruments of a loving God. Their mission was originally established as a community effort. Louise's leadership often focused on building a community, a unity of spirit among the sisters. Her letters often advised sisters to support each other in all things. She applied this to everyone, sisters in positions of leadership and companions[20] alike. For example, she wrote to the sisters at Brienne in 1652, "What He asks of you at the moment, my dear sisters, is great union and great support for one another. He also asks that you labor together at God's work with great gentleness and humility, and that what goes on between you remain there so that everyone may be edified."[21] And to Sister Jeanne Lepintre, who had entered the Company of the DC around 1638 and became Sister Servant at Nantes in 1647, she wrote, "I hope, Sister, that you are very careful not to show more affection for some than for others. If some are more faithful to you than others, do not give them any reason to believe that you want them to report the faults of their sisters to you. Just listen without reacting and without commenting on the failings of the others."[22] The sisters were obliged to offer respect to all.

Louise told the DC that they must be united to fulfill God's expectations. She explained that:

> since sin separates us from our unity which is God, following the example of the Blessed Trinity, we must

have but one heart and act with one mind as do the three divine Persons. We must do this in such a way that, when the sister in charge of the sick requests the help of her sister, the sister who instructs the children shall readily comply. And, if the sister in charge of the children requests assistance from the sister in charge of the poor, she shall do likewise since both tasks are equally the business of God. Considering themselves both chosen by Divine Providence in order to act in unison, we hope never to hear the words, "That is your business, not mine."[23]

They imbibed the gospel-based spiritual values of Vincent and Louise, who had taught in the seventeenth century that the *spirit* of the "Company" would "stay alive" if it consisted of charity and "to love Our Lord and to serve Him in a spirit of humility and simplicity."[24] Service to the sick poor provided the environment for the inculcation and ongoing nurturance of the virtues of humility, simplicity, and charity in new members during their initial formation and also in sisters who had already made vows for the first time.

Each DC was to initiate the practice of the three virtues. Louise taught that if the "holy practices" were not "universally in use, let each of us be the very first to start."[25] She summarized the virtues that provided the spiritual structure for the Company's works: "Assembled by Divine Providence: Gentleness, cordiality and forbearance must be the practices of the Daughters of Charity just as humility, simplicity, and the love of the holy humanity of Jesus Christ, who is perfect charity, is their spirit."[26] She suggested that while the sisters knew that their work was important in the sight of God they should begin all acts of service with self-reflection on their own "faults and infidelities."[27] True humility, Louise de Marillac wrote in 1639, would "regulate everything."[28] According to Vincent, the cornerstone of ministry was humility because this virtue provided a lens to recognize and acknowledge both personal talents and limits.[29] Embracing human limitations empowered the sisters to place greater trust in God than in self. Placing talents, skills, and knowledge at the service of the human family connected the DC to people at risk and in need, drawing them into relationships of caring and compassion. In so doing, service evolved into person-centered mutuality and value-based ministry.

The Company of the DC was formed in gospel values that inspired them to "perform all their actions corporal as well as spiritual in a spirit of humility, simplicity, and charity, in the same spirit and in union with those Our Lord Jesus Christ performed on earth."[30] Their spiritual motivations led them to "abhor the maxims of the world and embrace those of Jesus Christ."[31] This was for them the spiritual foundation for responding with compassion to human misery. Striving to live up to these high standards could require nearly heroic virtue at times as the following excerpt illustrates.

> They shall suffer cheerfully and for the love of God inconveniences, contradictions, scoffings, calumnies, and other mortifications which may happen to them even for their good actions, remembering that our Savior, who was very innocent, endured for us far greater ones and prayed even for those who crucified Him and that all this is only a part of the cross which He wills them to carry after Him on earth to deserve the happiness of living forever with Him in heaven.[32]

In her writings Louise likened charity to knowing God. She wrote that "this practice of charity is so powerful that it gives us the knowledge of God, not as He is in Himself, but we penetrate so deeply into the mystery of God and His greatness that we may say that the greater our charity the greater our participation in this divine light which will inflame us with the fire of Holy love for all eternity."[33] Louise's participation in divine light as a result of charitable service to humanity suggests the possibility that a deep spiritual experience of God, often referred to as "consolation," could be found in the simple, humble acts of nursing the sick poor. Nursing was charity, the spiritual essence encompassed in the name of a Company of sisters so deeply devoted to its physical expression.

Vincent de Paul held the virtue of simplicity in such high esteem that he called it his "gospel." He admonished the DC to strive to approach their work in the spirit of simplicity, to be transparent in word and deed—to speak and act "without embellishment or guile."[34] Embodying simplicity was a spiritual act and did not mean that the sisters were to provide a nursing care that was simple. Some have judged the early nursing care of the nineteenth century "from what the practice of medicine was at the time."[35] Doyle wrote for the *American Journal of Nursing* in 1929, "It is reasonable to suppose that it was very simple, and was confined to procuring cleanliness, nourishment, and safety for the sick, and the administration of simple medication. Thus the work of the sisters was confined to the kitchen, the laundry, supervision of the wards, and taking care of the spiritual welfare of the patients."[36]

As will be shown throughout this history, the work of the DC Nurses and the American SC who followed in their footsteps was anything but simple. For example, the sisters cared for patients dying from cholera in hospitals without the benefit of modern plumbing. Cholera is a disease characterized by excessive diarrhea, and caring for patients with this disease under these conditions would certainly not have been simple. Louise clarified in 1656, "We certainly must simplify our intentions by abandoning ourselves to the guidance of His Divine Providence and to the direction of our superiors."[37] The virtues of humility, simplicity, and charity were foundational to the sisters' spiritual intention as they went about their missions. The expression of that intentional, virtue-based care and comfort of others is exemplified throughout this book.

Poverty and Obedience ⌒

The DC were called to a life of poverty and obedience. Each year the DC made simple vows privately, while their Vincentian Brothers made perpetual vows of poverty, chastity, obedience, and stability.[38] The DC took simple, private vows to distinguish themselves from cloistered orders of nuns such as the Visitandines. Vincent and Louise's careful construction of a "Confraternity" of apostolic women helped to ensure that the women could navigate public circles without fear of rebuke from church leadership or social scandal in a time when the only vocational option for women was in their own home or the cloister. The DC Community and its resulting nursing tradition, founded upon vows of poverty, chastity, obedience, and service to the sick poor, both corporally and spiritually,[39] was unique in its design in seventeenth-century France. Although the DC were and continue to be religious women, they were established by the founders as a "secular" community in that they did not belong to a religious order or congregation.[40] The Community of DC were apostolic servants of the sick poor who lived among those whom they served.

Louise was very strict that the Daughters of Charity express themselves when working in community in a way that equated them with the poor rather than distance themselves from the poor. The DC were only allowed to own the food and clothing "God provided them gratuitously."[41] They were also not to act in any way that would suggest superiority to the poor. Their own poverty helped them understand the suffering of the poor, who in the seventeenth century were thousands of French people, and to enter into a life that they believed Jesus Christ had "practiced perfectly."[42] Their own poverty also helped them identify with the poor, who, as the object of their devotional service, were referred to in their annual vows as their "true Masters."[43] Under the guidance of Vincent and Louise, the DC learned how the vow of poverty would enable them to build a unified Community in which all sisters contributed to earning the monies necessary to fulfill the mission to the sick poor. The DC also learned the spiritual purpose of their vow of obedience.

Under the guidance of Louise, the DC defined the boundaries for their spiritual service within the societal context of the time, especially in terms of the role of women. Day-to-day issues surrounding the care of the sick poor would arise, such as what cares the women could provide to men and when they could or could not provide certain treatments, such as blood letting, to the poor. Obedience was the foundational practice that set the sisters' social boundaries and established order within the developing Company. Obedience was an opportunity for externalizing the virtues of the Company. Acts of obedience, the sisters believed, fostered their growth in humility and simplicity.

Obedience, especially when referring to the history of apostolic women who valued humility, simplicity, and charitable service, can be easily misinterpreted, especially when viewed through present-day eyes. Obedience was defined by Louise for the DC as a *conscious* act of yielding. She wrote, "I think obedience should be cheerful, prompt, and uncritical, with submission of our own judgment and a faithful observance of whatever we may have been ordered to do."[44] She instructed the sisters to obey all who had a right to command them as if God was the one commanding them. She wrote that a condition for "true and meritorious" obedience was not to "influence our Superiors to order us to do what we ourselves desire but to desire that we may be ordered to do what they know God demands of us."[45] The DC recognized a connection between obedience and attention to God by serving Christ in the person of the poor. Most importantly, the sisters were taught to discern true, spiritual obedience from a blind obedience that would cause them to deviate from their spiritual course of service to the sick poor. The Company was obedient to God first and foremost. They saw God in the sick poor and demonstrated their obedience to God by providing nursing care as well as other services. Their obedience to God demanded the renunciation of self-love for the choice to embrace the "holy will" of God as "the directing force" in their lives.

It was also the responsibility of the leadership of the Company to be attuned to the will of God that they might lead in such a way that inspired obedience in their companions. One of the most important and highly studied relationships of the Vincentian-Louisian tradition is that of the founders of the DC, Vincent and Louise.[46] In Catholic tradition the phrase typically used to identify the history of the DC is "Vincentian tradition." Louise de Marillac played a critical role in the establishment of the DC, and her writings hold historical relevance in establishing the nature of the early nursing work. Therefore, the term chosen for use throughout this book, Vincentian-Louisian tradition, refers to the reciprocal mutuality and collaboration between Vincent de Paul and Louise de Marillac, who formed the DC Community and established the DC nursing tradition as spiritual work of women in the Catholic Church.

Louise had extensive knowledge and expertise in the care of the sick poor that she had developed over many years when first caring for the sick in Paris while under the spiritual guidance of Vincent de Paul after the death of her husband. She may have reported to Vincent at first as an inferior, but she very soon began to demonstrate a "co-ownership" for the mission.[47] Louise's "relational, developmental" leadership style differed from Vincent's "strong, principled approach." While she may have deeply respected Vincent, it is well documented that her own spiritual integrity and discernment would lead her to question and disagree with him on matters.[48] In her relationship with Vincent, Louise modeled the definition of the "obedience" expected of the sisters.

The collaborative relationship between Vincent and Louise is a historical prototype for the affiliation between the DC and the Congregation of the Mission (CM) or Vincentian priests who provided their ministerial direction and spiritual formation and also between the DC and the administrators of institutions in which they served the sick poor throughout the world. The possibility for collaboration between women and men in the apostolic work of serving the sick poor was initially made possible by the efforts of Vincent de Paul. He used the influence of his role, and the knowledge gained from his earlier relationship with Francis de Sales, to reinstate women in the public ministry. He wrote of his vision:

> It has been eight hundred years or so since women have had public roles in the Church. Previously there had been some, called deaconesses, who were charged with grouping women together in the churches and instructing them in the ceremonies which were then in use. However, about the time of Charlemagne, by the secret plan of Divine Providence, this practice ceased and your sex was deprived of any role and has had none since. Now this same Providence has called upon some of you, in our day, to supply for the needs of the sick poor of the Hôtel-Dieu.[49]

Obedience was further defined by Vincent and Louise in both the *Common Rules* for the Company of the Daughters of Charity and the *Particular Rules* for various offices and duties that they crafted over the course of several years as the Community developed and their missions expanded and diversified.

Common Rules ⌣

The DC tradition began as a parish-based model of apostolic service founded on the gospel of Jesus Christ, the teachings of Vincent de Paul, and the practical preparation of Louise de Marillac in the care of the sick poor. The lived experience of the DC was preserved in a document known as the *Common Rules*.[50] The *Common Rules* not only represented a "revolutionary change from the status quo" in Catholic women's service but was "Spirit-inspired and, therefore, lasting."[51] When speaking to the early sisters on love of vocation and assistance to poor persons, Vincent de Paul explained that "communities are not formed all at once" because their founders, "those great servants of God whose Orders are so flourishing, never dreamed of doing what they actually accomplished; but God acted through them."[52] The DC considered God as the ultimate author of their Company.

The charism[53] of the founders and the spirit of the Company are still the guiding principles for service of DC today, according to *Constitutions and Statutes* updated to address the needs of today's world. The *Common Rules* originally served for directing communal apostolic life in the Company of the DC and ultimately became a prototype for many religious communities and nursing leaders. In 1996 a genealogical study of the Vincentian-Louisian heritage showed that eighty Roman Catholic institutes "substantially followed" the *Common Rules of the Daughters of Charity*. In addition seven Anglican institutes were "rooted" in the *Common Rules*.[54] Their rule outlined the protocol to be followed in taking remedies to the homes of the sick.[55]

Protestant lineages were also inspired by the *Common Rules*. Nurse Amelia Wilhelmina Sieveking of Hamburg, Germany, who was called to care for the sick poor in 1830, adopted St. Vincent de Paul as her "special saint" and "model for setting about her special duty."[56] Sieveking unsuccessfully attempted in the 1830s to procure the *Common Rules* of the French DC, who had missions in Germany beginning in 1852, but ultimately drew up her own to be utilized in the training of her "Association" of nurses, which she named the Protestant Sisters of Mercy. In 1831 Sieveking worked in a temporary cholera hospital. She was approached in 1837 by Pastor Fliedner of Kaiserwerth to accept a head nurse position for his hospital. She declined because she believed that the success of his institution would continue and that she was needed by her family and her visiting-nurse association much more. Sieveking met Fliedner face to face for the first time in 1843; she recommended one of her students for a position he was trying to fill. That student became Fliedner's second wife and a worker at the Institution at Kaiserwerth.

Florence Nightingale had a three-month period of training at Kaiserwerth in 1851. She subsequently trained with the DC in France. In an 1852 letter to the Reverend Henry Manning, Nightingale wrote: "There is nothing like the training (in these days) which the Sacred Heart or the Order of St. Vincent gives to women."[57] During her short periods with the DC in Paris, she may have studied all or some portion of the DC *Common Rules*. Her "papers" from the early 1850s demonstrate that she had read French instructions for novice nurses while in Paris.[58] Nightingale, like Sieveking, was aware that the DC were experts in the care of the sick poor. Nightingale was so moved by the DC that she was on the brink of conversion to Catholicism when she wrote, "The daughters of St. Vincent would open their arms to me. They have already done so, and what should I find there. My work already laid out for me instead of seeking it to and fro and finding none; my home, sympathy, human and divine."[59] But Nightingale did not convert; instead, from her sick bed she became the leader of the nursing-reform movement in Britain that ultimately led to the secularization[60] of nursing practice and nursing education both in Britain and in America in the latter part of the nineteenth century.

The DC found comfort in the structure provided by their Community's *Common Rules* and regulations. Regulations were created for the physical safety of the sisters, as well as for the protection of the integrity of the spiritual mission. The regulations were established rituals of spiritual practice that became part of the identity of the DC and ultimately the American Sisters of Charity (SC) as apostolic religious women and as professional nurses. The regulations of the American SC were called "*The Rule of 1812.*"[61] Louise instructed the DC who nursed in hospitals to be careful that nothing in the hospital experience be "contrary" to the humility and simplicity of the Community or interfere with their ability to adhere to their "strict observance" of their *Common Rules*.[62] In other words, the DC Nurses were sisters first, women dedicated to a calling from God, and nurses second.

Their *Common Rules* represented the values and virtues of the members of a Community from which the image of DC was constructed and made recognizable for the public. Louise led the sisters in a life of service dedicated to grateful conformity to God's will. She wrote, "I pray that the force of Your [God] love, by its gentle power, may compel the acquiescence of any of my senses which may continue to oppose You [God]."[63] This foundational, cultural belief in God's will is important to understand as the history of the nursing work of the DC and SC is explored because it provides the framework for understanding the sisters' intentions and choices and, ultimately, their contributions to nursing and women's history.

The sisters' *Rules* and regulations as an expression of their devotion to religious service led them into ritual practice in nursing care that became integral to their work among the sick poor. For example, the *Regulations at Angers* outlined the most basic protocols for the DC morning routine in caring for the sick:

> At six o'clock they will go to the ward of the sick, empty the chamber pots, make the beds of the patients, clean the toilets, and administer the medicines. Before going there, they will take a little bread and a finger of wine when they first enter the hospital. On Communion days, they will sniff a little vinegar or rub some of it on their hands. At seven o'clock they will serve the sickest patients some broth or a fresh egg for breakfast, and a little butter or stewed apples for the others. After that, they will assist at Holy Mass, if they have not done so at five o'clock, and will be very careful to see that broth is served at the appointed times to the patients who have been purged.[64]

These model schedules were followed by Nightingale, Sieveking, and others who learned them from the DC. Louise also highly valued and modeled the importance of attention to the details of good hygiene and cleanliness. She frequently sought to instill these values in the Company. She once wrote to Sister Élisabeth Martin at Nantes asking if she would keep clean towels at the bedside of the sick.[65] She wrote to Sister Cécile-Agnès Angiboust of Angers: "I do not know if you regularly wash the hands of the poor. If you do not, I would ask you to begin this practice."[66] Hand washing, a valued seventeenth-century nursing practice found in one of the earliest documents for the Confraternity of Charity at Châtillon-les-Dombes (1617)[67] and also in the *Particular Rules for the Sisters of the Hôtel-Dieu of Paris* (1672),[68] continues to be the chief deterrent to infectious disease today.

The corporal and spiritual traditions of the French DC were preserved in the writings of the founders, in the education of the newer nurses, and in the ongoing and evolving practice of the nurses. One scholar of French history states that "the Company's greatest accomplishments were in the field of nursing, and they became France's most important nursing community."[69] The DC faced significant challenges to their work and existence especially during the French Revolution (1792–1800), when they were suppressed. Authorities issued a decree of suppression, which included all teaching and hospital congregations by name, on April 6, 1792. Although the Daughters of Charity were not specifically named, the Company was included among the other associations of piety and charity. In 1792 there were 4,500 Daughters of Charity in France and approximately one hundred novices, known in the community as "seminary sisters." Those who had not made vows for the first time returned to their families. The members of the Company dispersed, but where feasible, the DC continued their ministry clandestinely until 1801. Napoleon reconstituted the DC on December 12, 1800, for the purpose of training nurses for the service of hospitals whose patients were primarily veterans of the Revolution. Throughout the eighteenth century the French DC nursing tradition gained sufficient momentum, and in the early nineteenth century, the mission traveled to America.

Migration of the Vincentian-Louisian
⁓ Nursing Tradition to America ⁓

Roman Catholicism was introduced to the tidewater region of Maryland when Lord Baltimore, a nobleman, was granted the state as a refuge in America for people of his religion from the penal laws of England. Rev. Andrew White and Rev. John Altham, both Catholic (Jesuit) priests, accompanied the first colonists to settle in Maryland in 1634. Revs. White and Altham were charged by Lord Baltimore to attend the Catholic settlers and convert Protestants and native peoples. Rev. Altham traveled with Governor Leonard Calvert twenty-five miles up the Potomac River and visited the native peoples near Potomac Creek in Virginia, where they landed before crossing over to the Maryland shore of the Piscataway Nation. Their chief, believing their peaceful intentions, gave his permission for the English to settle in Maryland. In

1635 a Virginian named Captain William Claiborne, who was angered by the grant of Maryland property to the settlers, succeeded in disturbing the friendly relations between the native peoples and the English. The colonists stayed close to their settlement of St. Mary's during this period of unrest. They also feared disease.

In 1639 Rev. White began to reside with the Piscataway people about fifteen miles south of Washington, D.C. A trusting relationship developed between Chilomacan, the chief of the Piscataway Nation, and White. According to the Catholic records, during the visit, Chilomacan contracted a disease and was near death. After exhausting all of his own people's remedies, he allowed Rev. White to administer one of his powders to him and to bleed him. Chilomacan's health was restored, and he subsequently converted to Christianity and began to adopt the culture of the English, such as their clothes, language, and marriage customs. Other settlers, led by Claiborne, continued their "holy work of rooting out the abominations of popery and prelacy in Maryland."[70] The colonists had endured religious persecution in England such as "confiscation of property, civil degradation, and those refined cruelties which operating upon the ties of blood and the laws of nature, sought to destroy their religion by extinguishing the affections of the heart, and with-holding the advantages of education."[71] While not at risk of penalty of death in America, they still endured the burden of religious prejudice from Protestants.

The first priests to work with the American Sisters of Charity on the formation of the Community, the Society of Saint-Sulpice (Sulpicians), arrived in Canada in 1657 and Baltimore in 1791. The first members of the Congregation of the Mission (Vincentian priests and brothers) arrived in Maryland in 1816 bound for the Missouri Territory. The early American Catholics also had their own prejudices. Many thought of Native Americans as "savage." The early Vincentian priests, although willing to adapt their clothes and religious schedules to the American lifestyle, often continued to use their own Italian language. They did not approve of whiskey or American dancing, and their relationships with non-Catholics, whom they called "heretics,"[72] varied. The beliefs of Catholic colonists inspired their religious mission and a fervent desire to convert others to those beliefs that they associated with the message of the true Church. They were very successful.

Catholics as well as Protestants marveled at the "astonishing rapidity" of the increase in Catholic members and institutions emerging throughout the country.[73] It was during this period of expansion that Elizabeth Ann Bayley Seton (1774–1821)[74] converted from the Protestant Episcopal Church to Roman Catholicism in 1805 as a result of a trip to Italy to restore her husband's health but that left her a widow. The Filicchi family of Livorno, Italy, who were friends and business associates of her husband, William Magee Seton, provided lodging and hospitality to the Setons. Exposed to the Catholic culture of Italy, the Widow Seton questioned the Filicchis about their religion and its practices. Elizabeth Seton, or Mother Seton as she would be called, was a wealthy New York socialite whose subsequent religious conversion in New York resulted in loss of support by her family and near homelessness and poverty. The Filicchis were also acquainted with Catholic clergy in the United States, particularly Rev. John Cheverus (1768–1836) and Rev. Francis Matignon (1753–1818) of Boston and John Carroll (1735–1815) of Baltimore. Their correspondence and counsel, along with the providential meeting of a Sulpician priest, Rev. Louis Dubourg (1766–1833), president of St. Mary's College, Baltimore, led her to remain in the United States instead of moving to Canada. Rev. Carroll, a Jesuit prior to their suppression in 1773, was elected the first American bishop headquartered in Baltimore, the seat of the diocese. At the suggestion of Rev. Dubourg and with the support of Bishop Carroll, Mother Seton moved her family of five children to Maryland and opened a school for girls, first in Baltimore, then in Frederick County.

She felt called to seek out and serve the needy, especially individuals and families living in poverty, by teaching children who lacked educational opportunities and by providing nursing care to the sick or dying in their homes. Rev. Dubourg, who with many other French priests had immigrated to America as a result of exile during the French Revolution, told Mother Seton of the charitable education and nursing missions of the DC in France. With Sulpician support, she subsequently founded the Sisters of Charity of Saint Joseph's near Emmitsburg, Maryland, on July 31, 1809. This was the first Roman Catholic sisterhood native to the United States for religious women. The Vincentian-Louisian tradition in America began with a vision expressed in these words of Mother Seton in a letter to Robert Goodloe Harper of Frederick County, whose daughters attended Saint Joseph's Academy:

> the promising and amiable perspective of Establishing a House of plain and useful Education, retired from the extravagance of the world—connected also with the view of providing Nurses for the sick and poor, an abode of Innocence and refuge of Affliction.[75]

They were legally incorporated as the Sisters of Charity of Saint Joseph's in Maryland (SC) in 1817, and their charter outlined their mission: "Works of piety, charity and usefulness and especially for the care of the sick, the succor of the aged and the infirm and necessitous persons, and the education of young females."[76] They established the first free Catholic school for girls staffed by Sisters in the United States (Emmitsburg, 1810). Mother Seton sent Sisters to Philadelphia in 1814 to manage Saint Joseph's Asylum, the first Catholic orphanage in the United States. The next year the SC opened a mission at Mount Saint Mary's College and Seminary near Emmitsburg to oversee the infirmary and domestic services. In 1817 Sisters from Saint Joseph's Valley went to New York to begin the New York Roman Catholic Orphan Asylum (later Saint Patrick's Orphan Asylum).

Mother Seton had personal experience of nursing care and the fundamentals of medicine from her years in New York, where her father, Richard Bayley (1744–1801), was a well-known physician, surgeon, and medical authority, particularly on yellow fever. A maternal uncle, John Charlton (1736–1806), was another prominent physician. Her brother-in-law, Wright Post (1766–1828), also practiced medicine. Mother Seton was a caregiver for her five children, her father in his final illness, and her husband and sister-in-law Rebecca, who both died of tuberculosis. She was sought by other sick relatives because of her compassion and nursing competence. She, like many women of the time, learned how to provide basic nursing care from many sources. In addition to growing up in a medical family, Mother Seton learned nursing from many of the women who joined the early Community of the Sisters of Charity. The

Fig. 1-2   *Mother Elizabeth Ann Bayley Seton*

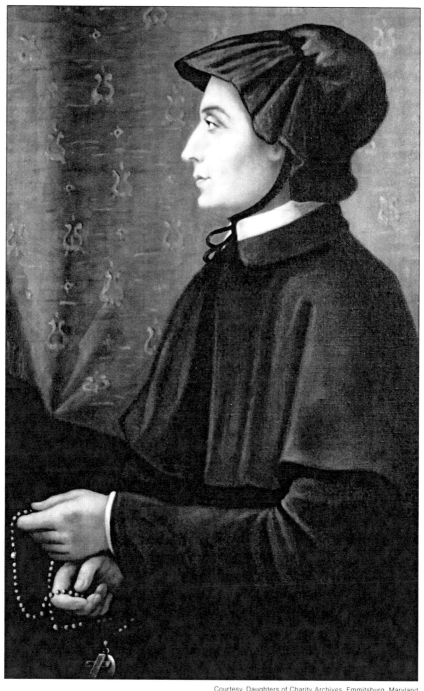

Courtesy, Daughters of Charity Archives, Emmitsburg, Maryland

correspondence of Mother Seton during her years in Maryland contains numerous references to the treatment of illnesses such as ague, fever, bleeding, blisters, boils, cholera, rheumatism, tuberculosis, and yellow fever.[77] Mother Seton and the SC nursed many at Emmitsburg, including Seton's son William, who recovered from near death; her daughters Anna Maria (Annina) and Rebecca, who succumbed to tuberculosis; and more than a dozen SC who died as young women.

"That the Sick Poor May Not Be Kept Waiting"~

Anticipating the establishment of the SC at Emmitsburg, Mother Seton wrote her lifelong friend Julia Sitgreaves Scott of Philadelphia, expressing her sentiments regarding her pending mission: "so far I can express, but to speak the joy of my soul at the prospect of being able to assist the Poor, visit the sick, comfort the sorrowful, clothe little innocents, and teach them to love God!"[78] She and the SC also knew of the challenges that lay ahead. Caring for the sick poor was a tremendously difficult task. Vincent had written of the challenges of hospital ministry to the poor in particular. He described the work to one of the brothers in Genoa:

> If you were to go and serve the sick, it would be in a hospital or in their own homes. If it were in a hospital, alas! Poor Brother, you would be going from the frying pan into the fire, for so many painful crosses and contradictions are encountered there that the ones about which you are complaining are nothing in comparison. The work is heavy, times of rest are short and interrupted, repugnance is certain, and reproaches and insults are frequent there. Almost all the poor grumble about things because they are never satisfied and usually complain to both the devout persons who visit them and the Administrators who are in charge of them. They even make false reports to them about those who serve them because the latter have refused them something. Those poor servants are harassed on all sides, having as many supervisors and critics as there are masters, chaplains, and persons who

have some responsibility in those houses. This is what our poor Daughters of Charity find the hardest.[79]

It would be a number of years before the American SC would take up their first hospital mission in Baltimore. In the meantime they provided nursing care for their own Sisters in their infirmary, supplied domestic and infirmary services for the Sulpician priests at Mount St. Mary's College and Seminary, and visited the sick poor in their homes. In 1811 the *Common Rules* were translated into English by Rev. John Dubois (1764–1842), a Sulpician,[80] who knew the Vincentians and had worked with the DC Nurses in France at the Hospice des Petites Maisons in Paris, where the nurses cared for the sick poor and the insane. There were differences between the French and the Americans, however. For example, he noted in the *Rules* that the American SC would educate female children of all stages of life, not only the poor. The calls of the Church as well as the needs of the poor were "the criteria upon which the Community would base its acceptance of new missions."[81] At the time of Mother Seton's death in January of 1821, the SC, fifty in number, were already serving in the

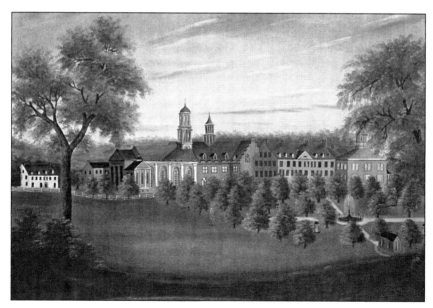

Fig. 1-3   *Sisters of Charity of Saint Joseph's, Emmitsburg, MD. 1848*

archdiocese in Baltimore and two of the five Catholic dioceses, New York and Philadelphia.

The SC constitutions approved in 1812 stated that "although this Institution is the same in substance as that of the Sisters of Charity in France, it will have no connection whatever with the Company or Government of the said Sisters in France or any European country, except that of mutual charity and friendly correspondence."[82] The American SC chose to have no connection with France in the early years. After the restoration of the monarchy in France and exile of Napoleon, Dubois was the first to have left a record raising the possibility of establishing connections between the Daughters of Charity and Sisters of Charity and also with the Congregation of the Mission (Lazarist/Vincentian) priests to take over the role of religious superior to the American Sisters.[83] Rev. Louis-Regis Deluol (1787–1858), a Sulpician, successfully concluded the negotiations in 1849.[84] Rev. Mariano Maller, CM (1817–1892), became the first Vincentian provincial director for the American SC in 1849. He oversaw the implementation of the union of the SC and DC, which became reality later in March of 1850.[85] The priests were responsible for giving the Sisters annual spiritual retreats in addition to celebrating Holy Mass and other sacraments in the SC chapels. They often served as chaplains to the Sisters and to the patients in the hospitals staffed by the Sisters.

Founded as a community of women for apostolic life, not a contemplative order, the life of the DC/SC was dedicated to a ministry in which Vincent de Paul said, "The service of the poor should be preferred to everything else according to their founding charism or spirit."[86] The Sisters were taught that when necessary they should prefer acts of service to the poor to saying their prayers. They lived by the principle of *leaving God for God* which had permeated the DC ministry from the beginning. The beliefs instilled by Vincent and Louise in the company of apostolic women helped them to understand that if they left prayer and Holy Mass to respond to urgent needs of the poor they would be "going to God" because they would "see" God in the sick poor whom they served.[87] They chose to be in solidarity with those who suffered, doing all they could "to provide them with a little assistance and remain at peace."[88] Despite their spiritual vision, the Sisters realized that they would also see a great amount of misery that might not be relieved by their prayers or nursing care. The focus of the Sisters' religious education and nursing preparation was to learn to care for those who were suffering in such a way that they would be able to joyfully sustain and ultimately fulfill their individual spiritual callings and the apostolic mission of the Community as a whole.

CHAPTER 2

⁓ ♏ ⁓

Holistic Education
of the Sister of Charity Nurse

Sisters who would care for sick or poor patients—body, mind, and spirit—had to be prepared for very challenging work. The DC and SC were called to a service modeled by the founders as an active apostolic life. Louise de Marillac taught that it was not enough for the sisters to "have a mind enlightened by the consciousness of our faults" but that "our wills must also be moved to correct them."[1] Forgiveness of sin and cleansing of faults was achieved through sacramental confession and living their vowed commitment through practice of virtues: fasting for chastity, almsgiving for poverty, and prayer for obedience.[2] Teaching children and caring for the sick poor and insane was the active expression of the sisters' spirituality and vocation—their way of life.

The sisters were formally[3] educated for nursing and ministry just as they were for communal apostolic life. The ideals and visions of the French healing heritage of providing charitable nursing care to the sick had to be translated, literally[4] and figuratively, by Mother Seton, the supporting clergy, and the Sisters of Charity themselves. In addition to the adaptation of the *Common Rules*, the SC's religious service had to be made compatible with nineteenth-century American society. The SC's nursing care was created within the framework of the values and ideals of their religious life and beliefs; however, they also wanted their community to grow and flourish. Therefore, societal norms and values had to be taken into account when designing their nursing practice and service.

The early SC designed and implemented a curriculum of nursing education. While mentorship and apprenticeship were part of the model for preparation of SC Nurses, it was not the foundation of their education. The early education of the SC Nurses, as will be described, is best characterized as vocational formation in the Vincentian-Louisian tradition of service. The word "vocation" comes from the Latin *vocare*—to call to live a life consecrated to God (as opposed to the call to an occupation).[5] That preparation was structured and formal. SC Nurses were formed first by the Community leadership, specifically the Mistress of Novices or Seminary Directress, prior to being sent on their first mission. After their initial formal vocational preparation, Sister-Nurses were given on-the-job nursing education in the corporal and spiritual care of the sick and dying. They were closely mentored by the Sister Servant and other experienced hospital Sisters who were instructed by their founders' teachings to have respect toward young nurses under their care, not look for faults in the Sisters, and to "not reprimand a Sister while she is in an emotional state" so that the Sister would learn from a mistake and not "feel shame."[6] The vocational path of the American SC Nurse was nurtured in a way that allowed for a deep connection with spiritual life and religious experience and a focused expression of fully grounded and intentional caring service.

The history of their early nursing missions reveals the struggle for balance between religious and societal expectations that the Sisters had to address when establishing themselves as professional nurses. The vocational education of the SC Nurses was holistic[7] in that it prepared nurses spiritually, to enter a devout life of religious service according to Catholic values and Vincentian-Louisian *Rules* for community; mentally and emotionally, to understand and carry out the healing traditions that had become characteristic of Vincentian-Louisian nurses; and physically, to become the instrument of healing that would provide excellent corporal care of the sick in collaboration with physicians. The desire to provide exemplary service to the sick poor led the SC Nurses to learn by gathering knowledge from many teachers.

⁓ *Contemplation in Action* ⁓

The enlightened charity of the American SC developed out of a deep, faith-filled, religious spirit nurtured by the teachings of the early founders and preserved in their writings and the *Common Rules* created for the DC. The body of the original teachings of Vincent and Louise, spoken and written in French, were not all translated into English initially. Mother Seton did speak and read French, as did some of the early SC such as French-speaking Sisters Madeleine Guerin and Mary Xavier Clark, who taught it to other Sisters and the children in the SC schools; however, early instructions to the DC found in the *Spiritual Writings of Louise de Marillac*, for example, were not fully and definitively published in English until 1991.[8]

One major work that had been translated into English and greatly influenced the SC was the book *Introduction to the Devout Life* by Saint Francis de Sales.[9] This book was on the reading list for all Catholic Americans in the nineteenth century.[10] It discusses soul purification, provides guidance in meditation on such topics as "how the soul chooses devout life" and "of creation." St. Francis de Sales wrote on the virtues of humility, obedience, poverty, and friendship, as well as issues of daily living such as marriage, modesty in dress, and conversation. He taught about emotions such as courage, anxiety, and sorrow and how to respond to spiritual consolation. The teachings in this book by St. Francis de Sales, a friend and director of Vincent and acquaintance of Louise, were compatible with the French and American missions. Nursing in the Vincentian-Louisian tradition was a devout life through service to the sick poor. As will be shown, SC Matilda Coskery was particularly inspired by St. Francis de Sales and his teachings on kindness.

The correspondence, Community documents, and writings of Mother Seton and other Sisters of Charity demonstrate the influence of founders Vincent and Louise. Hugh O'Donnell, CM, a Vincentian scholar, describes Vincent's "way" as emanating from his experience and connection with people and events. "Events called him to respond and showed him the way in which God was leading him," writes O'Donnell.[11] Vincent's way was intentional action in which he believed God was present. Vincentian observation on experience, discernment, and reflection encircle action determined by response to the pivotal question: "What must be done?"

Vincentian priests moved from village to village preaching and establishing Confraternities of Charity. The DC, characterized by flexibility and mobility, went on short- and longer-term missions educating and nursing the sick poor. Vincent modeled his way of practical wisdom in three rules for his followers: The first rule was to "act always with purity of intention and singleness of purpose."[12] Followers were to strive to internalize faith in God's care and not allow their purity of intention to be compromised by their own concerns. The second rule was to "consider an action as manifesting God's way when it effectively embraced the extremes."[13] For example, Vincent brought together rich and poor in society, inspiring the rich to know the poor through compassionate service and generosity. Vincent's third rule was to "mirror God's fidelity to his own being, and his great flexibility toward human beings. Vincent's rule of action was to be always firm and persevering in regard to goals, flexible and gentle in regard to means."[14]

Perhaps one of the most practical gifts Vincent gave the sisters was an understanding of his process of discernment. The sisters, filled with desire to serve the sick poor, still had to determine the rightness and wrongness of their actions. Although each sister came to the Community with a willing heart and a desire to care, Vincent and Louise knew that a spiritual fervor to care for the sick poor had to be grounded in an understanding of the stark realities of providing day-to-day care for the myriad of sick and destitute people. Their task was at times monumental, and therefore the sisters were taught discernment, a very spiritual praxis and yet also a practical one too. Vincent taught that discernment was a three-part process: unrestricted readiness, weighing the evidence, and taking counsel.[15] Unrestricted readiness meant that the Sister would be open to the will of God and be listening in a way that was detached from any personal agenda. Readiness could be achieved through prayer, meditation, and reflection on life events. It was in this state of readiness to listen that the sisters would weigh the evidence of a given situation and determine the pros and cons of action. Vincent was a person molded by his reflection on his life experiences. He viewed events in his life as signs sent by Divine Providence to reveal God's plan. Vincent, like Francis de Sales, believed that God's will was revealed during the process of taking counsel with a wise person. The sisters were encouraged to discuss their concerns with Community leadership, such as the Mother, Sister Servants, and the clergy who were their directors. Vincent often took counsel with others, in particular Louise de Marillac, when matters of the DC were at stake. He believed that Louise had a high degree of prudence, a quality necessary for developing the ability to discern. "Prudence, my Sisters," said Vincent, "consists in discerning the proper manner, time, and place of comporting ourselves in everything."[16]

Some have noted that while Vincent's teachings typically inspired the heart and spirit, Louise's teachings addressed the intellect.[17] The nurses in Community received the benefit of a holistic education of heart-inspired spiritual conferences from Vincent woven with correspondences from Louise that detailed instruction in nursing and community service. Louise was initially a very reasoned person who followed a more rigid structure in her spiritual life. Vincent, as her spiritual guide, urged Louise to find moderation, peace, and calm, for he feared that she "would become anxious if she were unable to maintain the rule that she had drawn up for herself."[18] Louise's desire for structure gradually matured into a very skilled talent for organizational leadership and community building centered on love. Louise's letters and conferences reveal the vision for a community that she shared openly with the DC. She was particularly attuned to the needs of the individual DC serving the sick poor and the importance of each one in the success and growth of the Community mission as a whole. "Her great flexibility in adapting to local needs was the key to her success."[19]

Louise prepared the sisters to teach as well as care for the sick poor. She educated "the whole person," which meant that her means of instruction helped the students to better understand life and their relationship with God.[20] The Louisian methodology of holistic education was centered on gentleness, respect, and availability.[21] In his July 24, 1660, Conference on the Virtues of Louise de Marillac, Vincent said to the sisters, "O mon Dieu, what a beautiful picture! What humility, faith, prudence, sound judgment, and always the concern to conform her actions to those of our Lord! It's up to you, Sisters, to conform your actions to hers and to imitate her in all things."[22] Louise laid the foundation for holistic education and nursing care that the sisters followed. She encouraged the sisters to look to Christ's life, birth to crucifixion, as the model of charity and exemplar of service to the poor that they would strive to emulate and teach.

In addition to learning from the French founders, the American SC were inspired by the lives of Mother Seton and the early Sisters of Charity who created their Community based upon the ideals of the French and the needs of the sick poor in American society. In collaboration with Sulpician priests, Mother Seton established the SC community. Elected four times as Mother until her death at the age of forty-six (possibly from consumption [tuberculosis]), she steered the Community through very trying times while the sisterhood and the physical community were being established. Mother Seton was canonized by the Roman Catholic Church in 1975 as the first native-born saint of the United States. Her vision of mission led to the creation of the Community near Emmitsburg, Maryland, in an area that she named Saint Joseph's Valley, where she inspired other women to take up the calling to live an apostolic life in community in order to serve people in need, particularly the sick poor and illiterate girls.

The women were courageous and highly committed to their mission in a country where anti-Catholic sentiment was growing. The SC established the first free Catholic school for girls staffed by religious women in the United States in Emmitsburg, in 1810. While their primary focus in the first years was caring for orphans and creating schools for their education, this early Community also provided nursing care in the homes of the sick. A glimpse of early nursing can be gleaned from Mother Seton's correspondence about the nursing care of some of the priests by her SC:

> That Mr. Duhamel has been two weeks home with many complaints arising from cold. Ma Farrell[23] nurses him. (O, most happy!) and Joanna[24] good Mr. Egan, who is almost gone. Mr. Hickey quite well. So embarrassed with the three minutes I stand by his table in the morning. I believe it is the plague of his life, yet I persevere, and often catch a word to show him what he is on the eyes of my Faith. Blessed soul! We have nursed him, and given him all the little cares we could. I give him a share of Martina's bitters, make him candy for his cough, etc. . . .
>
> Ma Farrell makes us laugh till we cry. She went to nurse Mr. Duhamel. 'I walked in Mother, with my cabbage leaves[25] in my pocket to dress the Reverend

gentleman's blister,[26] and he refused my services because he had some old woman he had sent for. So I told him, Mr. Duhamel, Mother sent me here, the Superior, I am sure wished me to come, Sister Betsy, I know wished it, and Margaret herself desired I should be sent; —(all the Council) and so, Mr. Duhamel if you will not let me dress that blister, at least, I will have a hand in it.' And so, Mother, I picked my leaves most carefully, and stayed it out. Then the Reverend Gentleman was so much better the next day, and Miss Polly so much better, we sat all to breakfast together, and the Lord forgive me!—in the middle of breakfast, I remembered there was no grace said, and up I got to say mine, and up got Mr. Duhamel to say his, but he was not offended for before I left him, I was the best old woman in the whole country, and he did not know how to part with me.[27]

In 1814 Mother Seton sent Sister Rose Landry White as Sister Servant and other Sisters to Philadelphia to manage Saint Joseph's Asylum, the first Catholic orphanage in the United States. The next year the SC opened the infirmary mission at Mount St. Mary's. In 1817 Sisters from Saint Joseph's Valley went to New York to begin the New York Roman Catholic Orphan Asylum (later Saint Patrick's Orphan Asylum). Sister Rose White, who was Mother Seton's assistant from 1809 to 1814 and then her successor after Mother Seton's death in 1821, led the Community into hospital service.

The "Mother's" role in the Community was that of Director, which according to tradition was the Sister who animated the Community. She delegated responsibilities and collaborated with the "Superior," a Sulpician priest appointed by the Superior of the Society of Saint Sulpice in Baltimore as ecclesiastical superior and religious guide to the Community. The priest Superior did not interfere with the governing of the Sisters any more than was necessary to assure that the constitutions were maintained. The Mother was the "soul and life of the whole body"[28] and keeper of the Vincentian-Louisian tradition as written in the *Regulations for the Society of Sisters of Charity in the United States of America*, an adaptation of the *Common Rules*.

Another very important role in the Community was that of "Mistress of Novices."[29] The Mother appointed the Mistress of Novices to serve as spiritual teacher for women entering the Community. The Novice Mistress was considered the primary carrier of the knowledge and wisdom of Vincentian-Louisian tradition. Sister Catherine (Kitty) Mullen (?1783–1815) was the first appointed by Mother Seton to the position in 1813. After her death it appears that Mother Seton took over the role again until 1818. Sister Mary Xavier Clark (1790–1855) followed for eighteen years, from 1818 to 1829 and 1845 to 1855. Many Sisters up to the year 1855 were influenced by Sister Mary Xavier Clark.[30]

⌒ Sister Mary Xavier Clark on the "Blessed Art" ⌒

Sister Mary Xavier Clark was born Catherine Eugénie Mestezzer in Saint-Domingue, a French colony on the Caribbean island of Hispaniola. Catherine's parents were quite prosperous at first but then fell into extreme poverty. Because of the family difficulties, she did not receive an education. Community accounts of Sister Mary Xavier's early history record that at a young age Catherine went to the nearest chapel to implore Mary, the Mother of Jesus, to teach her to read. "Full of confidence in our Blessed Lady, and opening a little prayer book she found near her, she began to read, never having the least difficulty afterwards."[31] After the murder of her father in San Domingo, her mother and family moved to New Orleans, where she met and married Captain Clark at the age of seventeen. Just months after the birth of their son, Captain Clark died, and nine months later their son died also. Catherine became friends with a French woman in New York who subsequently engaged her as an assistant to teach at her academy in New York City. While she was in New York, Catherine met Sister Rose White, the Sister Servant of the SC New York orphan asylum in Manhattan. She was so impressed with the works of the Sisters that she joined the Emmitsburg Community where she became Sister Mary Xavier.

Her friendship with Mother Seton was said to have been like that of Francis de Sales with Vincent.[32] Sister Mary Xavier became Mother Seton's assistant in 1820, and when Mother Seton died, Sister Mary Xavier became comforter as well as beloved teacher to the Community. Her classes primarily comprised women ages sixteen to twenty-five. "Many of them have been heard to say that they would rather listen to her than to the most eloquent sermons of the clergy, because she knew so well how to adapt her instructions to the uncultivated minds of the country people."[33] She was also elected Mother from 1839 to 1845. She was dedicated to the mission of the Community and the life she had chosen of humility, simplicity, and charity. The focus of her instruction for novices was the "counsel of Saint Francis de Sales," as well as St. Vincent de Paul and St. Louise de Marillac. She "impressed upon the minds" of the novices the importance of simplicity in words and actions. She is remembered as often quoting the Bible: "He that despises small things shall fall by little and little."[34]

Sister Mary Xavier was very strict in the observance of the *Rule*. She was remembered as saying often that "when God calls a soul to a Community

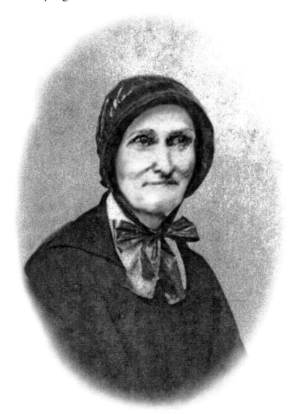

Fig. 2-1   *Mother and Novice Mistress, Sister Mary Xavier Clark*

Courtesy, Daughters of Charity Archives, Emmitsburg, Maryland

43

life He gives her the requisite qualifications to adapt herself to the *Rules* and customs of it. . . . She exhorted the Sisters to mortify themselves daily in something that would not injure their health or attract attention."[35] For example, she suggested that the Sisters practice simple and inconspicuous tasks of self-denial, such as being silent when having the inclination to speak or refraining from eating a desired food.

In addition to religious formation, Sister Mary Xavier provided the first vocational nursing instruction for novices before they were sent to their missions. Nursing was a service that was a fully integrated part of the corporate identity of the DC and SC Community. Throughout the early documents of the Community, it is clear that nursing, even the smallest acts of kindness and comfort, was important to the fulfillment of the mission. As was stated by Rev. Simon Gabriel Bruté, (1779–1839), chaplain to Mother Seton and the early SC Community, "Let us bless, love, serve with great joy, and expansion of heart, in the smallest things.

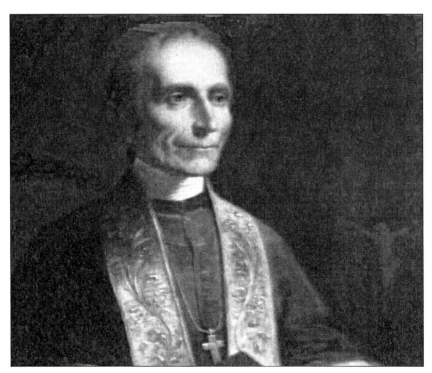

Fig. 2-2   *Rev. Simon Gabriel Bruté*

Courtesy, Daughters of Charity Archives, Emmitsburg, Maryland

Alas! What great things we can do for this Sovereign Master of Heaven and earth, this King of Eternity! What? Anastasia, a broth—Sally, the washing,—Jane, some ciphers,—Augusta, some crochets and quavers,—Xavier, the medical syrup,—Catherine, her bread,—Barbara, and Marina their milk and butter,—what more?"[36]

Sister Mary Xavier did make medicines for the sick, and her "solicitude for the sick knew no bounds; she was always planning for their comfort, any little delicacy sent to her was immediately given to the infirmary."[37] Some of her empathy for the sick may have been due to the fact that she was physically weak and often sick herself, subject to hemorrhages of the lungs. She was also an accomplished caregiver, as demonstrated in one of the rare pieces of written evidence of the formal, vocational instruction given by Sister Mary Xavier Clark to Sister-Nurses. The handwritten, pocket-sized booklet containing two sets of copied instructions is archived at the DC Marillac Provincialate in St. Louis, Missouri.

The first part of the booklet includes instructions in French, *Instruction pour les Filles de la Charite et les autres Religieuses Hospitalieres en 1796*, followed by the English translation. This was the spiritual instruction that the French DC provided the public during the French Revolution when priests were forbidden to perform their usual duties. The responsibility for ministering to and "instructing" the sick poor in spiritual matters fell to the DC and others. The translated French instructions are primarily focused on the needs of the soul because the "detail of what concerns the body" is "sufficiently explained in the Constitutions and Rules."[38] However, this should not be construed as meaning that the Sisters did not value the body. The author wrote that the body was "an object worthy of the greatest respect & most tender care: first because after the soul of man, his body is the most admirable and perfect work of God; being sanctified by baptism, consecrated by the body of Jesus Christ in the holy Eucharist, and, according to the expression of St. Paul, the temple of the Holy Ghost."[39]

The three duties that the Sisters were to fulfill in terms of soul work were to "instruct" the sick poor in the Catholic religion, to "press them gently and prudently towards their conversion" and "to help them die well."[40] The Sisters were to explain in simple terms the Catholic dogma of the "Holy Trinity, the Incarnation, and the Redemption."[41] Sisters were also instructed in the "Motives of Contrition"; specifically, the notion of "sin," which according to Catholicism is a "disobedience to the law of God—a revolt of the creature against the Creator."[42] The instructions guide the nurse who was expected to help each patient make "good use of his suffering."[43] While it is not entirely clear why this eighteenth-century instruction was included in the booklet, it can be surmised that the French DC tradition of religious ministry to the sick poor was also valued, taught, and recorded by the American Sisters.

The second part of the booklet, entitled "Instruction on the care of the sick. By M.X.," is attributed presumably to Sister Mary Xavier Clark because she was the only Sister in Community at the time whose name correlates with the initials found in the booklet and because in her office as Mistress of Novices (1845–1854), she might have either written her instructions or been recorded by others. The booklet is dated on the final page as October 26, 1846. Sister Mary Xavier's instruction begins on page 32 with a foundational teaching on the demonstration of *charity*:

> As we have, for the love of God engaged ourselves in the care of the sick, we must be generous and do so with every possible care and attention. 2ⁿᵈ Our charity must be extended to all;[44] all are the redeemed souls of our Saviour. It is true that we cannot treat all alike & must proportion our cares to the wants of each one as the case before God requires it; but it should never be because we like this one more than that one; or because we feel more interest or compassion for this or that one. To act in such a manner, would indeed be a sin, and a great breach of our engagements with God, for whose sake we have promised to serve the poor sick.
>
> A Sister who would be actuated by such bad motives, would indeed render herself unworthy of God and her blessed vocation. . . . What a misfortune after spending perhaps a long life in the most painful and arduous duties of exterior charity to die without merit because we had not purity of intention, which consists in doing all things for the love of God![45]

Mary Xavier carefully placed the religious instruction of the first pages within nineteenth-century American context. The instruction was particularly important for those who worked in hospitals where, as she noted, there were different denominations of patients. The SC Nurse was expected to first address the "corporal aid and comfort" needed upon admission before asking about the patient's religion. If a patient was Protestant, the Sister was to "not say a word about the Catholic religion." The spiritual instruction states clearly, however, that SC Nurses not try to convert patients to Catholicism. Nurses were not to show preference for Catholic patients, and the nurse was not to proselytize. She is quoted as teaching, "Her charity towards the body, will more easily gain the soul than pressing exhortations."[46] Sister Mary Xavier taught the nurses that they should even be careful in discussing religion with confirmed Catholics because "there are some Catholics who are even worse than infidels and heretics; therefore an imprudent urging to go to confession might put the person in a passion and even draw from him words of imprecation & blasphemy . . . remember one thing—never begin to speak of religion before you have afforded them all the little relief & comforts you can to the poor body: by these you will find the way to the soul. Your charity to their bodies will aid them to raise their minds to God."[47]

It was suggested that a Sister-Nurse offer "silent supplications" for a dying patient not of the Catholic faith to have a "death bed conversion," but otherwise she was certainly capable of working with the priests to be sure that the Catholic patients received the last rites known as "extreme unction" and the "last indulgence." Sister Mary Xavier pointed out that some priests forgot the "last indulgence," and therefore she instructed the Sister-Nurse to prepare her patient for the rites and be sure that the priests supplied the opportunity. Sister-Nurses were to light a candle at the head of the patient's bed, pray for the patient, and sprinkle holy water around the bed and very lightly on the face of the patient so as not to arouse his nervous system.[48] She also instructed the nurses not to disturb the pillows of a dying patient, stating that if they took any of the pillows away with the purpose of lowering the head they would cause the person to expire. Pages 89–95 of the booklet are examples of prayers that Sister Mary Xavier suggested be said on behalf of the dying patient. Her final instructions are about the nurse's attendance to the body of the dead.

In her instructions Sister Mary Xavier referred to nursing care of the sick poor as the "blessed art."[49] She gave detailed accounts of the basics of patient care such as what a nurse should do when receiving a new patient. The way she differentiated an experienced versus an inexperienced infirmarian is that the experienced nurse knew that a new patient must be assessed immediately, and if she was not able to attend to the newcomer, "she should at least show her good will towards the person . . . she should give orders at least, for the person to be put to bed, and go herself as soon as she can."[50] Sister Mary Xavier stressed the importance of an orderly approach to care and complete attention to the proper preparation and administration of remedies. She admonished the Sisters to know the "signs" used by physicians in writing prescriptions. She also differentiated "mixing" from "boiling" remedies and stated that the Sisters must thoroughly clean each mixing vessel after each use. She specifically mentioned her personal experience of observing a nurse who misread the label on a bottle of medicine and gave a patient calomel instead of magnesia.[51] She instructed the nurses to purchase "the best" ingredients for a remedy and never get "indifferent things because they are cheap: nor even when given them free of cost" when preparing remedies.[52] Sister Mary Xavier was known to "go herself to the kitchen to show the Sisters how to prepare little delicacies for the weak and infirm."[53] She taught by example, as had Mother Seton and Louise de Marillac, demonstrating in simple acts of daily life how one would embrace the Vincentian-Louisian tradition of spiritual life and humble service to God by nursing others.

After the passing of Sister Mary Xavier, many of the Sisters whom she had helped enter religious life wrote letters to the Central House at Emmitsburg telling of their memories of their teacher: "I never met one so interiorly enlightened. A brief interview with her sufficed to banish all fear and dispel the clouds that darkened the mind."[54] Another wrote, "She was truly a guiding star to all who sought the path to perfection; her kindness, gentleness, and affability, won all hearts."[55]

⁓ *Gathering Nursing Knowledge in Public* ⁓

Women have historically formed community as the social framework for the exchange of ideas, resources, knowledge, and recipes for both culinary and healing purposes. Nursing care and the education of nurses has, as Vincent and Louise knew, been inextricably linked to community. It was not possible for Louise to care for the sick poor of Paris completely on her own. She created and nurtured a community. The Community of caregivers that Vincent and Louise envisioned and inspired existed because they shared resources within their own Community as well as with others in the Catholic Church community. The Community comprised an interdependent healing network of women. They systematically expanded their social network of healing people and resources wherever they went. While non-Catholic women may have had initial concerns about the religious aspect of the Sisters' nursing work, they often supported the need for the Sister-Nurses' caring work.

Forming a sisterhood and expanding domestic duties into charitable work in community was often the goal of a nineteenth-century American woman who did not have to labor as a domestic servant or a worker in the factories emerging in urban areas. The model of community-based vocational nursing education developed by the Sisters at Emmitsburg resonated soundly with the gender roles and ideals that permeated middle- and upper-class American society. The philosophy of female education in the early and mid-nineteenth century "inclined women to see their destiny as a shared one and to look to one another for similar sensibilities and moral support."[56] Female education typically took place in ladies' societies, "dame schools," and "academies" that focused on Christian beliefs. Historian Nancy Cott writes that "when academy education was combined with religious revival the impulse toward female friendship was doubly forceful."[57] The Vincentian-Louisian community model mirrored the conclusions about the results of sisterhoods of religious women and the fruit of their gatherings.

The difference between the Protestant academies and the Catholic sisterhoods was in the structure provided the women for the release of their religious fervor. The structure established in the DC *Common Rules* was the basis for the SC's *Regulations*. These *Regulations* were used to conceive their religious vision fully channeled into an organized nursing service carried out not only with and for Catholics but also with Protestants in Protestant-administered hospitals. American middle- and upper-class Protestant women of the period were neither educated nor inclined to move beyond their local network to nurse the bodies of the sick poor as publicly as did the Catholic Sisters. When they did decide to work for public reforms, they often focused on women's social issues; for example, the Female Temperance Societies aimed to convert women to Christianity and move them to abstinence from liquor for the betterment of female solidarity.[58] Sociocultural belief during the period also included the notion that because women were united by their "preeminent susceptibility of heart" and their "correspondent obligations" only they could fully understand and relieve the needs of women.[59]

The Sisters managed the gender issues associated with nursing care as well as with their Community much in accordance with the mores of the period and the customs of their heritage. For example, while the SC referred to priests as "Father," signifying the hierarchical structure of Roman Catholicism, the title "Sister" that they used to refer to themselves individually and collectively suggested an equality that characterized their spiritual relationship. Because they were excluded from the clerical status assigned to men in the Catholic Church, the Sisters formed close bonds with each other in community.

When women joined the SC Community, they brought ideas, knowledge, experiences, and talents. The nursing care that emerged in the American Community was as much a product of the American Sisters who created the Community as it was a product of the heritage that inspired the work in the first place. The growth of any community depends upon the ingenuity and resourcefulness of the people involved. When Mother Seton began the Emmitsburg Community she attracted resources: funds, land, food, and people; some of the Sisters came to the Community with extensive nursing skills. The ingredients for the creation of Vincentian-Louisian nursing in America included physical space for the gathering of the Community, the founders' vision as described in the *Common Rules*, the French DC momentum of success, and the nursing experience and skills of American Sisters.

In the nineteenth century, American women were expected to be able to nurse their families and to a certain extent their communities. But early diaries, journals, and community records such as the records of the Ladies Physiological Institute[60] reveal that some women were identified and supported, often financially, as experts in nursing the sick, pregnant, or infirm in their local communities.[61] Charitable nursing work in particular opened the door for women to enter what has been defined as the "public sphere." While some in Europe and America, such as Herbert Spencer, believed that "society was evolving towards the point when all women would be able to stay at home" and the separation between the male-dominated public sphere and the female-dominated domestic sphere would be "complete,"[62] some women argued that domestic talents should be applied to local government and public institutions such as hospitals. The general cultural recognition of the importance of women's domestic expertise and the perceived predilection of women for religious experience set the stage in America for the emergence of an organized, holistic, and enlightened nursing profession in the hospitals of the public sphere.

By the nineteenth century Vincentian-Louisian nurses in Europe had been providing professional nursing care in the public sphere for centuries. The American SC's Community provided the means for women to enter public life in a way that was not only nonthreatening but most welcome. Nursing the sick poor in hospitals allowed the Sisters of Charity to exercise their familial and community charitable influence more broadly. The early Sisters' partnership with the male Sulpician and Vincentian priesthood enabled them to broker relationships with male hospital administrators in the public sphere that they might not have been able to accomplish had they negotiated on their own.

The SC wanted to move among the people, in particular the sick poor. Their mission was to be *in public*, not in the cloister. The demand for nurses for the sick poor was and perhaps always will be immense. Joining an apostolic community to serve the sick poor was a natural consideration for the single or widowed nineteenth-century American woman, especially if she was Catholic. Many came from patriarchal religious homes, and therefore the transfer to the culture associated with religious life would have been relatively easy. What was perhaps more of a challenge was the *work* that brought the Sisters, the religious women, outside the home and the grounds of the emerging Emmitsburg Community. While the early

Sisters of Charity, like other nineteenth-century American women, may have first entered the public sphere as benevolent women visitors caring for the poor in their homes, the SC quickly moved into the male-dominated public sphere of hospitals, where they worked beside male physicians under the constitutional protection of priest ecclesiastical Superiors.

Indeed, the Sisters needed protection. The very establishment of a women's Catholic community in the nineteenth century was a form of religious activism on two accounts: first, the religious Community comprised and was administered by women in collaboration with male Church leadership, and second, the Sisters provided public service in a period of rising anti-Catholic sentiment from nativist Protestants. It was societal understanding of the necessity of the expert level and scope of the Sisters' benevolent work among the sick poor and insane, who were some of the most marginalized individuals of American society, that may have best protected them from religious ridicule, persecution, and the destruction that was the result of nativist riots during the period. The early SC history of nursing care, entrepreneurialism, and enlightened charity takes place within a strong anti-Catholic, particularly anti-Irish-Catholic, sociopolitical climate.

By 1830 the population of Maryland was 446,913 whites and 102,878 slaves.[63] Baltimore was the largest Catholic city in the nation. The *Catholic Almanac* approximated the American Catholic population to be 1,300,000 in 1840. It was during this period that rising numbers of immigrants were viewed by many white, native-born Americans as posing a crisis for the country. Between 1830 and 1840 immigration into Baltimore, which included many Irish Catholics, was 55,322; from 1840 to 1850 it was 68,392.[64] The formation of the Native American—that is, the American-born—political party, also referred to as "Know-Nothings," drew tens of thousands of supporters, including women. Although they did not have the right to vote in elections, native-born American women joined the movement against "popish" Catholics, especially Catholic foreigners.

While nativist women might have supported the work of the SC because of their belief in the spiritual superiority of women, they were also "outspoken proponents of the ideology of true womanhood and domesticity,"[65] a view that would not have conjured the image of a woman's life demonstrated in that of the Catholic SC Community of teachers and nurses. Many Americans would have viewed the benevolent work of the SC solely as a means of proselytizing. Winning the trust of Americans was not easy for the Sisters. Their decision to create a Catholic community of women during the early and mid-nineteenth century was quite bold, and the protective relationship with priests was important to the physical survival of the Community during the early years. While perhaps not the focus of their intention, the Sisters' acts of community building were in fact part of the religious reform that occurred in America during this time. The power of the Catholic Sisters' nineteenth-century public statement in a nativist environment might be analogous to the impact the establishment of a twenty-first-century Muslim nursing service in midtown Manhattan following the attack on the World Trade Towers might have had on native New Yorkers.

It is questionable whether the Sisters could have achieved their goals without the support of the male priesthood who worked with them. According to one antebellum historian, religious activism was one of the "rare arenas of nineteenth-century life where men's and women's lives and identities very closely intersected."[66] This was certainly true of the SC, but as was discussed earlier, the relationship was not something newly invented to further the Catholic agenda. The sister-priest relationship was foundational to the Vincentian-Louisian heritage and community. American-based priests were instrumental in helping the SC carve out public opportunities for their missions, such as nursing the sick poor. The first such occasion for hospital service came to the Sisters in 1823.

The First Hospital Mission at the Baltimore Infirmary ⌒

The Baltimore Infirmary was established in 1823 by the physician faculty of the College of Medicine of Maryland, now the University of Maryland. Adjacent to the medical college, the infirmary was described by the Sisters as "small and inconvenient"[67] in the early years. There were four wards, one specifically for ophthalmic surgery, and an operating theatre that would be converted in 1852 to a chapel. The capacity of the building was said to be 160 beds, an "exaggerated statement," according to a University of Maryland historian.[68] In Arthur Lomas's early history, the infirmary was established under the "immediate control" of the professors of the college, "with a view of affording to the medical students an opportunity of witnessing the practice of their future profession and attending clinical lectures."[69] Rev. John Dubois, the director of Mount St. Mary's College and Seminary near Emmitsburg and Superior for the SC, negotiated the contract between the SC and the faculty of the college, led by Dr. Granville Sharp Pattison. As mentioned in chapter 1, Dubois was very familiar with the DC Nurses' work in France and was therefore well aware of the potential for success the Sisters could have in America given the right environment. Some were concerned and hesitant, however, to enter into hospitals administered solely by Protestants. In 1818 Ambrose Maréchal, archbishop of Baltimore, spoke of the Emmitsburg Sisters in a report to Cardinal Litta:

> Sisters who live according to the rules of their holy founder, the exception of the modifications demanded by American customs and dispositions. They do not take care of hospitals, nor could they since the administration of these hospitals is Protestant. Their principal work is the pious education of Catholic girls, those of the poor as well as those of the rich.[70]

Mother Seton, much like Louise de Marillac at first, favored education, care of orphans, and some home nursing, rather than the movement of the SC Nurses into the hospitals. While Bishop Carroll agreed with Mother Seton's stand, some of the Sulpician priests disagreed and took steps to import French DC to Maryland to help establish the hospital-nursing aspect of the mission. Bishop-elect Benedict Flaget (1763–1850), who brought the *Common Rules* from France that Dubois translated and who originally favored the importation of the French DC, wrote, "I dread the arrival of the religious women who are to come from Bordeaux. . . . Their hopes will be frustrated. . . . I would wish at least that they be informed in detail of the spirit which reigns in the house at Emmitsburg, of the slight hope of serving in hospitals."[71] Napoleon prohibited the French DC Nurses from going to America.

The Sulpician priests were the protectors of the spiritual mission of the SC. Dubois's letters negotiating the mission at the Baltimore

Infirmary demonstrated his desire to establish proper authority as well as responsibility for the Sisters so that they could follow their *Regulations* and serve society in a manner in keeping with their tradition. He wrote to Mrs. Pattison in May 1822 that the Sisters felt that, having accepted the hospital mission, they were "true Sisters of Charity."[72] Dubois also wrote in his letter that the Sisters were educated before being assigned to their Baltimore Infirmary mission: "Prudence does not permit us to turn out young Sisters, until sufficiently tried and instructed."[73]

Dubois made specific demands on administrators. He stressed, for instance, that the Sisters would report only to Dr. Pattison:

> He may depend upon their exertions, their economy, their human attentions to the sick, their cleanliness in every department of the house, but on his part, he must put an unlimited confidence in their management. . . . They must be at liberty to follow the rules of their institution which so far from interfering with their duties as nurses of the sick, will enable them to fulfill them with greater facility as this is the first trial of the kind.[74]

Dubois was also quite clear that the men servants would be selected by and report directly to the Sisters, so that the men would pay them the "respect and obedience necessary for good order."[75] To ensure the success of the Sisters' mission, Dubois set out to establish institutional "rules" that he felt would secure respect for the Sisters. His comments to Dr. and Mrs. Pattison showed that Dubois did indeed have vision, experience, and knowledge regarding the way in which missions for women nurses should be carried out:

> It will be also necessary, according to the nature of Mr. Pattison's institution, to establish certain rules in the beginning which will secure for the Sisters from the patients admitted there that respect, that modest deportment in language and behavior which in Catholic countries is never departed from, but which might easily be forgotten here where they know nothing of the dignity

and purity of those religious women who with so much
charity stoop to the meanest offices of servants.[76]

Bishop Dubois and Dr. and Mrs. Pattison negotiated terms of the
management of the infirmary, including such things as the Sisters' board
at the facility. The agreement with the infirmary provided for "medical
insurance" of sorts for the Sisters who served there, and the Sisters' burial
expenses were also to be paid by the infirmary administration should a
Sister die while in service to the institution. The Sisters were required to
keep a register of patients and an inventory of supplies, furniture, and
money. They had the ability to hire male attendants to perform tasks such
as carrying coal, wood, and water to the wards; carrying messages and
provisions and transporting sick male patients. Most importantly, the
male attendants were to "render services repugnant to female delicacies
or propriety."[77] The *Regulations of the Baltimore Infirmary* included
instructions for patients and the duties of medical students.

By 1834 the infirmary had eight wards and ninety beds: three wards
for seamen, three wards for white male citizens, one ward for females,
and one ward for blacks.[78] Patients were required to pay $3.00 per week
to the medical students. There were two resident students who lived at
the infirmary; the *Regulations for the Baltimore Infirmary* state that at
least one medical resident student had to be present at all times in the
infirmary and that all patients had to be visited at night before the student
retired. In addition to collecting all fees, the student also kept a record of
all prescriptions and "did all the dressings."[79] The students were to be in
the infirmary after nine o'clock p.m. in the winter and ten o'clock in the
summer.

Students were not allowed to approve leave for patients without
supervision by the Sister Servant, the attending physician or surgeon,
or a senior student. They were also to expel any patient who returned
intoxicated or "disorderly." The Sister Servant could also expel patients
who violated infirmary regulations. The regulations were established
to provide the structure necessary for the facility as it embarked on a
pioneering endeavor in medical education. The program of bedside
instruction at the Baltimore Infirmary was said to be the first of its kind:

The Hospital department of the University, in the immediate vicinity, and nearly opposite the Medical College,
from its proximity, offers advantages for Clinical studies
not to be found elsewhere. Here the student can, day by
day, watch the progress of disease and the operation of
remedies, and become familiar with the aspect of both
acute and chronic complaints—can not only witness
surgical operations, but also what is equally important,
the nature and result after treatment—advantages not
to be obtained, where the Hospital is at a distance and
visited only at long intervals.[80]

In January 1824 Bishop Dubois wrote a lengthy letter to a Mr. Smith at
the infirmary (presumably the senior student) about difficulties with the
students. The students were not obeying the ten o'clock curfew and were
not giving the Sister Servant the key to the infirmary at night. Dubois
wrote of the students, "They want to unite the pleasures of life with the
serious studies of the medical art—and spoil them both. . . . I lay aside
all the scandals, irregularities which the privilege claimed by the young
students of returning to the Infirmary at any hour in the night might
introduce in the institution."[81]

The Sisters, with Dubois's help, created a new public role for women
in America in 1823. They were able to design a work environment at
the Baltimore Infirmary that was safe for women nurses as well as for
patients. Sister Joanna Smith (1768–1841) was selected by Mother Rose
White to be the first Sister Servant or local Superior for the mission. Sister
Joanna was born in Frederick, Maryland, and entered the Community
in 1812. Prior to 1802 SC Community records state that she had joined
the Discalced Carmelite Nuns residing in Port Tobacco, Maryland, but
she left the Carmelite order and was "in the world" for ten years until
she became a Sister of Charity. She was described in Community records
as a "rigid disciplinarian"[82] and very devoted to the care of the sick. The
records continue that Sister Joanna:

possessed in an eminent degree that holy liberty of the
children of God, doing what her conscience dictated, wholly

regardless of any human consideration of this, she once gave remarkable example in the following circumstance:

Being appointed as Sister Servant of the Baltimore Infirmary, she found that some of the arrangements entered into by the Most Rev. Archbishop [Samuel Eccleston] and Trustees, compromised the interest of the Community. She repaired in company with one of her companions, to the residence of that Archbishop and very simply and candidly told His Grace what she thought it a duty to say. Then knelt down and said: Archbishop, I have spoken plainly, if I have offended you I humbly ask your pardon.[83]

Sister Joanna trained Sisters Ann Gruber (1799–1840), Adele Salva (1785–1839),[84] and three new sisters who entered the SC in 1821: Veronica Gough (?–1804), Appollonia Graver (1799–1838), and Ambrosia Magner (?–1841), who were the first among many SC to be missioned to the infirmary.[85] Sister Joanna died of dropsy (edema) in January 1841 at the age of 72 after a ten-year bout with the illness. She left the Baltimore Infirmary in failing health in 1827, at which time Sister Ambrosia, who had pronounced her vows for the first time, was named Sister Servant.

The Baltimore Infirmary served as a prototype nursing mission for other SC work. Many of the Sister-Nurses rotated through the Baltimore Infirmary to be educated and gain experience. Sister Ambrosia Magner,[86] who was Sister Servant until her death in 1841, was born in Philadelphia. Her birth date is unknown, but she was the elder biological sister of Sister Josephine Collins (1801–1850), who was also born in Philadelphia. Sisters Ambrosia and Josephine both entered Emmitsburg in 1821. Sister Ambrosia was considered a "natural" at nursing the sick and was quite revered in Baltimore, as demonstrated in the obituary printed in the *Catholic Almanac*:

The death of this excellent Sister of Charity was a public calamity. Not only were her services invaluable to the hospital, over which she so wisely and vigilantly presided for so many years, her generous charity was felt far and wide, while the amenity of her disposition and her sweetness of manner gave it a tenfold charm in the eyes of the world.[87]

According to community records, Sister Ambrosia had a "weak stomach." When she began caring for patients, she felt great repugnance at dressing sores and ulcers and would generally throw up her meals after being engaged in this kind of nursing duty. She was considered:

> a brave soul who so much loved the suffering members of Jesus Christ, that she determined to overcome herself in this point, and so admirably she succeeded, that she has been heard to say, that she would sometimes forget to wash her hands after one of these operations, before going to meals. Ever after to the end of her life, though Sister Servant, she took as her duty, the dressing of the worst and most disagreeable sores and blisters.[88]

The Sister-Nurses cared for the patients at the Baltimore Infirmary at all hours, every day of the year. They willingly took on the "most menial or disgusting offices" asked of them so that the infirmary services could be performed with more "propriety, regularity, and union."[89] It took only five years for the Sisters' expertise to become well known.

Bishop Joseph Rosati, CM (1789–1843), one of the first Vincentians to come to America from Italy, requested Sisters to staff a new hospital in St. Louis that was to be the first hospital owned and operated by the diocese and the Sisters. A wealthy man, John Mullanphy, who was funding the building and staffing of the hospital would not, according to Rosati, "leave it in the hands of mercenaries; if we do not get the Sisters of Emmetsburg [sic], this establishment will fail, for I see too many difficulties to obtain any from France, and those of Kentucky[90] do not understand hospitals."[91] Sisters Francis Xavier Love (1796–1840),[92] Martina Butcher (1800–1849), Rebecca Dellone (1801–1848), and Francis Regis Berrett (1804–1862) opened the establishment in St. Louis. Bishop Rosati wrote the Mother[93] in Emmitsburg:

The hospital is on the footing of all the institutions of our State. It is but an embryo. I have no doubt it will grow into perfection, but before this time comes, we shall do what we can. Mr. Mullanphy has made over everything to me, and I have given *carte blanche* to the Sisters. They will have the advantage of not being under any other control than that of the Bishop of St. Louis who will never be in the way of their doing what they think proper, conformably to their customs and rules. I have been highly pleased with them, and edified at their conduct. I have discovered with pleasure that the Daughters of St. Vincent in America have perfectly succeeded in acquiring the virtues which he transmitted as a precious inheritance to his Daughters of France. St. Joseph's School must be acknowledged to be as proper as that of Paris to transmit the amiable spirit of their holy Founder to the Sisters of Charity.[94]

The Sisters realized that they would experience hardship associated with starting a new hospital. The original buildings were "poor and the furniture not brilliant," but the Sisters courageously kept their focus, as was their preparation, and raised the hospital in St. Louis into an esteemed institution. The nursing care provided by the Sisters in St. Louis carried the mission, just as had the Sisters' care in Baltimore. It was the expert nursing as well as the medical care that made each institution, such as the Baltimore Infirmary, a success. In the case of the Baltimore Infirmary, however, the Sisters' presence was not only important to patients; they also made the bedside learning opportunity for medical students of the University of Maryland's School of Medicine[95] possible.

Learning from Doctors and Disease

Some of the best resources on medical science to the Sister-Nurses were physicians. The Sisters had direct, didactic instruction from physicians: Community leadership paid faculty from the medical school at the University of Maryland to speak to them at Saint Joseph's in Emmitsburg from time to time. For example, William Aiken (1807–1888), a doctor and a chemist, who represented the medical faculty as one of the organizers of the Maryland College of Pharmacy in 1840,[96] gave a lecture on chemistry to the Sisters. His services were brokered through Rev. John Purcell, the president of Mount St. Mary's College and Seminary in Emmitsburg, who was to speak to the Mother on his behalf. In February of 1833 Aiken sent a letter offering his services to do a series of lectures on chemistry for the "very attentive and interesting audience at St. Joseph's."[97] The series would "occupy 6 or 8 weeks at the rate of three a week and would of course be accompanied by all the experiments necessary to illuminate the Science." Aiken also offered to give a lecture on botany once a week during the Sisters' recreation period, as it would be "recreation" for him to do so. He even agreed that for $100 plus room and board while teaching he would bring along his chemistry "apparatus."

More often, the Sisters learned through dialog and observation of physicians with whom they collaborated in the care of the sick. The Sisters also had direct access to the knowledge of physicians who attended the Community of Sisters when they were ill. During the early years, the Sisters may have also learned from physicians connected with the Community through Mother Seton's brother-in-law, Dr. Wright Post. One of the earliest notations listing the physicians who attended the Sisters is found in a chronology of the Community. It states that Dr. Robert Moore was appointed attending physician to the Sisters on June 27, 1820, at the death of his brother Dr. Daniel Moore.[98] The early SC also had access to the knowledge of Dr. Pierre Chatard (1767–1848) and Rev. Bruté. Mother Seton was very good friends with Dr. Chatard, a French physician residing in Baltimore, and his wife, Marie Francoise. Chatard, an eminent physician, midwife, and ophthalmologist, was a member of the Medical Society of Baltimore beginning in 1804 and was a consulting physician to the Board of Health and the Public Hospital in 1812.[99] Chatard, a Catholic, sailed to Baltimore in 1797 from Saint-Domingue, a French colony in the West Indies, to the southern United States with others, including Archbishop John Carroll, who was given ecclesiastical duties in the West Indies in 1804 and the Louisiana Territory in 1805.[100] Carroll, born in Maryland, was the first bishop in the United States, the first archbishop of Baltimore, and the Superior who witnessed the vows of Mother Seton and gave her the title of "Mother" in 1809.

Sister Mary Xavier also emigrated from the French colony to New Orleans during the same period, but her surname, Mestezzer, is not listed.[101] Two of Dr. Chatard's grandchildren entered religious life: Julianna became an SC, and his grandson Francis Silas trained as a physician at the University of Maryland in 1856 and then entered Mount St. Mary's Seminary. He became the fifth bishop of Vincennes, Indiana, in 1878, following in the footsteps of the first bishop, Rev. Bruté, who like his grandfather Pierre had been instrumental in supporting the mission of the SC.

Rev. Bruté was personally aware of the work of the French DC Nurses. His maternal aunt, Sister Françoise le Sanier de Vauhello (1740–1802), had been a DC at the Hospital Saint-André at Bordeaux, and a DC named Sister Magdalen lived with his family for a number of years after the French Revolution. Sister Magdalen had been a nurse for the inmates of the Prison of St. Michael's Gate for forty years when the prisoners were set loose by the new government.[102] From his description of her devotion to "her prisoners," one can imagine the nursing stories she might have told.

Bruté received his formal education and medical degree in Paris before being ordained to the priesthood. In 1799, at the age of twenty, he was a student of the renowned physician Dr. Philippe Pinel.[103] In 1802 Bruté was given the Corvisart Prize by the president of the School of Medicine.[104] Rev. Bruté had been in healthcare as an official medical doctor in France before entering the seminary of the Society of Saint Sulpice in 1804, after which he moved to Baltimore in 1810 and then Emmitsburg in 1812. Bruté was appointed spiritual director (pastor and confessor) to the Sisters in 1818. After entering seminary, Rev. Bruté did not practice medicine per se, which may have been due to a Church prohibition against priests shedding blood.[105] Bloodletting played a large role in the practice of physicians at that time.

There was continual correspondence between Rev. Bruté and Mother Seton. He was loved and respected by Mother Seton and the SC, as his spiritual instructions seemed to inspire such religious fervor. Mother Seton in a letter to her friends in Europe introduced Rev. Bruté as "a most distinguished soul . . . esteemed as an inestimable treasure in the Church."[106] He addressed the Sisters as "true priests of Charity" and admonished them to "save souls: be not selfish; be truly priests yourselves;

priests of mercy and charity."[107] He often prayed all night for a Sister in trouble and gave the SC "the full benefit of his spiritual and intellectual accomplishments."[108] Bruté's medical dissertation, titled "On the History and Advantages of Clinical Institutions," traced the development of clinical institutions from the time before Hippocrates to the year 1803. It is quite possible that he would have shared this historical knowledge of clinical institutions and his medical expertise with Mother Seton and the Novice Mistress, Sister Mary Xavier, who spoke French.

In 1814 Bruté returned from France to Emmitsburg with his personal library, which included his medical books and one very small, pocket-sized reference book written in 1767 entitled, *Description Abrege des Plantes Usuelles. A vecleurs vertus, leursufages & leurs proprietes. Par l'Auteur du manuel de Dames de Charite & pour server au suite au même Ouvrage. A Paris Chez Debure pere, Quai des Augustrus, a l'Image Saint Paul.* The French translation of this title indicates that this pocket-sized herb book was written by the same author who wrote the nurses' botanical manual for the French Ladies of Charity, Royal Physician Louis Daniel Arnault de Nobleville. Bruté's collection is housed today at the Library and Museum of the Old Cathedral of St. Francis Xavier in Vincennes, Indiana. Because the nursing work of the Sisters was part of their religious life and mission, it also seems probable that Bruté would have shared his medical books and provided medical consultation to the SC Nurses as he did religious instruction.

Rev. Bruté held counsel with physicians who treated seminarians and the SC when they were ill. One example appears in his notes about the "Seminary of Mt. St. Mary's, 22nd. 8bre, 1829:"

> Monday 12. I met just in the street Jerome Bonaparte, who stopped his gig to speak the first to me, remembering well his old stay at the Mountain. He promised to call on me. I have seen Mr. Kensey this morning with Mr. Hughes and Mr. Pise. I have conferred with M. Chaoan about Caroline Livers. He sees 'No need of prescription (nor I)' . . . Exercise and 'Ointment of opodeldoc' is sufficient.[109]

Another example occurred on June 20, 1826: "I have not been to the Sisters since the 29th of May. That day I did not see Sister Benedicta.[110] I do not remember having seen her. I had never examined the character of her malady, nor had I any conversation with the Doctor concerning it. I confined myself to believe her generally in consumption."[111] Sister Benedicta's "cure" was considered "supernatural," a term commonly used by the Community to refer to what they perceived as miraculous and divine intervention. The Sisters believed Sister Benedicta's cure to be related to Bruté's prayers. Bruté became a doctor of the spirit as well as of the physical body. He was the "favorite doctor" of Mother Seton's child, Bec,[112] who died in 1816 of tuberculosis of the bone.

On rare occasions, Bruté did treat patients when a physician was unavailable. He once treated a Mount St. Mary's student's broken arm when the college physician was not there. Bruté was also known to have traveled long distances to minister to the sick and dying. An avid walker, he once walked thirty miles in one day.[113] In light of his personal history with the DC and given the ecclesiastical prohibition against priests practicing medicine, Bruté's care of the sick might be better described as "nursing." In fact, one historical account of his work during the cholera epidemic of 1832 does describe his work as that of "nursing" the sick.[114] During the cholera epidemic in 1832, Bruté walked to Baltimore from Emmitsburg to volunteer his services after receiving authorization from James Whitfield, archbishop of Baltimore. Two years later in 1834 when he was named bishop, Rev. Bruté left the Mount and the SC for Vincennes, Indiana.

Cholera Victims and Victors

While the Vincentian-Louisian tradition was well known throughout Europe, the Sisters' hospital work was still new to Americans in the 1830s. The major event that served to solidify the SC's reputation as professional nurses was the cholera pandemic of 1832. Cholera is a deadly disease discovered by Robert Koch in 1883, caused by bacteria that lodge in the intestines. The onset of the disease is rapid, with death occurring in approximately half of the victims within a day, even within hours, of the first symptoms of diarrhea, vomiting, and cramps. Victims turn cyanotic from severe, rapid dehydration, and their extremities become cold. The disease is most often spread through contaminated water but also by unwashed hands and raw vegetables and fruits. While Americans in the 1830s did not know the bacterial cause of disease, they did have understanding that filth, contaminated water, and fruits and vegetables were probable causes.

Although cholera claimed fewer victims than malaria and tuberculosis, its shocking, rapid onset and death spurred many to call for sanitation reform and better public health standards. It also changed medical belief. Many adopted a more "positivistic" approach to medicine and public health, calling for evidence that could be expressed in numbers and tables.[115] The Sister-Nurses collected much of the data on cholera in Philadelphia and Baltimore because they staffed the cholera temporary hospitals during the 1832 outbreak.

The Sisters began their cholera service in Baltimore during the summer heat of August. According to reports by the Baltimore Commissioners of Health, the city had been unable to procure "suitable persons" to attend the sick at Temporary Hospital Nos. 2 and 3. They appealed to Rev. Deluol and a Rev. Elder[116] to request Sister-Nurses from Emmitsburg.[117] Seven Sisters were missioned to the temporary hospitals: the County Almshouse (Hospital No. 2) and the old meeting house (Hospital No. 3). The commissioners praised the Sisters highly:

> The zeal with which these important duties were performed, entitles those pious ladies to the highest praise from all humane persons, and has deeply impressed upon the members of this Board feelings of high respect, and obtained their most sincere thanks. [The following appears as a footnote] Note—The fact is so well known, that it is almost needless to state, that those truly benevolent ladies refused, absolutely, to receive any compensation whatever for their services.[118]

One can only imagine the environment in which the nurses performed their care: managing copious amounts of bodily fluids without the benefit of modern plumbing. They entered the cholera hospitals knowing the risks, and two of the Sisters did die from cholera: Sister Mary George

Smith (1811–1832), age 19, died in Hospital No. 2 while working with Dr. Edward Carrere, and Sister Mary Frances Boarman (1804–1832), age 28, died in Hospital No. 3 working with Dr. Augustus Warner. The two Sisters were mourned by the Catholic Community and by Protestants as well. The mayor of Baltimore eulogized the Sisters' courage and sacrifice, and the city paid $600 to erect a monument in their honor. Perhaps the most poignant account of the work of physicians and SC Nurses and the compassion they had for each other during the 1832 scourge is depicted in the journal account of Dr. Warner:

> At 15 minutes before 11 o'clock A.M. I left the Hospital for the purpose of recruiting myself from an attack of cholera—I left Sr. M Francis at the bed of a patient just admitted in a state of Collapse. She complained of feeling weak—Upon a strict examination by interrogation I found, agreeable to her assurance that her bowels were as usual—Not more relaxed than she was accustomed to—I advised her; Nay! Urged her to desist from duty a day or two and rest herself—she persisted however and I went home—At 11 o'clock I was summoned to the Hospital to see Sister Mary Francis and was at her bed side 15 minutes after the attack. She had fainted a few minutes after I left the Hospital and remained in a state of exhaustion when I saw her.[119]

Warner (1807–1847) described his treatment of Sister Mary Frances in detail. He even called in his "friend," Dr. R. H. Thomas, to help. They tried treatments such as "Pulv. Ipecac z," warm brandy toddy, cupping of the abdomen, and "Magnesia jalap and enemas." When it became clear that the Sister had cholera, Mother Augustine Decount (1827–1870) was called to the hospital. She and Sister Mary Francis sent for the Superior, Rev. John Hickey and Dr. Baker, the "old physician" who attended the Sisters. Numerous other treatments were tried, to no avail. At 7:30 P.M. she was dead. Warner wrote, "Life's taper dies in the socket. Dead. My life! What a figure!!!"[120] The tenor of his notes demonstrated his anguish.

His relationship with the Sisters did not end after the close of the cholera hospitals; he would contact them again from Virginia. In the meantime, news of the lives saved[121] by the noble work of the physicians and Sister-Nurses in the cholera hospitals and the deaths of the two Sisters spread throughout the state and the country. While it may not have been their intention, the sacrifices made by the SC—who chose to enter cities suffering a dreaded plague when many ran the other direction—proved to create a legacy for the Community. Their skill and character was broadly known among Protestant and Catholic circles alike. Numerous other successful nursing missions spread south to New Orleans as well as many other American cities after the cholera outbreak of 1832.

By aligning themselves with medical programs and physicians such as Drs. Augustus Warner and William Aiken at the College of Medicine in Baltimore, the SC Nurses gained access to a segment of the traditionally male-dominated public sphere where physicians pursued the "cutting edge" science of the day. Although women were not allowed to enter medical programs until later in the nineteenth century, the SC Nurses had recourse early on to medical knowledge through their professional relationships with physician colleagues, particularly the students at the college with whom they lived and worked at the Baltimore Infirmary. By 1833, just ten years after entering the infirmary for the first time, the American Sisters of Charity had firmly established their expertise in hospital nursing, especially in the care of patients stricken with cholera, a disease that baffled physicians. Although their physician colleagues were unable to find the keys to unlock the mysteries of all diseases, the Sister-Nurses continued on their journey of building their skill in the "Blessed Art." In 1833 they took up the cause so near and dear to the heart of Vincent de Paul: the nursing care of the insane.

⌒ Called to Nurse the Insane ⌒

Vincent de Paul had strong beliefs about the importance of the care of the insane to the spiritual mission of the DC. He instructed the Sisters who were sent on mission to a hospital in Paris called *Les Petites Maisons* that God

> willed to give those Sisters another ministry, namely . . .
> those poor persons who have lost their minds. Yes, my

> Sisters, it is God Himself who willed to make use of the
> Daughters of Charity to look after those poor mental
> patients. What a happiness for all of you. What a great
> grace for those Sisters engaged in this work to have such
> a beautiful means of rendering service to God and to His
> Son Our Lord."[122]

Vincent had personal experience with people who were suffering from emotional imbalance and mental illness. When reflecting on the early years of the Congregation of the Mission at their motherhouse on the outskirts of Paris, Vincent recalled that when his Community assumed ownership of the former priory of Saint Lazare in 1632, originally built as a leprosarium, there were a few insane persons living there. Vincent assumed responsibility for their care, but when faced with litigation about the property, he recalled asking himself the question, "If you had to leave this house right now, what would you find hardest about leaving? And it seemed to me, then, that the worst thing would be to have to abandon these poor people and not be able to look after them and serve them."[123]

During Vincent's lifetime, people with mental illness lived in a small asylum in one of the buildings on the property of the priests' motherhouse called Saint Lazare. Young people with delinquent behavior whose families had committed them there as to a reformatory were confined in another area. Vincent oversaw the care of both groups of inmates. He was dedicated to the humane treatment of the insane, and patients were served the same food as the priests and brothers. Failure to do so resulted in a grave reprimand.[124] His firsthand experience of emotional pain and mental suffering sensitized Vincent to instructing the DC in nursing ministries, which in his day included the care of galley slaves, beggars, the homeless, prisoners, and the violent mentally ill.

Although Mother Seton and the American SC had intentions of nursing in hospitals, as had the DC in France for nearly two centuries, anti-Catholic sentiment precluded their entry in the early years. As stated previously, out of necessity for educating their medical students, the physicians at the Baltimore Infirmary recruited the Sisters. The SC also provided nursing at the Marine Hospital in Baltimore for a brief period in 1827. By the conclusion of their heroic service during the 1832 cholera epidemic, the American Sisters had successfully turned the tide of prejudice. In 1833 the Sisters were asked to staff the Maryland Hospital for the Insane in Baltimore, situated on Broadway.[125]

In December of 1833 Mother Mary Augustine Decount missioned Sister Olympia Boyle McTaggert (1802–1869), who had nursed cholera victims in Philadelphia during the 1832 epidemic, as Sister Servant to the Maryland Hospital. She sent two Sisters with Sister Olympia: Sister Octavia McFadden (1813–1853), who had been missioned at the Baltimore Infirmary since 1831, prior to making vows for the first time in 1833, and Sister Matilda Coskery (1799–1870), who in a very short time would be recognized by the SC Community, patients, and physicians as an expert in the care of the insane.

Sister Matilda Coskery, 1828–1833 ⌒

Sister Matilda Coskery was born Anastasia on November 21, 1799, to Irish-American John Coskery (1766–1834) and English-American Jacoba Clementina Bathilda Spalding (1772–1850), daughter of Anne Elder and Henry Spalding of lower Maryland, probably either Prince George's County or Saint Mary's County.[126] Anne and Henry were believed to

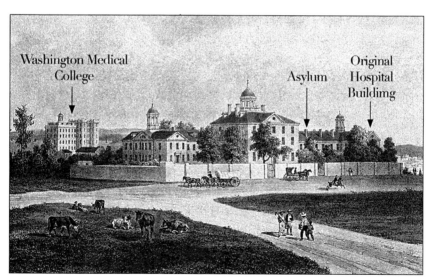

Fig. 2-3   *The Maryland Hospital (1827-1836)*

have been married in 1792 by Archbishop John Carroll.[127] At the time of Anastasia's (Matilda's) birth, the Coskery family was living in the vicinity of Taneytown, which was then located in Frederick County, Maryland. John Coskery may have been employed as both a hatter and a teacher. There are few records of the life of Jacoba, but she had been the eldest of a family of eight children of Taneytown, Maryland. She also became mother of a family of eight children. Anastasia, as second to the eldest, would have assisted her mother, Jacoba, in managing the household and caring for the younger children.

When Anastasia's brother, Henry Benedict (1808–1872),[128] was born, the family lived at the Haines Farm by Middleburg in Frederick County near Taneytown. A deed dated May 20, 1805, recorded in Frederick County between John Coskery and Rev. Nicholas Zocchi and the Trustees of the Roman Catholic Congregation of Taneytown, shows that the Coskerys sold land to the parish. Two Coskery girls, first cousins to Anastasia and about the same age, attended Saint Joseph's Academy in its early years, soon after Elizabeth Ann Seton established the school for girls in 1810. Their names, Catherine and Elizabeth (Eliza) Coskery, daughters of Bernard and Anastasia, appear in the ledger as early as 1813; they were enrolled soon after the death of their mother. Their father married again in 1816. Rev. Zocchi witnessed the marriage vows between Bernard Coskery and his second wife, Elizabeth, of the prominent Taney family for whom Taneytown was named.

It is not exactly known how Anastasia, who was raised in a Catholic home and town, was first drawn to religious life. She may have had opportunities to be introduced to Mother Seton and the new order of American SC through Rev. Zocchi. Or she may have inherited the "Spalding Spirit" to join a religious community from her mother, which had already inspired one of her cousins, Catherine in Kentucky, to establish a new SC Community there. Anastasia's maternal grandfather, Henry Spalding, was the brother of Edward, who is believed to have been the father of Catherine (1793–1858).[129] In 1813, fifteen years prior to Anastasia's entry into Saint Joseph's, Catherine helped to found the Sisters of Charity of Nazareth in Kentucky.

Catherine was born in Maryland but moved to Kentucky after her father died. Her mother died soon after, and she was reared by her

Uncle Thomas and Aunt Elizabeth Spalding Elder. The SC Nazareth was formally established by Rev. John David (1761–1841) and Bishop Flaget in Nazareth, Kentucky, near Bardstown using the Vincentian-Louisian *Rules* translated for the Emmitsburg Community. Catherine was elected the first Mother and was subsequently reelected many times over the course of her lifetime, serving as Mother for a total of twenty-five years in the Community. Mother Catherine was known for her "pioneer spirit" that infused all that she did in Community.[130] She led the SC of Nazareth to found schools and nurse cholera victims during the 1832 epidemic. Mother Catherine was adept in financial matters and brokered the purchase of land and buildings for the Sisters' missions. In 1836 Mother

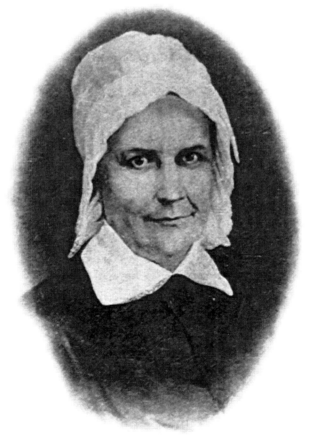

Fig. 2-4   *Mother Catherine Spalding*

Courtesy Sisters of Charity of Nazareth, Nazareth, Kentucky

Catherine opened the first privately owned hospital of the Sisters of Charity of Nazareth in Louisville, called St. Vincent's Infirmary.[131]

Whether Anastasia ever met and was prompted to religious life and her work in nursing by SC leaders Catherine Spalding or Elizabeth Seton is unknown. She was impressed by some of her friends' piety and felt drawn to devote herself more earnestly to the service of God. She told a friend that when visiting Baltimore during her youth she had attended daily Mass, a privilege not typically available in more rural areas in the early part of the nineteenth century.[132] One of Anastasia's favorite activities was reading, particularly popular works. As she moved toward religious life, she resolved to change her reading habits by curtailing light reading and choosing devotional and inspirational titles instead. Anastasia's enjoyment of reading may have led her to assist her father in his teaching duties at a neighborhood school, but there is no record of her employment or whereabouts prior to joining the SC in Emmitsburg.

In 1828 Rev. Nicholas Zocchi, pastor of the Saint Joseph Catholic Church in Taneytown, recommended the twenty-eight-year-old Anastasia for entrance to the Sisters of Charity of Saint Joseph's at Emmitsburg. At the time that Anastasia was discerning her vocation to be a religious woman, the SC had been functioning for almost twenty years. According to a personnel roster maintained by Sister Margaret Cecilia George (1787–1868), SC treasurer, approximately 178 women had joined the Community by the time Anastasia submitted her application. In 1828 Mary Augustine Decount (1786–1870) was Mother of the Community. She was assisted by Sisters Fanny Jordan (1793–1867), Anna Maria Hartnett (1802–1852), and Ann Gruber (1799–1840). Rev. Deluol was the ecclesiastical Superior of the Community at the time (1826–1830), followed by Rev. Hickey. Rev. Bruté was chaplain for the SC in addition to his teaching responsibilities at Mount St. Mary's Seminary and pastoral obligations to Saint Joseph's Parish in Emmitsburg.

In their meeting of July 7, 1828, the Council of the Sisters of Charity, the Community's governing body, approved Anastasia for admission as a candidate. She must have arrived sometime before the end of September, because on October 1 the council decided that she was "allowed to return if she comes [back] within a month & [the] constitution [is] unbroken."[133] The records provide no detail or explanation for Anastasia's leave of the Community, but homesickness or family need would have been plausible reasons. Whatever the circumstances, Anastasia complied with the stipulation, completed her candidacy, and on August 11, 1829, the council approved her entrance into the seminary[134] under the instruction of Mary Xavier Clark. On August 15, 1829, Anastasia was admitted to the seminary and given the name Sister Matilda. At the end of her seminary Sister Matilda exchanged the brown dress and cap of a novice for the Mother Seton–styled black cap, cape, and dress, patterned after the attire of Tuscan widows.[135]

After about fourteen months in the seminary, on December 9, 1830, Mother Mary Augustine sent Sister Matilda on her first mission[136] to the infirmary at Mount St. Mary's College and Seminary, less than two miles from Saint Joseph's House. The Mount's infirmary was the location of the American Sisters' first nursing mission. Mother Seton, who was indebted to the Sulpician priests for their kindness and service, was concerned that Rev. John Dubois was having difficulty retaining qualified personnel for support services. She had established the Sisters' mission at the Mount under the direction of Sister Ann Gruber, Sister Servant,[137] in 1815. The Community provided Sisters as nurses, sacristans, catechists, and managers of the domestic department for the college and seminary until 1852. Sister Benedicta Parsons (1797–1876), who had fourteen years of experience in children's asylums and infirmary services and was highly esteemed, was the Sister Servant at Mount St. Mary's when Sister Matilda arrived. In the Vincentian tradition the Sister Servant played a key formative role among the Sisters, particularly for those who had not yet made vows for the first time. Although they intend a commitment for life, the SC, like the DC, made vows annually for one year at a time on the feast of the Annunciation.[138] This action of making vows ratified their commitment to the mission of the Company of the Daughters/Sisters of Charity, which was service of Christ in persons who are among the sick poor.

Sister Benedicta instructed Sister Matilda and prepared her to commit herself by pronouncing vows for the first time. Sister Matilda and two other novices, Sister Valentine Latouraudais (1812–1895)[139] and Sister Mary Domitilla Fanning (?–1865), made their vows for the first time on Christmas of 1831 in the little chapel of Saint Joseph's House, later referred to as the "White House." Sister Matilda was described by the Sisters who knew her as one who was "small, slight, rather pale with piercing black eyes, a quick and often abrupt manner of speech [and] whose lips were often moving in prayer."[140]

In 1831 Sister Benedicta was replaced as Sister Servant by Sister Martha Daddisman (1797–1889), who had served at Saint Joseph's Asylum in Philadelphia before assuming a role of leadership in the Community. Sister Martha was described as "short, stout, blonde, frank in disposition, cheerful and stirring to everybody who knew her, and everybody liked her."[141] For the remainder of that year, Sister Matilda, now thirty-two years old, worked with Sister Martha, Sister Servant, and Sister Perpetua Shannon (1806–1868), who had arrived at Mount St. Mary's in 1827.

The formative influence that Sister Mary Xavier, Sister Benedicta, and Sister Martha had on Sister Matilda may have been the genesis of her clinical expertise. Like Sister Mary Xavier, Sister Benedicta and Sister Martha had both joined the SC during the lifetime of Mother Seton; Sister Martha Daddisman entered in 1813, followed two years later by Sister Benedicta Parsons. Sister Benedicta had experienced a healing from a life-threatening illness in 1826.[142] Both had nursed the sick for some time. Some of their initial nursing skills were probably learned from Mother Seton and other older women in the Community, such as Sister Bridget, "Ma" Farrell, and Sister Joanna Smith. Ultimately, Sister Martha and Sister Benedicta transferred what they learned about caring for members of their own Community to other settings, such as Mount St. Mary's Infirmary, where they were missioned to provide nursing skills. In keeping with Vincentian-Louisian nursing tradition, Sisters Benedicta and Martha would have instilled in Sister Matilda a spiritual and compassionate concern for patients as well as a sound basic knowledge of nursing techniques.

Sister Matilda replaced Sister Mary Magdalen Councell (1808–1865) in the infirmary at the Mount, where she served in the role of Infirmarian until 1833. According to Vincentian nursing tradition, the Infirmarian-Nurse worked under the supervision of the Pharmacist-Nurse, who called the doctor when necessary and was "most exact to prepare the prescriptions." The Pharmacist also made sure that the Sister-Infirmarian "carried out her duty well; that she gave nothing to the sick which could cause them harm; that she did not tell them anything which could sadden them, or anything which is said at the House; that she gave nothing which was served at the sisters' meals."[143] The Pharmacist also had to "punctually obey, for others as well as for themselves, the prescriptions of the physician in every thing proper to his office and not contrary to their rules. They also obeyed in the same manner the infirmarian or nurses given to them, according to the extent of authority given to them by their office or their Superiors."[144]

Sister Matilda made her first annual spiritual retreat at Saint Joseph's in 1831, along with the other Sisters. Rev. Bruté, who preached during that retreat, also proved influential in the development of Sister Matilda, both as a religious woman and a holistic nurse. Bruté opened by preaching from the text, "Working together, then, we appeal to you not to receive the grace of God in vain" (2 Corinthians 6:1). He then went on to inspire the Sisters with thoughts on the grace of God, referring to "plans of peace—I have loved you with age-old love" (cf. Jeremiah 29:11 and 31:3). He concluded by exhorting the Sisters to have proper dispositions, a good intention, and confidence in God and to maintain and nurture a fervent life of prayer, characterized by both punctuality and perseverance.[145] Records of the SC Community state that Sister Matilda was a "timid and scrupulous" young woman at first who was prone to anxiety and subjected to "inner conflicts and interior struggles of a spiritual nature."[146] With the five years of education she received and the guidance of Mother Mary Augustine Decount, Mother Mary Xavier Clark, Sister Benedicta Parsons, Sister Martha Daddisman, and Rev. Bruté, Sister Matilda developed the self-confidence needed to express the nursing expertise for which she would soon become known.

Serving the Insane at the Maryland Hospital, 1833–1838 ⁓

Sister Matilda left the Mount and Saint Joseph's in Emmitsburg for the first time in 1833 to live and work in Baltimore. She continued to live in Community with experienced SC Nurse mentors such as the Sister Servant of the Baltimore Infirmary, Ambrosia Magner, and the Sister Servant for the new mission, Olympia McTaggert.[147] Sister Matilda's assignment was to nurse the patients at the Maryland Hospital for the Insane,[148] a public city hospital with a mental department. According to the report of a committee of the Maryland General Assembly assigned to conduct an inspection in 1837, the hospital had upon its recovery by the state in 1827 been "dilapidated, without furniture, and in debt." By 1837, just four years after the arrival of the SC, however, the establishment and its equipment were partially renovated, its debts were paid, and the nursing care of the patients had improved significantly. While the committee recognized the need for serious renovation to the west wing of the facility and recommended that the state allocate $30,000 for the task for the betterment of the care of patients, they were still very complimentary of the work the Sisters had already done to improve care. They wrote, "The committee feel it a duty incumbent on them, to extend to the ladies engaged in the management of the institution much credit, not only for the systematick [sic] neatness which characterize[s] its condition and operations, but also for their charitable zeal, in extending to those unfortunate beings every comfort and consolation."[149] According to the report, the Sisters had cared for 842 patients in three years. The biggest concern about the care of patients was that there was no wall surrounding the facility, and many patients had escaped. This was most likely due to the nature of the insane patients' illnesses rather than a lack of supervisory staff. At the time of the inspection there were seventy-four patients and twelve Sister-Nurses who administered the care with the aid of two men and six assistant women.

The Sisters typically drew little compensation for their missions, though receiving what they needed for clothing. At the Maryland Hospital for the Insane, each of the female attendants and the SC were paid five dollars per month and each of the male attendants ten dollars per month.[150] Five dollars per month was a low wage even in the nineteenth century, especially for the kind of work the Sisters did. In the 1830s the Maryland Hospital had two areas for care. They treated diseases such as epilepsy, fever, syphilis, dysentery, typhus, gangrene, and wounds. Beginning in 1834, however, they were not allowed to admit "contagious diseases." Another area was dedicated to the care of patients with mental disorders such as mania a potu (delirium tremens), intemperance, and melancholia, as well as diseases that in the nineteenth century were referred to more generally as insanity and idiocy.[151]

The Sisters were also responsible for the domestic duties of the institution. The Sister Servant collected all payments from patients and handled legal and business matters pertaining to admissions. Upon a patient's admission, she had to collect from the patient the certificate of insanity issued by the Court of Competent Jurisdiction or two "regular"[152] physicians, except in the case of those suffering delirium tremens or drunkenness, who could be admitted as long as they furnished a certificate soon thereafter.[153] The Sisters kept a ledger of all admissions and attended the insane under the direction of the medical attendant.

They executed medical prescriptions and were to make every effort to "soothe the patient's mind."[154] The Sisters worked with physical therapeutics, such as tea made from hops (*Humulus lupulus*), an herb that calms the nervous system. For example, it was given hourly to patients with delirium tremens who found it hard to sleep. If the hops tea was "not sufficient to produce sleep," the Sisters might administer forty drops of opium tincture.[155] Working with the hospital physician, Dr. William Stokes, until he resigned in 1836, the Sisters implemented a moral-therapy approach to treatment of the insane. This type of treatment will be explained further in chapter 3. It is a philosophy and practice of psychiatric care based on humaneness. The Sisters were to "engage the patient's affections and thoughts—amusing him—affording him exercise, by light labor, walking, riding, music, dancing—with wholesome diet, and cheerful conversation as the chief materia medica."[156]

It was neither their work nor their salaries, however, that caused the Sisters to withdraw from the Maryland Hospital on September 30, 1840, and open their own psychiatric hospital. It was the lack of authority granted them by administrators regarding the care of the patients. According to a "History of the Maryland Hospital" recorded in the front of the Maryland Hospital Patient Register for 1834–1872, the "Board dissolved its engagement with the Sisters, having found them good and faithful nurses but claiming more authority in the management of the patients than was deemed compatible with the rights and duties of a Resident Physician whose opinions the Board deemed paramount. From this period the Medical moral and financial conduct of the house had been under the direction of the Residents and Resident Physician subject alone to the supervision of the Board."[157] But according to the Sisters and their representative, Rev. Deluol, Dr. Richard Sprigg Steuart (1797–1876),[158] the Superintendent, was not keeping his end of the original agreement that he and the Sisters had made in 1833. Rev. Deluol wrote a follow-up letter threatening to contact the Board of Managers after having waited three months for Dr. Steuart to construct a new document of rules that the physicians would abide by. He suggested that

> if they wish to keep them [the Sister-Nurses] on the same conditions on which they were asked from the agreement will be written and they will remain. If not, they will go home. I might take them with me next week. When you requested me to use my influence for the Hospital you assured me repeatedly that they should have entire control of the Institution. It was with great difficulty that I prevailed upon the Council to send them. But they were sent upon the express condition last mentioned above, and it is only on the same condition that they will stay.[159]

Dr. Steuart responded to Rev. Deluol's letter, stating that he was surprised at Deluol's "tone" and that it was an "absurdity" to think that he would have made a "concession" to give the Sisters "entire" control over the institution. He wrote that the Sisters would have "entire control in the Domestick [sic] affairs of the House, and sh^d participate largely in the moral management of the patients, in fact exercising any degree of moral influence that did not directly conflict with medical principles which of course must always have precedence."[160] Dr. Steuart continued, stating that the Sister-Nurses were like "children" when they began their mission at the Hospital, and yet when they became more experienced he:

> allowed them and encouraged them to exercise more moral management. It was then for the first time I discovered that difficulties w^d occur between them and the Regular Physician of the house [Note: Would refer to Dr. William Fisher who succeeded D. Stokes] . . . medical dignity requires certain privileges and no medical man of character will dispense with these rights.[161]

One biography of Dr. Steuart described the man as performing his work with a "systematic fidelity, which showed a disciplined mind, and a high moral sense" and as a "pioneer" in the care of the insane; he is also said to have had a "temper exceeding quick and an honor equally sensitive."[162] It is not clear why Dr. Steuart was not able to negotiate a compromise that would suit both physicians and the Sisters. He was not a "professing Christian," and it is possible that there may have been religious differences between him and the Sisters.

Sister Servant Olympia's reason for pressing authority for the Sisters was chiefly her concern for the safety of the Sister-Nurses. She wrote to Rev. Deluol, "We are subjected to much inconvenience from the Patients, without having the Doctor to contend with & if Drunkards can go in & out without the Sister's permission, I think it a very improper place for us to be."[163] The power struggles between the Sister-Nurses and the resident physician were not resolved, but the historical records show that their service was exemplary. The SC left the Maryland Hospital because their differences with the administrators could not be reconciled. But the Sisters did not go away easily; they knew the importance of perseverance. Some of the same safety and authority issues had happened at the Baltimore Infirmary too, but the Sisters were able to resolve the differences with those administrators, at least until 1876, when they decided to leave after fifty-three years of service.

The historical records at the Maryland Hospital for the Insane do not detail the contributions of each Sister, and the SC Community records about the mission are scant. From the initial corps of three SC, the number of patients and subsequently the number of Sisters assigned to the Maryland Hospital ministry rose to nine by 1837, suggesting that the Sisters were indeed successful in creating an environment for the care of the insane that had the approval of patients or their family members. Sister Matilda was part of that successful mission until 1838, when she received her first leadership role as Sister Servant for a new hospital. Her collaboration with Dr. Stokes, with whom she had worked at the Maryland Hospital for the Insane, was not over, but before the next mission with him, she was missioned to Virginia. The SC Community was asked by one of Stokes's colleagues from the early days in Baltimore and friend of the SC from cholera hospitals, Dr. Augustus Warner, to help establish another infirmary associated with a new college of medicine, this time in Richmond.

Sister Servant in Richmond, Virginia, 1838–1840 ⌒

In response to an application from the faculty, the council sent Sisters to open the infirmary at the Richmond Medical College in Virginia. Mother Rose Landry White (1784–1841) missioned Sister Matilda, age 39, as Sister Servant for the new ministry in 1838. This was the first of several leadership roles Sister Matilda would fulfill in the Community. Sister Matilda left her family, the Sisters at Saint Joseph's, and her Baltimore medical and nursing community for the Commonwealth of Virginia on August 25, 1838. In her new role as Sister Servant, Sister Matilda had administrative as well as patient-care duties. Just as she had proven adept in the care of the insane, she exercised business skills with prudence and shrewdness, as was demonstrated in her reports on financial matters to Sister Margaret George (1787–1868), the Community treasurer at Saint Joseph's.

In 1840 her nursing team included Sister Romana Hemmell (1814–1835), Sister Mary Catherine Edward (?–1843), and Sister Priscilla Tuke (dates unknown). Sister Matilda most likely knew Dr. Warner, also of Baltimore, who was the founding physician at the Richmond Medical College. He graduated from the University of Maryland Medical School in 1829 and practiced in Baltimore until 1834, during which time, as mentioned previously, he worked at the Cholera Temporary Hospital No. 3 with the Sisters. He then accepted a position as professor of anatomy, physiology, and surgery at the University of Virginia. Warner was described by one of his students as:

> a man of medium stature, handsome face, brilliant blue eyes, possessed of 'soft musical voice, easy and graceful manners, great fluency of speech, a mind of great penetration, grasp, and logical power, a vivid imagination, and refined poetical taste. . . .' Both his lectures and his 'bold and dexterous operations' fascinated students. Dr. Warner's philosophy of instruction was summarized in a statement to at least one of his classes: 'Facts, opinions and theories will be passing in review before you. Theories will be discussed, errors must be exposed, and truth made triumphant.[164]

Dr. Warner left the University of Virginia in 1837 because of a salary dispute and the inability to obtain dissection "material."[165] He moved to Richmond, where he and other practicing physicians organized their own medical school under the Charter of the Hampden-Sydney College[166] in 1838. An infirmary with a capacity of 200 beds was opened in the remodeled Union Hotel.[167] The Sisters managed and staffed this infirmary as they had done for the medical college in Baltimore. It is understandable that Dr. Warner would have contacted Emmitsburg for a contingent of nurses to be sent to Virginia. His relationship with them in Maryland had been highly collegial. The SC had a reputation for proficiency if not expertise in the opening and management of infirmaries affiliated with their colleagues' medical schools. The Sisters of Charity are not mentioned, however, in Richmond Medical College's history of the medical department and its infirmary written in 1976.[168]

The role of the Sister Servant at the infirmaries was to run not only the business aspects of the nursing mission on behalf of the Sisters of Charity of Saint Joseph's but also to coordinate the community life of the Sisters. Sister Matilda's mission must have been successful; one history of the early years of the medical college states that "the infirmary which had opened in October, 1838, about a month before the Medical Department, had proved popular with the patients," and five years after its opening, the physicians were petitioning the state general assembly for a new building.[169] The SC nursed hundreds of sick and insane patients every year. Some hospitals were better staffed than others, and these staffing levels were published in the *Catholic Almanac* for review by the public. In 1840, for example, Sister Matilda reported that the Richmond Infirmary had forty patients on average and three Sisters attending them, a 1:13 nurse-patient ratio. The Sisters at the Maryland Hospital reported ninety patients on average and fourteen Sisters; a 1:6 ratio. The Baltimore Infirmary had fifty patients and eight Sisters, also a 1:6 ratio, and Charity Hospital in New Orleans had 360 patients on average with sixteen Sisters, a 1:22 nurse-patient ratio.[170] Just as is the case today, nurse-patient ratios were a concern to nurses, patients, physicians, and the public in Sister Matilda's time because ratios are one indicator of the level of attention paid to the patient.

Sister Matilda liked Richmond. But by November of 1840, the SC council had replaced Sister Matilda with Sister Josephine Collins (1801–

1850)[171] so that Sister Matilda could return to Emmitsburg for a new mission. Given the content of the correspondence between Sister Matilda and Sister Josephine, their time in Richmond must have overlapped, perhaps to ensure that Matilda had time to "pass the reins" to the new Sister Servant. Sister Josephine stated that Sister Matilda "insisted" that the views in Richmond were "beautiful."[172] Sister Josephine, however, did not think much of Richmond's hills and determined to "keep indoors as much as possible."[173] Sisters Matilda and Josephine were both happy with their dealings with Dr. Warner, the physician from whom the Sister Servants received reimbursement for the Sisters' expenses, such as clothing and travel. Sister Josephine reported to the Motherhouse that she "always got what she asked for"[174] from Dr. Warner. When discussing "money business" in her letters to the leadership at Emmitsburg, Sister Josephine mentioned that she and Sister Matilda had dealt successfully with the Sisters' travel expenses to and from their missions and Saint Joseph's. She also described the success of the first Catholic fair in Richmond to raise funds for painting the church. Although the Catholic fair was held the same days as were two Protestant fairs, Sister Josephine reported that their fair "took in more than the other two together."[175] Sister Matilda's Richmond experiences with fund-raising and establishing a new hospital's nursing services would prove useful in the not-so-distant future, when she would lead the Sisters in an entrepreneurial endeavor to open their own hospital for the insane.

CHAPTER 3

⁓ ♏ ⁓

Sister Matilda
⁓ Moral Entrepreneur, 1840-1849 ⁓

During the time that Sister Matilda Coskery was in Virginia opening the Richmond Infirmary, Sister Olympia McTaggart and the SC who remained at the Maryland Hospital[1] for the Insane were going through a major transition. In 1839 the Sisters and Dr. Richard F. Steuart, administrator and attending physician, had serious disagreement over the level of authority the Sisters should have in managing the hospital and its patients. As it began to appear that they might reach an impasse in negotiations, the SC, during a Community Council meeting at Emmitsburg, voted to purchase a hospital in Baltimore in case the Sisters "decided to leave the Maryland Hospital."[2] After all attempts to reconcile the differences failed, the SC withdrew on September 30, 1840, to forge a new path in the care of the insane. Only this time they determined to own and manage the institution themselves.

The Sisters moved temporarily into a building located on North Front Street beside the new Saint Vincent de Paul Church. The two-story, small-frame house was located among Irish immigrants in Jonestown, one of the oldest neighborhoods of Baltimore, and was owned by Rev. John Baptist Gildea, pastor of the parish. During the Sisters' withdrawal from the Maryland Hospital, the relatives and guardians of eighteen patients asked to transfer their family and friends for whom they promised to be financially responsible to the Sisters' care. The Sisters informed Community leadership in Emmitsburg about the prospect of continuing asylum care for the patients.

By 1840 the Community of Sisters had been incorporated as the "Sisters of Charity of Saint Joseph's" for twenty-three years, and with a surge of entrepreneurial spirit, they decided to create their own asylum. They would capitalize on their expertise in the care of the insane for the benefit of patients and their Vincentian-Louisian mission. The Sisters found a property on Harford Road in Baltimore, and at the annual meeting in July, "it was then moved and seconded, at the suggestion of Rev. L. R. Deluol to purchase the property . . . and there to commence an Asylum for the Insane, the motion was carried."[3] The property was purchased for $7,000, and an additional $3,000 was spent for furnishing and provisions. This was the beginning of the SC-owned asylum mission in America; the first name of the asylum was Mount St. Vincent's.

The newly purchased property on Harford Road included ten acres on which stood an old frame building with a capacity of about fifty patients. By 1841 it was ready for occupancy by the Sisters and their patients. Sister Mary Xavier Clark, Sister Matilda's Novice Mistress, had become Mother of the Community, and she missioned Sister Matilda to Mount St. Vincent's to replace Sister Olympia, who was recalled to Emmitsburg in January. Sister Matilda, in her role as Sister Servant, led the Sisters of Charity into a new phase of ministry with the insane that built upon their earlier experience as nurses for the insane at the Maryland Hospital.[4] Although she had not been the Sister Servant at the Maryland Hospital, she had demonstrated that she was particularly adept in the care of the insane:

> Sister Matilda was admirably suited for the management of this class of afflicted beings that the entire care of them devolved on her, and so wonderful were the benefits derived from her kind and judicious treatment of the Insane, that the Physicians were in admiration and considered her a real treasure. God certainly gifted her in a remarkable manner for the comfort of these poor bereaved creatures. They [the patients] loved her as a Mother, a benefactress and a friend; many of them attributed their restoration to reason to her gentle influence.[5]

Sister Matilda began the mission at Mount St. Vincent's with six Sister-Nurse companions; within two years however, the patient population had grown sufficiently to warrant adding three Sisters to the nursing staff. Of the original six Sisters, four nurses had transferred from the Maryland Hospital, including Sisters Francenia Bigham (?–1857), Mary Baptista Douds (1814–1871), Jane Frances Higgins (1808–1879), and Sister Octavia McFadden, with whom Matilda had worked from 1833 until 1838. The other two SC Nurses were Sister Ann Elizabeth Corby (1776–1869) and Sister Thaddeus McGowan (?–1883).

At first the Sisters admitted both sane and insane patients to the "house." The patients called the new facility the "boarding house" because it had "nothing of the 'Hospital' appearance about it."[6] The Sisters knew that the Harford Road facility would be temporary because they had pressure from Archbishop Samuel Eccleston (1801–1851) and some of the supporters of their care of the insane who objected to the asylum's location. The Sisters did not plan to erect a permanent building on Harford Road, but the large old house soon became overcrowded and required expansion, so a two-story frame wing was added to the old building at a cost of $700. This allowed for the admission of at least twenty-five more patients. Staff and residents were constantly wary of fire, which could devastate their establishment, constructed entirely of wood. Within about two years patient numbers had grown beyond the capacity of Mount St. Vincent's, and Sister Matilda and the SC began to plan for a larger facility. In the meantime, the Sisters rented the house next door for expanded patient care.

The details of the early days of the SC's first asylum for the insane were documented by Sister Matilda in her journal, *Mount St. Vincent Hospital, Cradle of Mount Hope Retreat.*[7] This historical account provides important insights into mid-nineteenth-century American healthcare culture through the lens of a psychiatric nurse and religious woman. Within the numerous stories of patients and their nursing care, some of which are recounted in this and subsequent chapters, the journal *Cradle* demonstrates some of the beliefs and practices of the SC in their care of the sick and the insane. The journal also provides an understanding of Sister Matilda's business expertise, for which she ultimately became well known in the Catholic and medical communities. Her ability to lead the SC into hospital ventures was the outer expression of her personal integration of the three qualities foundational to Catholic spirituality and Vincentian-Louisian nursing tradition: Sister Matilda was a woman of *faith* who created a place of *hope* to fulfill her mission of *charity* to the sick poor and insane.

⌒ *Foundational Faith in Mission and Business* ⌒

News spread about the good quality care received by patients at Mount St. Vincent's, and within months of its enlargement, the facility was crowded again. To meet the increasing demand for services, more space was needed. The Sisters were stressed; they were not able to offer suitable programming and diversionary activities in the house or on the grounds because of the overcrowding. They desperately wanted to improve the situation for their patients and to welcome new admissions from among the many applicants for their services. Sister Matilda recalled:

> A few months after this enlargement, we were again crowded down, more room was still wanting, and applications being made for Patients better calculated to aid the new work, the Sisters became restless under their inability to improve the condition of those already with them, or to receive new pensioners. They were not able to afford suitable amusements in the house or on the grounds. They therefore importuned the Superiors for a better house, even there, or a removal, saying; "none can be cured under these circumstances, and the hard-earned success we have had at the Maryland Hospital will be lost, or attributed to what would not benefit Religion, as indeed it might be benefitted, could we continue to exercise our experience under similar auspices."[8]

Although the council understood the situation, they saw no alternatives or opportunities on the horizon to alleviate the problem. Their advice to Sister Matilda and the Sisters was "Pray, pray; - the providence of God is obtained by prayer."[9] In response, Sister Matilda prayed to the "Saints of

Heaven and their mighty Queen," Mary the Mother of Jesus, whom she invoked with "renewed devotion."[10]

The Washington Medical College, located on Broadway and Fairmount Avenue, was on the market at the time and presented an attractive deal. The Sisters decided to seize the opportunity and acquire the property. As the deal was about to close, they discovered an intricate maze of legal and financial complexities involving title and debts on the property. Rev. Deluol, acting on behalf of the SC in the transaction, withdrew the offer. He and Sister Matilda attributed the timeliness of discovering the problems to the loving vigilance of Divine Providence and St. Vincent de Paul, who watched over the charitable works of the Sisters. Sister Matilda was so relieved to have been spared the legal and financial nightmare that she and the Sisters were moved to accept their present facility constraints with greater calmness and courage and "to bear up quietly under our many grievous disadvantages."[11]

But admissions continued to increase beyond available space, and the Sisters' concerns about crowded conditions and patient safety grew. They did indeed have a fire in the asylum during the summer of 1843. After saying their prayers one June evening, the Sisters, who succeeded one another in spending time in the chapel, left a candle burning on the altar. Each supposed the next one would want to read by the candle. Unintentionally, the candle was left to burn throughout the night without supervision. When the Sisters awoke the next morning, they smelled the smoke. Sister Matilda's account of the fire provides another glimpse of the nature of her faith:

> On opening the parlor door the ceiling was in a cloud of white smoke, and on reaching the door of the chapel it seemed to be only a little mountain of smoke; – presently the fire appeared, creeping along through every thing; best vestments and flowers, laces, albs, altar-lines, all brunt; and the Altar itself just ready to fall: the Tabernacle still unhurt but one corner of it began to burn. . . . As quick as possible we adjusted every thing, and again the little lamp was lit up, before our Bountiful Reserver [the Blessed Sacrament]. Yes, for all night long that fire was

working, but a most tender Father had watched it while
his children slept. . . .[12]

Sister Matilda, faith buoyed, searched for meaning in the event. She
described a healing that had resulted. A woman patient, "whose insanity
was supposed to be from pride & passion, considered this event as a
warning for her, and it effected in her a cure both in soul and mind."[13] The
woman had been confined in a secure room adjoining the chapel, and had
the fire burst out, she would have been a victim. The experience enabled
her to respond with insight leading to the improvement of her mental
health and also to religious conversion.

The escape from fire heightened the Sisters' realization that change
was desperately needed. They pleaded with their superiors in Emmitsburg
for either a safer facility or relocation; but both alternatives seemed
impossible at the time. Attempts at bank loans failed. Sister Matilda, with
her indomitable faith and confidence, continued to represent the situation
and advocate for safer patient conditions to Rev. Deluol:

> Indeed my Father, we could not, in case of fire, save our
> dear Insane, all locked up as they are, and our entire
> building, inside and out, of a most igniting material,
> and exposed to unavoidable accidents in waiting on
> such patients. Suppose, my Father, we discontinue the
> establishment until you can do better?[14]

Again the religious superiors encouraged prayer. Rev. Deluol said
emphatically: "Pray, pray, my child, let the Sisters' prayers be unceasing!"[15]
This response served to motivate the Sisters to renewed fervor in prayer for
improvement of the situation. They decided to make a novena, nine days
of consecutive prayer ending on March 25, with the intention of finding
a solution for all who might be benefited by their success and prosperity,
especially the poor and needy.[16] Prior to the novena, Sister Matilda spoke
with tremendous faith in Divine Providence to the Sisters. She said, "My
dear Sisters, it seems, that all things human have combined against the
work assigned us to perform; let us then have recourse to our loving
God, whose power, is most manifested, when human efforts fail."[17] Their

faith in intercessory prayer proved powerful. On the termination of the novena, the Sisters of Charity became the proprietors of the Mount Hope College, which was considered the very best and most desirable facility in the vicinity of Baltimore.

The gentleman who owned it subsequently declared that he never had an idea of selling it until the very day he advertised it. Three Sisters missioned at the Mount St. Mary's Infirmary in Emmitsburg had been shown the ad about the sale by the vice president of the college. They told Sister Matilda about the ad, who then mentioned it to Dr. Stokes. Stokes also had "seen the ad in the Sun-Paper" and told her that he thought Mount Hope College would be a "fine location."[18] Its seventeen acres included a solid brick building, capable of accommodating eighty or ninety patients. The original terms were $15,000, with $3,000 to be paid in cash. Dr. Stokes went to see the property to confirm the occupancy, and when Rev. Deluol heard the confirmation from Dr. Stokes, he had the $3,000 down payment within one hour. Although the sale price to the SC was $12,000, after allowing for the improvements on the building and the furnishings, the total expenses increased to $80,000, all financed by loans.

Rev. Deluol, who had arranged for the financing, signed for the facility on behalf of the SC.[19] Mr. Oliver W. Treadwell, the owner, was shocked at his own decision to sell. At one point he tried to be released from his contract and to annul what he termed his "rash act." The articles of agreement were drawn up in such a manner, however, that there could be no retraction. Sister Matilda, Dr. Stokes, Rev. Deluol, and the Sisters established Mount Hope without one dollar of capital for the undertaking. Sister Matilda acted in accordance with her belief that "the treasury of God's Providence is inexhaustible, and belongs to us, unless God closes it in punishment of our infidelities."[20]

During the first three years, the Sisters were not able to pay the interest, and Rev. Deluol continually struggled to meet payment due dates and preserve his credit. Occasionally, this meant borrowing from another source to meet obligations on the first loan. The Sisters also struggled to make ends meet, sometimes having to borrow funds for groceries. Sister Matilda recorded that "through all this, our good Father was not at all discouraged. He firmly believed that Mount Hope was the work of God, and that it would eventually succeed. His prediction did come true."[21]

The SC Nurses believed that there was meaning not only in their work with the insane but also in the experience of insanity for each patient. Sister Matilda often recorded patients' spiritual experiences and religious conversions to the Catholic faith in her journal about Mount Hope. For example, Sister Matilda wrote about the "remarkable conversion" of a Protestant woman who had been at Mount Hope for a year due to suicidal thoughts and violence. "Her mind became suddenly restored," and she converted to Catholicism. She stated later that had she not become insane, she would not have found Mount Hope nor "had the opportunity to find the true religion."[22]

Patients also found a level of comfort in the care of the Sisters at the Mount Hope asylum that they might not have received had they been admitted elsewhere, such as a state-run institution or almshouse. One historical work, *The Mad Among Us*, provides a thorough account of life in the nineteenth-century American state asylum as a significant improvement on the previous options of entering the almshouse or "wandering aimlessly in community."[23] Living in a state asylum, however, was quite different from the experience at Mount Hope. A visiting physician from a model (public) psychiatric facility, Worcester Asylum for the Insane, summarized that difference in comments he made upon his departure from a visit at Mount Hope. He stated that "the house should rather be called 'Home' than Hospital, so much of home-comforts did he observe in every room. And this opinion was confirmed in him by the smiling, happy faces he met all around."[24] Creating an atmosphere of healing and hope when caring for the insane—those who were suicidal, depressed, psychotic, anxious, verbally abusive and physically violent— was not a simple task, however.

⁓ *Leadership, Vision, and Hope* ⁓

By May of 1844 the SC Nurses had completed the move of their furnishings and equipment to the new site, which Matilda referred to in her history as the "Mount Hope House."[25] Like the visitor from Worcester, patients stated that they felt the hospital was more like a home than a hospital. This is not surprising, for two reasons.

First, Sister Matilda and the other nurses lived at Mount Hope. They treated patients who came to the asylum with the dignity and respect that they would if those persons were entering their own home. Sister Matilda welcomed each patient to Mount Hope, saying, "You are in your Heavenly Father's own house, for Hospitals are not man's invention but God's, therefore you are as much at home here as we are. He makes you sick, and leaves us well that we may take care of you; so we are all His children, and as far as may be in our power we will supply the place of your other friends."[26]

Second, establishing the asylum's homelike ambience was very important to the realization of the model of care that the Sisters planned to implement at their institution for the insane. They planned to expand upon the works of European physicians and asylum administrators, who for more than a century, with the assistance of such nurses as the French Daughters of Charity, had developed what they deemed a more humane system of institutionalized care of the insane called "moral treatment." Sister Matilda, with the support of her physician colleague, William Stokes, whom she had known since her mission at the Maryland Hospital, used her business savvy to enter the world of *moral* entrepreneurship, as had French physicians of the insane, who pioneered moral therapy beginning in the eighteenth century.

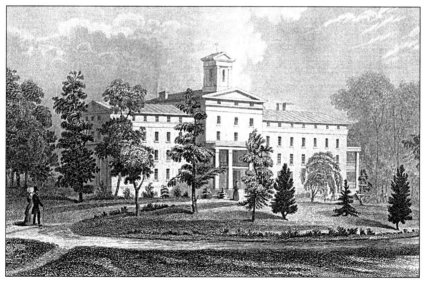

Fig. 3-1   *Mount Hope Retreat 1849*

Courtesy, Daughters of Charity Archives, Emmitsburg, Maryland

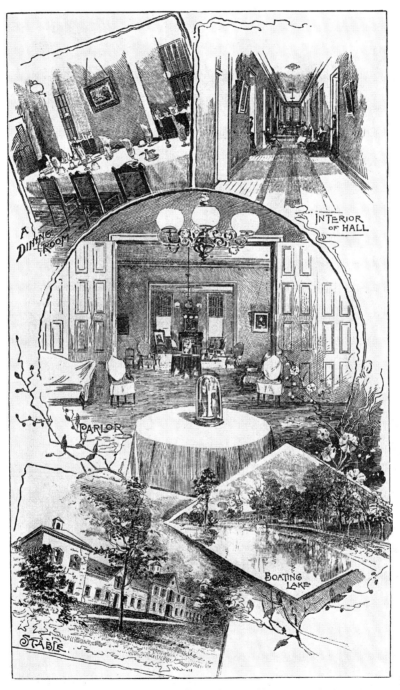

Moral Therapy and Social Justice ⌒

At the time that the Daughters of Charity Community was formed in France, few people believed that the insane could be cured, and the curability of insanity continued to be a question into the nineteenth century. Over time, however, the Daughters' care proved that, despite some peoples' belief in the impossibility of a cure, the insane were in fact persons who were ill and in dire need of help. The DC's attention to the insane illuminated the need for social justice in regard to the care of the mentally ill.

Vincent de Paul is recognized as the "director of the first hospital in France which was devoted to the treatment of the insane."[27] Le Grand Bureau des Pauvres sponsored a large hospital in Paris known as Les Petites Maisons. More than four hundred poor women and men were patients there including old people and the mentally ill. As early as 1639 Vincent had visited there, preached a mission, and written *L'exercice du chrétien* ("The Exercise of the Christian"), a leaflet for distribution to its patients. Filled with compassion and pastoral zeal, Vincent inspired priests who attended the Tuesday Conferences, a formation and support group for clergy, to become involved in pastoral care at Les Petites Maisons.

As a result, Le Grand Bureau des Pauvres requested that the DC staff the infirmary of that hospital. Les Petites Maisons stood on the site occupied in modern-day Paris by the chic Bon Marché Rive Gauche. It was originally the Saint-Germain-des-Prés Hospice for the Sick. Cardinal de Tournon transformed it into a hospital in 1557. Later, the board of the Grand Bureau began to operate it as a hospital for poor persons, including "old and decrepit men and other incorrigible and chronic cases, crippled persons, sick women and the insane."[28] Despite the challenges of providing quality care at Les Petites Maisons, Louise de Marillac wrote to Sister Barbe Angiboust (1605–1658) that she hoped there would be "sisters at the *Petites Maisons* to care for the insane and the poor sick women in whatever way they can."[29]

The ministry of the DC among the mentally ill involved domestic as well as direct patient-care duties. One of the earliest DC Nurses sent to

Fig. 3-2   *Mount Hope - Collage of Images 1893*

this mission later remarked that "when they were sent to the Hospital of the *Petites Maisons,* which up to then had been badly organized, Vincent "instilled into them such a high idea of the grace which God bestowed upon them, that they felt inflamed with zeal and encouraged for having given themselves to the service of the poor insane, in spite of the troubles and difficulties involved."[30] Bishop Louis Abelly (1604–1691), a companion of Vincent, described how considerately and charitably the DC cared for their patients to the satisfaction of the administrators, who "acknowledged that the Daughters had put an end to many disorders, including the serious financial loss of the institution, but especially the lack of care of the patients themselves. The administrators were most edified and satisfied with their contribution to the welfare of the hospital."[31]

The DC pioneered asylum-based psychiatric nursing at Les Petites Maisons, and they endured many of the hardships associated still today with the care of the insane, particularly the violent insane. Sister Nicole Lequin (1626–1703) entered the Community in 1649 and worked at Les Petites Maisons until her death. She was injured several times and maltreated by patients but did not show resentment. Sister Nicole calmly accepted the patients' negative behaviors and often expressed her hope to care for mental patients until the end of her life. A surgeon examined a newly admitted patient abandoned by an attendant who had found the patient's condition offensive; soon the surgeon also tired of caring for him because of the offensive odor of his infection. On observing this, Sister Nicole assumed the patient's care with great devotion and attention to him. She used simple remedies that she had available, and he healed perfectly in no time.

Sister Nicole delighted in instructing her associates and companions and gave them practical lessons in dressing wounds and preparing herbal remedies. She endeavored to train them in best practices and impart to them all the knowledge of nursing she possessed in order to make them competent servants of the poor.[32] The DC who served in the insane asylums of France were "renowned bloodletters and some possessed profound pharmaceutical knowledge."[33] The DC Nurses' ministry and work in the seventeenth and early eighteenth century brought a new level of humanity and expertise to the nursing care of the insane patient. Later in the century physicians contributed greatly to that progress as well.

In 1793 Dr. Phillipe Pinel, Rev. Bruté's teacher in medical college, ordered the release of insane inmates in Paris' Hôpital Général from the chains used to restrain them in their cells. He instituted a period in psychiatric care that focused on the humane treatment of patients. French physicians and hospital administrators, until Pinel, had considered insanity to be a social or hereditary rather than an "organic" problem related to cerebral hyperemia or hardening of the nerves. One historian of the period wrote:

> Protection of the community from damage at the hands of the unruly or pyromaniac lunatic, the maintenance of family honour and name in the face of the insanity of a close relative, the upholding of traditional codes of conduct which risked subversion by the social deviant, along with the real financial benefits to be reaped from caring for the insane: all these factors bulked larger than a care for the well-being of the individual lunatic or a desire to fit him out for reintegration into the wider society.[34]

Pinel and his student Jean-Étienne Esquirol (1772–1840), who had created one of the most successful Maison de Santé or private asylums in Paris, believed that the cause of mental illness lay in the passions of the soul and that insanity did not always affect one's ability to reason. Esquirol, however, insisted on the definitive medicalization of the care of the insane. The physician was to be the principal of a lunatic hospital; it was he who should "set everything in motion. . . . The physician should be invested with an authority from which no one is exempt."[35] Later a physician named Henri Rech studied the works of Pinel and worked with Esquirol. Rech, in his *Clinique de las Maison d'Aliénés*, argued that the doctor was the "moral entrepreneur" within the asylum rather than the dispenser of medical therapy.[36] He did use medical therapies such as drugs but for their tranquilizing (i.e., symptomatic) rather than curative effect. As moral entrepreneur, the physicians of the insane applied "moral therapy," a system of care that stressed kindness to patients and the employment of the patient in meaningful activity.

Medical treatment, such as bloodletting and drugs, was considered secondary, and therefore great importance was assigned to the quality of the attendants, nurses, and supervisors who created and maintained the therapeutic environment of the asylum and administered the moral therapy. England's York Retreat, a Quaker hospital led by Daniel Tuke and George Jepson, who pioneered moral therapy in Britain, was under the control of lay therapists rather than physicians, as was advocated by Esquirol in France until the adoption of the Lunatics Act in 1845. This act required the asylum to be run by a medical superintendent. Prior to 1845 Tuke and his followers believed that the "key to moral therapy lay in the quality of personal relationships between staff and patients."[37] One did not need to be a physician to implement the tenets of what had come to be known as the successful treatment of the insane.

In England after 1845 moral treatment was assimilated into the area of medical expertise. The assumption of "medical monopoly over moral as well as medical treatment was a general feature of mid-nineteenth-century asylums"[38] in Britain. An editorial was printed in the 1853 issue of the new *Asylum Journal* in Britain stating that the moral system of treatment could only be properly carried out under the constant supervision and continuous assistance of a physician.[39]

In America there was at least one asylum, however, where moral therapy was fully implemented by nurses—the SC's Mount St. Vincent Hospital (Mount Hope). Dr. Stokes served as consultant physician, for which he was paid $250 every quarter.[40] He had visited the Hanwell Asylum in England in 1841, where he witnessed the operation of the asylum under the direction of Dr. John Conolly, who had become well known for his application of the moral system of nonrestraint treatment. Stokes returned to America in 1842 to his new post as physician to the Mount St. Vincent Hospital under "the inspiration of the grand ideas embodied in this new system and with an abiding faith, that a new era was destined to dawn upon the treatment of the insane in this country."[41] Stokes's *Eleventh Annual Report* of 1853 contains one of the most vivid descriptions of the moral philosophy and practices at the institution that were influenced by Esquirol and Pinel.

Stokes also listed the causes of his patients' insanity that were treated under the system of moral therapy. The major diagnoses included "hereditary predisposition, family affliction and trouble, anxiety of the mind and too close application to business, ill health, intemperance, pecuniary losses and reverse of fortune, jealousy and inordinate pride, disappointment, epilepsy, masturbation, and unknown."[42] From his experience of eleven years at Mount Hope, Stokes validated the findings of physicians before him that "the influence of moral agency is great upon men and women and moral causes, primarily reversal of fortune, was the primary cause of insanity.[43]

Moral causes were more difficult to identify because, as Stokes noted, people did not typically talk openly about their family member's odd behaviors. But when the doctor and nurses at Mount Hope were called upon by families and friends to help, they inspired patient confidence in their services, which Stokes believed was the "very keystone of all moral treatment."[44] And they offered hope. They believed in the power of the healing environment, especially in the asylum created specifically for the moral management of mental diseases. In their counseling of patients, the Sister-Nurses aimed to "politely manage" rather than contradict the insane person's thoughts and feelings, as will be discussed further in chapter 5. Treatment was administered through personal interaction with the SC, day and night.

Dr. Stokes believed that the Sisters were particularly "qualified" to engage in moral treatment. He may have made this statement in light of what he had witnessed in Europe. There were a number of attendants of a lesser quality at Hanwell Asylum, for example, where drunkenness was the "commonest reason for disciplinary action."[45] Intoxication was not an issue with SC Nurses. If it was suspected during their Postulatum, the initial period of experience and observation, a candidate would not have been admitted to the Community. Hanwell administrators, like other asylum directors of the period, had to deal with high turnover rates; their nurses were not "missioned" as were the SC, and therefore committing to the staffing levels needed to implement moral therapy was more difficult than it would have been for Sister Matilda and the SC, who owned and staffed their own asylum.

Despite rules of celibacy among staff at Hanwell, pregnancies did occur. The Sisters also had vowed a life of celibacy; nevertheless, Sister Matilda and other Sister Servants were careful to follow social decorum and their Community's expectations for the expression of "holy modesty,"[46] especially when the Sisters were to care for male patients. As was typically done in the nineteenth century, the Sister Servants segregated and monitored relations as necessary between the SC Nurses and the male attendants and patients. Mother Mary Xavier Clark advocated for the hiring of male attendants to care for the male patients. The Sisters were to "teach" the male attendants how to make the beds of male patients and dress their blisters and sores.[47] She did add that the Sisters would attend (e.g., take the pulses of males) as well as supervise the care of male patients if "the urgency of the case is such that there is no medium. In such peculiar circumstances, charity is above all things, & God who sees the heart and knows all our secret thoughts & motives will in such cases give his special grace aid."[48]

Rech, Esquirol, and Pinel influenced the adoption of moral therapy well beyond the confines of hospitals in Paris. Their books and papers on creating a humane and healing environment for the care of the insane were highly read in America as well. By 1840 when the Sisters and Dr. Stokes opened their institution, many of the trials of their predecessors in France and England surrounding the establishment of an ordered, humane environment for the insane had been noted and remedied. One of the biggest issues for those engaged in moral therapy and its foundational philosophy of kindness was how to manage violent behavior in the asylum. In the past violent patients could have been stripped of their clothes, chained to walls in dungeons, shackled, and beaten. Pinel and his followers had achieved a level of care in which the most violent act of punishment administered by staff towards an insane patient was submerging the patient in a cold bath. Staff hired previously to enforce the institutional rules with physical violence were removed and replaced by domestics who were trained to be more tolerant of patients suffering mental illness. In French asylums physical restraint in the form of a straightjacket was also used. Unfortunately, the larger state institutions, such as Rech's Clinique des Aliénés, that admitted a number of highly violent patients were only able to demonstrate a 5 percent cure rate in 1838. When he opened his own small private asylum in the 1840s where he was able to restrict admissions, his cure rates soared to 25 percent.[49] Because of their size and high demographic of violent insane patients, state hospitals often continued to be holding tanks for the confinement of the insane rather than therapeutic institutions.

American asylum care in the early and mid-nineteenth century was defined in terms of the needs of the community and social and economic conditions. The roles of asylums differed from state to state and asylum to asylum. Some were created for the care of orphans, widows, and elders and others for the insane. The reputation of the DC for the care of the insane had first been established in Paris, yet it was the American SC who took the mission with the insane to a new level of importance in Community. The first noticeable change was that in the 1812 *Regulations*, the American adaptation of the *Common Rules* translated and written by Rev. John Dubois (the priest who had cared for the insane with the DC Nurses at the Hospice des Petites Maisons in Paris, as discussed in chapter 1), Rev. Dubois specifically mentioned the care of the *insane* in the *Regulations* as a part of the SC mission.[50]

The SC's Mount Hope mission required much courage, intelligence, and skill. In the beginning days of the founding of the Community, Vincent de Paul had warned about the challenges of caring for the insane. "Then, too, all the patients are mentally ill, extremely unbalanced, always sullen, and there are constant quarrels. Oh! There's nothing like it! I can't describe it to you. Lastly, there's so little social contact that two persons can't even get along together but have to be separated. Each does his or her own thing."[51] Like the DC, the American SC were grateful for the opportunity to nurse the insane. Their belief was that in serving the insane they could better understand how varied human misery was and what it meant to suffer.[52] In understanding human suffering, they were better able to address the needs of humanity through an expanded realization and internalization of the compassion and charity of Christ.

In nineteenth-century America, moral treatment was defined as care that focused on the rational and emotional rather than the organic causes of insanity. American physicians, like many of their mentors in Europe, adopted moral therapy as essential in the treatment of the insane, particularly those whose disease was not related to organic causes such as birth trauma. "Insanity" was the proper term used in the nineteenth century to describe those with mental diseases. It was defined by the editor of the *American Journal of Insanity* as "a chronic disease of the brain, producing either derangement of the intellectual faculties, or prolonged change of the feelings, affections, and habits of an individual."[53] The term also was used when referring to "idiocy," defined as the "total want or alienation of understanding"[54] and a "defect of development of the brain." Mental disease was generally organized under four classifications: mania, melancholy, demency (dementia), and idiocy. Hallucinations occurred in the manic or melancholic patient. Suicide and "drunkenness" or "intoxication," both of which were prevalent in early and mid-nineteenth century American society, were often the topic of discussions about insanity in the *American Journal of Insanity* and in meetings.

In his 1844 report in the *American Journal of Insanity*, Pliny Earle, superintendent physician at the Bloomingdale Asylum in New York, wrote that the causes of insanity included heredity, a predisposition in the nervous system (not blood as thought by Rush), and cerebral disease (some organic) that was mostly functional as in a sympathy of the brain with other organs that were diseased. Previous to their mental illnesses, patients were often noted to have sustained injuries or other harm from falls, masturbation (in men), fever, ill health and dyspepsia, parturition, or pregnancy and amenorrhea (in women). He also noted as possible causes of insanity chronic inflammation, such as occurred in the liver and mucous membrane of the alimentary canal when tobacco was smoked. Earle stated a belief that rheumatism and gout "undoubtedly" caused insanity due to metastasis to the dura mater of the brain. Idiocy was not caused by any external influence; the person was born with the condition.[55] Common moral causes of insanity included pecuniary difficulties, religious excitement, death of a relative, disappointed affection, domestic trouble, fear, and anxiety. The extreme tension that resulted from "excitements" in the environment caused by such situations as the constant shifts in population and the hectic pace of urban life in particular was the focus of mental health promotion.[56]

Some believed education to be a major contributing factor in the emergence of insanity. Spending too much time cultivating the mind was thought to lead to excess stimulation and therefore overexcitement, a state that threatened well-being. This belief had its roots in Dr. William Cullen's (1710–1790) theory of disease. He wrote that all disease was due to excess or deficiency of excitability, the biological capacity to react to external stimuli.[57]

Common medical therapeutics that were considered "depletive" or draining of excess excitability included bloodletting and emetics, and those who suffered deficiency of excitability received stimulants such as opiates. Cullen was the teacher of Dr. Benjamin Rush (1746–1813), who took depletive therapy to the extreme in his recommendations of massive bloodletting.

Religious fervor was thought to be a common cause of excess excitability and therefore was related as a cause of insanity. Some psychiatrists, such as Amariah Brigham, the superintendent of the Utica State Lunatic Asylum in New York, quoting Esquirol and Pinel, attributed another major cause of insanity as thinking too much. Brigham would have suspected the works of the SC in Catholic education, especially in young children, as a possible source for the disease of overexcitement that potentially led to insanity, which was spawned from excess study and religious fervor. Insanity, according to Brigham's assessment of statistics in some states such as Connecticut, was on the rise. He calculated that 1 in 262 people in the United States was insane.[58] He differentiated insanity from idiocy in the statistic and also noted that Americans were two to three times more likely to be insane than in European countries such as England. He suggested that Americans, living in a free society with representative government, had more opportunity to think and therefore a greater chance of becoming insane.

Brigham was highly critical of the infant-schools movement, in which children in the 1830s were beginning schooling at the age of three or four. He believed that such focused, structured education was "unnatural" and therefore not in keeping with Enlightenment beliefs in fostering the physical and what many people of the period knew as the "natural."[59] Brigham's call for education reform was published in his 1832 work *Remarks on the Influence of Mental Cultivation on Health*, in which he called for change in early childhood education to the study of the anatomy and physiology of the body rather than the cultivation of the mind. The idea that children became insane through education peaked in American society in the 1850s and 1860s—about the same time that people were becoming pessimistic about the ability of moral treatment to cure the insane. By the 1870s the notion that the etiology of insanity had something to do with some aspect of environment creating a state of overexcitement in the body crumbled.

During the peak years of its promotion, moral treatment was aimed at engaging the mind and exercising the body. The essential components of moral treatment included removal from one's home and former associations, respectful and kind treatment in all situations, manual labor (not a cure and best applied after achieving convalescence), religious worship on Sunday, established regular habits, self-control and diversion of the mind from morbid thoughts.[60] The Sister-Nurses assigned activities for each patient appropriate to his or her mental and social abilities. Interventions included conversation and recreational activities, such as sewing and taking walks. The new facility enabled the Sisters to offer their patients a greater range of activities and allowed them to better manage patient behaviors, including the risk of patient escape.

Striking a Balance between Freedom and Restraint ⌒

To be successful at moral treatment by increasing attentiveness to patient need and thereby decreasing the call for physical restraints, the number of nurses and attendants to patients needed to be significantly higher than that of the almshouses and state institutions. At the York Retreat in England in the 1840s, the number of nurses or attendants to patients was one to eight. While this ratio was an improvement, it was still higher than at expensive private asylums, where the ratio was typically one nurse to two patients or even one to one.[61] The purpose of "coercive" treatment or use of restraints was to protect the patient and other patients and staff from violent behavior. But the use of restraints needed to be weighed against the risk of creating excitement or irritation and therefore inflammation, which, as mentioned previously, was considered a significant contributor to insanity.[62] Free motion was one way the body discharged excitability, and when restrained, the insane person was unable to do this. The four most common restraints in use were seclusion, strait-waistcoats, force, and strapping to the bed (at all four points).

Ascribing to the philosophy of moral treatment did not mean that coercive means were never used in an institution. Patients were restrained by staff when their behavior posed imminent danger to others. Patients who could not control self-destructive acts could also ask to be restrained or to be put in seclusion for a period of time. While use of padded seclusion rooms was infrequent, confining patients to their bedrooms was a form of seclusion that was used quite commonly.[63] It was the *intention* behind the staff's use of restraints that set apart the institutions that were implementing moral therapy. Restraints were used not as cruelty or punishment but as the last resort to help a patient reestablish his or her self-control, that part of social conduct that was emphasized in treatment at the asylums.

Stokes wrote of his mission with the SC, "We have endeavored, by our united efforts, to establish in this State a model Asylum, in which the patients should enjoy the utmost freedom, consistent with their own welfare, and the safety of others."[64] Because of their serious attention to developing their skills of nonrestraint, the Sisters did not have to hire as many men for their brute strength to enforce coercive treatments. They were also able to participate in what Stokes referred to in his report as "a new departure."[65] The SC Nurses at the Mount Hope Retreat developed their skill in the moral care of male patients, which by 1880 would total 160 cases occupying eight halls presided over by two nurses and one male attendant for each hall. Stokes wrote that the "crowning merit" of the institution was that male patients enjoyed the services of the SC and that, in so doing, the SC had introduced in American healthcare "a new era in the practice of nursing male patients."[66] In forty years Stokes and the Sisters demonstrated that the Sister-Nurses were capable of handling even some of the most violent of patients with kindness rather than the brute force exerted by a hired male attendant. Stokes wrote:

> Both the Physician and nurses should feel that the affliction of mental disease does not necessarily block up the avenues of the humane heart, and that, however clouded may be the powers of the understanding, and however erratic the processes of thought and action, *the human heart,* with its tender susceptibilities, is still mercifully spared them, and is ever ready to respond to the voice of kindness and sympathy.[67]

The Sisters not only crossed nineteenth-century American gender boundaries when providing nursing care for the sick and insane. In keeping with Vincentian-Louisian tradition, they were observed by Stokes, other physicians, and the public as being consistent and impartial to "every class, to the rich or poor, Christian or infidel, Catholic or Protestant, Jew or Gentile."[68] They embodied the tenets of moral therapy, a model that sufficiently mirrored their holistic philosophy of care. Stokes was clearly appreciative of the services of the Sisters, which he called "pious and priceless"[69] and described as "enlightened and universal charity."[70]

The Sisters treated their patients as if they were rational beings; they did not reprimand them. It was only when the safety of the patient, other patients, the staff, or the property was at risk that they would use coercive therapies of any kind. The Sisters were inventive when it came to using restraints and creating a safe environment for patients. Their work was described in a report written in 1841 by a W. G. Read, who had been commissioned by the Committee of the Trustees of the New York State Lunatic Asylum appointed under an act of the Legislature to visit asylums to observe their methods for the management of the insane. Read wrote that he had interviewed the "Sister in charge of the institution," who would have been Sister Matilda Coskery. He ascertained that:

> The Sisters never *"permit the infliction of blows,* nor subject their patients to the strait-jacket, which they consider extremely harassing; and which, in one case at the Maryland Hospital (if I remember aright). Nearly caused the death of a frantic sufferer, by strangulation; the collar having, by his struggles, been drawn tightly across his windpipe, in which condition he was found by the Sisters. Neither are they partial to the 'mits,' which they consider insecure, and therefore dangerous both for patients and attendants. When they do employ them, they prefer linen ones, as less liable to stretch than leather. The Sister tells me, patients will almost always contrive to slip their hands out of the mits, when alone, and replace them when they hear some one coming. Their most usual mode of restraining the violent is, with a sort of sleeve, invented by themselves, as I understood, and which is attached to a frock body, made to lace up behind, like a lady's corset. The sleeves are some inches longer than

the arm, closed at the end and drawn around the body and fastened behind. . . . Having in the rapid glance I cast over the Worcester report, observed that solitary confinement, under due precautionary restraints, had, at the Massachusetts Hospital, been found preferable to the irritation produced by the perpetual surveillance, I directed my inquiries to that point, and learned that the experience of the Sisters was different; they find that the mind of the maniac, when deserted, preys upon itself. They therefore prefer, as far as their circumstances will permit, the restraint of their own presence and intercourse to actual bonds. . . . It is further the policy of the Sisters, of which they never lose sight, to elevate their patients in their own self-esteem.[71]

Sister Matilda, as will be shown more explicitly in chapter 5, taught the SC Nurses how to de-escalate patient behavior using communication techniques and directed spiritual intention. The Sisters sought to achieve a balanced and harmonious environment that would promote the same qualities in the life of the insane person, patient by patient.

A Healing Environment

When a patient was first admitted to Mount Hope or was entering an acute phase of his or her chronic illness, such as in the case of a patient suffering from mania, the patient was encouraged to rest in a calm environment in which every external source of excitement had been removed. Admittance to an asylum was considered a form of social seclusion in which the patient was removed from the home and work environment thought to have instigated or promoted the illness in some way. Seclusion in a specific room within the asylum environment might also be used, but Sister Matilda and the Sisters "preferred the restraint of their own presence."[72]

During the convalescence phase, staff provided activities that would employ both the body and mind of the patient, without which, according to Dr. Stokes, "neither mental nor physical health can be maintained

CASE STUDY 3-1 **Propriety and Restraint**

Patient Account at Mount Hope as Recorded by Sister Matilda

A woman was admitted for "Mania a Potu" [acute temporary insanity, "crazy drunkenness"]. With the exception of this fault she was a very worthy person; industrious in her family, & charitable to every body. She was a Catholic. We told her husband that there was no hope of her recovery, and he might call the Priest. In the meanwhile we tried to get her on the bed, as being a more easy position, against [sic] the priest would arrive; for although we thought she would die before more morning, we hoped that the presence of a priest might arouse her to her senses, for she showed none at all.

Five or six of us were ready, having bandages at hand, to fasten her gently on the bed as soon as she could be lifted to it: but she was so strong & furious, that we were obliged to call a man to aid us. "Now; Daniel" said we, "whilst we hold her by the arms & waist, do you grasp her by the feet, and we will all lift together." Two Sisters were on the bed to drag her in, two more by the side to lift her by the waist. After a vain effort, Daniel let go to take a fresh grapple, and once she seemed light as a feather. We were all astonished at this, for we had begun to think, that if with a man's assistance, we could not be able to lift her, surely she must be possessed. Well, the man went away: we tied the woman gently to the bed & told her that a priest had come to hear her confession: but she was unconscious of what we were saying. It was now 9 p.m. and we were resting a little before we could commence Night Prayers, for we had been a long time with her. We expressed our surprise that she had been so exceedingly heavy, & became all at once so light. "Why!" interrupted a grave, sober-minded Sister, "Daniel took hold of one of my ancles, [ankles] and one of the woman's, instead of her two; and I was obliged to hold down the woman as hard as I could, and myself too, to keep us from being both lifted up together." We expressed our surprise and asked why she did not tell Daniel of his mistake. "I'm sure you would not have the man to know that he had hold of my foot." --

We had to postpone our prayers a little longer. Presently the poor Priest came: – it was a terrible stormy night. We took him up stairs & told the patient that he was now ready to hear her Confession. – We then retired along the passage. After some while he returned to us & told us that she was perfectly herself and knew then as well what she was doing, as ever she had known. She recovered her soul and body and became an exemplary Christian, making her family quite happy around her.[73]

Courtesy, Daughters of Charity Archives, Emmitsburg, Maryland

or improved."[74] Stokes and the Sisters thought that fresh air was of "transcendent interest" and was an "anodyne." Patients were encouraged to take walks in all seasons of the year. They also had patients engage in domestic labor, which they defined as such activities as sewing, knitting, playing dominoes, attending vocal and instrumental music at social meetings, and reading books such as biography, travel, and history.[75] Manual labor was, for some patients, very important to relieve them of stagnation of mind and body. Stokes described the fatigue that the patient felt after working hard as the "best of opiates."[76]

It was typical of moral treatment to engage convalescing patients in daily work in the "house" to prepare them for reentry to their own family life. For example, some of the milder and more compliant patients assisted the Sisters and the hired asylum help with the process of relocation of Mount St. Vincent's to Mount Hope College in 1844.

Patients often accompanied the Sisters when they left the grounds to go shopping, but some insane patients, who really needed to be confined for safety reasons, would at times try to leave the property on their own. This was a common concern of mid-nineteenth-century asylum administrators and nurses, private and public.[77] Sister Matilda was highly attentive to the security features of the new Mount Hope building that would increase patient safety and decrease patient attempts at escape. Dr. Stokes and two of the Sisters visited other institutions before designing the necessary improvements that would add to the "comfort, security and neatness" of the new building that would house the insane, some of whom would be "excitable or dangerous."[78] The new building had to be secured before the most disturbed patients could be transferred safely. Sister Matilda's notes provide some insight into the type of construction used to create a secure as well as a healing asylum environment that could receive people at various levels of insanity:

> The large Study room must be partitioned off into small &
> secure apartments: All the windows must be secured. All
> the small wood cellars must be thrown into one or two
> large apartments, for kitchen, refectory &c. Many of the
> cellar rooms must be floored & more light thrown into
> them. In many parts excavations must needs be made.

A cemented cistern must be prepared near the kitchen door &c. &c. Many, many conveniences were absolutely needed even in this lowest department. . . . As the old wing needed being raised one story higher directions were given for the roof to be carefully removed to serve in covering a "Lodge" or building then in contemplation for the more excitable or dangerous patients.[79]

Sister Matilda and the Sisters had endured four years in a crowded building prone to fire where the ideal setting for the implementation of peaceful asylum care could not be fully implemented. They wasted no time in preparing the Mount Hope building and grounds to serve as the hospital milieu for the enactment of the principles and practices of moral therapy that they had learned over the years from Dr. Stokes, Rev. Bruté, Rev. Dubois, and others.

The healing power of nature was considered a key component of moral therapy, as it was throughout the healthcare arena of the early and mid-nineteenth century.[80] In addition to securing parts of the building to house some of the more violent patients, the grounds also had to be prepared to support convalescing patients. The grounds were landscaped and gardens were laid out so that patients could get plenty of fresh air and could exercise if they were able. The Sister-Nurses' focus on a healthy lifestyle for patients was in agreement with a number of physicians of the period, such as Edward Jarvis, who promoted the importance of exercise, occupation, and amusements to "keep patients' minds away from their delusions and vagaries, to calm their excitement, and raise them from their depression."[81] Sister Matilda had a large spring-fed pond constructed in a meadow on the seventeen-acre property. They dubbed it "Lake Oregon" and placed a miniature island in the middle, which they named "Washington's Island." They purchased a boat for the patients' enjoyment that ladies used in the morning and gentlemen in the afternoon. Lake Oregon was stocked with fish so that the ladies "could brag of catching fish."[82] Sister Matilda provided a detailed description of the Mount Hope grounds:

Our lot was 17 acres long, and narrow, with a deep ravine kind of meadow dividing it midway in two. The front part opposite the city was high ground on which the house stood, surrounded thinly by forest trees; the back hill, across the meadow was still higher and on this the forest trees were growing more thickly, leaving some acres for cultivation, for garden, potatoes &c. The back grounds afforded delightful promenades for such as might be able to go there. The little hills abounded with flint stones, and occasionally the convalescents and harmless insane patients would be invited to come out and amuse themselves by gathering these into piles, so that the place might be cleared and prepared for vegetation. . . . This harmless amusement gave them great delight, and made them forget for the time-being, their little pains & sorrows. No walls were around the house, and this together with the adornment of lovely trees, shrubs, flowers, and winding-walks, gave the place a very pleasant appearance.[83]

The twelve Sisters on staff were quite satisfied to retain the name of the property, "Mount Hope." However it was no longer referred to as a "college." Dr. Stokes's 1845 *Annual Report* provides the first reference to Mount Hope as an "Institution." By 1846 the number of Mount Hope nurses had increased to twenty. Of these, a core of six Sisters had worked with Sister Matilda over several years, including Sister Jane Frances Higgins and Sister Octavia McFadden, who had been with her at the Maryland Hospital for the Insane and at Mount St. Vincent's Hospital. Though creating, administering, and staffing an asylum was hard work, the Sisters and Dr. Stokes were very enthusiastic about the impact they were having, not only on patients but on the system of psychiatric care in the state and the country.

When the SC stepped forward in the early and mid-nineteenth century to create their own hospital to care for the insane, they were essentially participating in the expansion of women's distinct political culture centered on the virtues of domesticity, nurturance, and benevolence that were highly valued by nineteenth-century American society.[84] During the same decade that Sister Matilda and the SC Nurses opened Mount Hope,

American women began to organize around other social and political issues, such as women's right to vote. The historic Seneca Falls convention, the first women's rights event held in America, occurred in 1848 in New York State. In addition, women sought to end slavery and the excessive use of alcohol. Those involved in the nineteenth-century women's rights movement also championed the rights of the mentally ill to receive better care.

Insanity occurred among the poor and rich alike, but the poor were more publicly visible. They were cared for in state asylums that often housed hundreds of inmates. The destitute insane occupied the almshouses of Baltimore and other major American cities. It was the reform of the state asylums and almshouses that caught the attention of women activists seeking to exercise what was socially perceived as the inherent virtues of their gender. State asylums employed "matrons" to run the establishments and supervise nursing care. One physician wrote in 1847 of the role of gender in asylum care for the insane:

> Men may construct proper buildings for the insane, investigate their diseases philosophically, and apply to them the rules of art and the lessons of experience; but it is the more peculiar province and power of woman to enter into the feelings of the unfortunate, and to console the afflicted; and her sympathy and kindness are more frequently efficacious in "ministering to a mind diseased" than the science of the physician, or the drugs of the Materia Medica.[85]

Although the SC may not have been formally affiliated with the women's rights movement, they were aligned with many of its values and were active in their own way. Following their *Regulations* and the tradition that led them to serve the sick, poor, and insane in society with simplicity, humility, and charity, they set a standard for the care of the insane that challenged the social, political, religious, and medical status quo. By establishing Mount Hope, the Sisters had already achieved what women's rights leaders promoted; they had moved outside the women's single-family-oriented domestic sphere into the public sphere of healthcare, asylums, and hospitals. Their work and their lives, even the way they dressed, exemplified what was believed by men and women of nineteenth-century society, to be the "special moral nature" of women.[86] Under Sister Matilda's leadership, the SC Nurses were unorthodox moral entrepreneurs who in collaboration with physicians and clergy designed and directed the care of the insane.

⁓ The Charity of Nurse Sectarians ⁓

In 1838 the Maryland legislature granted what many other states had done: it sanctioned the rights of sects of unorthodox physicians, other than "regulars" (those educated at medical programs at universities who typically employed heroic therapies),[87] to be paid for their services. These sects of doctors included Thomsonians,[88] other botanic physicians, homeopaths, water curists and phrenologists.[89] Sectarian health reformers aggressively opposed the attempts of some regulars to secure what they perceived as medical monopoly in the state. Physicians in Europe and America had been vying for cultural authority and professional dominance for some time. Historian Colin Jones researched not only the eighteenth-century climate in which the DC practiced; he also analyzed numerous medical histories that mention the French sisters. His view was that the Daughters were *medical* practitioners who were typically "lumped together with all sorts of cranks and quacks, who were to be lined up to be medicalized into neutrality or oblivion"[90] in hopes of assuring that their work would not impede the flow of medical progress. During the period that Sister Matilda and the SC were pioneering Vincentian-Louisian nursing and moral therapy, sectarianism was highly popular, self-care and domestic medicine were widespread fixtures of American culture, and physicians were struggling to establish their right to lead American healthcare and be paid for their services.

Americans were very attentive to health reform and were ultimately supportive of well-meaning, knowledgeable, and experienced caregivers, whether or not they had a university medical diploma. Regular physicians and medical colleges were scrutinized by the public for their study of anatomy and dissection because the public had experience with physicians and medical students justifying "body snatching"[91] and grave robbing for the sake of medical students' anatomy education. In addition, Americans had become skeptical of the university-educated physicians who were attempting to establish medical dominance. With the election of Andrew Jackson, a populist president, regular physicians' practice became suspect. Many of the emerging sects, most notably Thomsonians, suggested that regular physicians were elitist. "Poorer people, in particular, were antagonized by what they saw as efforts by a professional elite to erode their medical choices."[92]

The opposition toward regulars influenced medical education. Doctors were concerned about public opinion, so they instructed their medical students in "basic professional and medical ethics, teaching them how to work effectively with other physicians and within their communities."[93] Regular or orthodox physicians had been prescribing and often overprescribing heroic therapies such as excessive bloodletting, administration of calomel, and blistering for decades without significant cures.[94] Accusation of excessive treatment by physicians was not a new concept to the SCs. As mentioned in chapter 1, Louise de Marillac had concerns about physician practice related to what she perceived as overprescribing. The SC's *Regulations* include instructions that Sisters should not describe their own ailments to physicians with whom they worked because the physician could, "by a heedless complaisance with their wishes," expose the Sister to "greater injury."[95]

The SC did not align with any of the sects typically identified in American medical history of the period. However, their attention to the care of the poor, their values of simplicity and spiritual life as expressed in their nursing care, and their unorthodox practices of care, as well as construction of their own facilities, certainly set them apart from mainstream orthodox medicine. The Sisters practiced nursing, a care that was distinct from the practice of the regular physicians. As their founders had established in the seventeenth century, the SC Nurses were neither religious nor secular, and it might be added that they were neither medically orthodox nor sectarian. While the Sisters used herbal remedies in the care of patients, there is no evidence that they ascribed to sectarian movements or the associated botanical, homeopathic, vegetarian, and lifestyle measures of movements such as Grahamism[96] that were highly popular alternatives to the medicines and treatments of the regular physicians. The antimonopoly rhetoric of the

Thomsonians and other sect leaders aimed at regular physicians may have actually been too strong for the SC, who had built positive relationships with regular physicians over the years.

Given the pluralistic, dynamic, and in many ways inclusive nature of early and mid-nineteenth-century American healthcare culture, the Sisters were able to carve out their own niche. In the nineteenth century, self-care was one of the foundations of American healthcare. Personal accountability associated with self-care was equated with the potential success of the newly formed democratic society. Every person was to be his or her own doctor. Every citizen was thought to possess the right to health, but each was also responsible for that health. Moral treatment was the modality in the realm of psychiatric healthcare that perhaps most reflected the self-care values of the period. It required the active participation of the patient. People's convictions about the superiority of self-care and hygienic practices over heroic drugs supported their loss of confidence in physicians. Thomsonians and others argued that self-care was safer than being doctored by regulars.

Health reformers emphasized the central role of women, wives, and mothers in supervising self-care regimens. Religious women in communities such as the SC also served to support the process of self-care and health promotion. The "investment of woman with a special responsibility in the spiritual regeneration of her family, and by extension, of civilization as well, was a recurring theme in their literature."[97] Women, nurses in particular, provided support for self-care, especially among women, who by being their own doctor could avoid the embarrassment and in some cases the potential risk of being examined by a male physician. Advocates for health reform, who grew increasingly frustrated with physicians' seeming inability to remove the causes of disease and render promised "cures," published their criticisms of regular physicians in popular advice journals. For example, Dr. Ellen Snow wrote in the 1856 *Water Cure Journal*, "They do not aim to enlighten mankind in regard to their physical well-being, but rather seek to envelop their processes of cure in deep and impenetrable mystery."[98]

During this period of sectarianism and health reform, medical treatment of the insane was also under scrutiny. Dorothea Dix was one of the most recognized health reformers on behalf of the insane in the mid-nineteenth century. In the 1840s, after touring various asylums throughout Europe, Dix petitioned superintendents of state institutions such as Amariah Brigham to support her vision of decentralization of care. She had constructed her model of care based upon a successful asylum program she witnessed in Geel, Belgium, where the patients formed a working colony. That model of care promoted a moral environment that "fostered tranquility without active medical intervention."[99] As will be discussed in chapter 4, the model of care that Sister Matilda designed with Dr. Stokes for the Mount Hope Institution was a lay, and in some ways a sectarian (i.e., nursing), program of care supported by medical consultation as needed. At the same time that Dix was attempting to move state asylums toward the lay model of moral treatment, the SC had already established moral treatment at Mount Hope. Dix did not receive support from Brigham or other superintendent physicians for her petition. Then in 1852, despite her notably anti-Catholic position, Dix's report on the state of Maryland's asylums described the SC's Mount Hope Institution as one of two successful asylums in the state.[100]

Dix noted that medical treatment of the insane often included the application of heroics and restraint. Mental illness among the poor was treated in almshouses, which were overflowing in cities like Baltimore, especially during the cholera epidemics in 1832 and 1849. A report of the Baltimore Almshouse in 1840 reported the employment of nurses who were "selected from among the temporary inmates of the house—few of whom can be expected to possess those qualities of mind and manner, with that experience and appreciation of their arduous and peculiar duties, which combine to form an accomplished, courageous and proper nurse."[101] Dr. Robinson, the attending physician to the almshouse and writer of the report, clearly knew about the benefits of moral therapy and attempted to make the argument to the trustees for more support for a better environment that promoted a cure in the insane pauper. He echoed what his colleagues all believed about insanity, that if treated early many patients were in fact curable. In 1840 he estimated that out of a total population of 467,567 people in the state of Maryland, there were 340 idiots and insane whites and 136 "colored" people in public and private "charge." Seventy-six were housed at the almshouse. He estimated that 90 percent of the inmates were curable.[102]

Just as had been occurring in Paris, the SC as well as state and consulting physicians and asylum staffs faced real challenges of caring for large numbers of sick poor and insane throughout the nineteenth century; many of these were African-Americans or women. The almshouses started segregating the sick poor from the well in the early nineteenth century, which ultimately led to the segregation of medical and mentally ill in the 1830s. Although the Sisters maintained a private institution for the insane, they accepted monies from the state of Maryland for the care of some of the more destitute patients. Mount Hope's administrators and staff were not at all shielded from some of the larger national and state healthcare issues surrounding the care of the insane.

Limits to Charity ⌒

Mount Hope continued to struggle financially. Sister Matilda cleverly invented "lotteries" (Note: these were like auctions) consisting of all sorts of articles priced in a way that families residing in the surrounding villages would be able to afford. She also went to Baltimore every year to solicit contributions from her acquaintances of financial means. Despite her innate aversion for begging, her goal of relieving the suffering of the families whom she assisted gave her the stamina for the cause and animated her pleadings. Upon her return from visits to her benefactors in Baltimore, she would exclaim that "this is the season of harvest," and her joy would be in proportion to the abundance of her harvest of charitable funds. Sister Matilda relied on some of the fund-raising strategies that had served the SC well in Virginia. She and the SC Nurses held a fair in 1847 to raise money to pay the Mount Hope debt. Although the Sisters had many "superb items" to sell, they were only able to make $1,000. Sister Matilda attributed the outcome to the public's false perception that the SC Community was wealthy and that Mount Hope, which belonged to the SC, did not need contributions.

In her journal Sister Matilda cited the cause of the financial challenges as "institutional expenses." There were too many patients for the resources of the house. Mount Hope was a private institution and according to Sister Matilda "received no contributions from any source whatever."[103] Patients typically paid $3 to $6 per week for care.[104] Rev. Deluol identified the cause of the excessive expenses as the admission of too many charity cases, and in 1847 he put in place a specific regulation for Mount Hope that forced Sister Matilda and the Sister-Nurses to reduce the number of charity patients. According to Sister Matilda, "He caused about ten of the charity patients to be sent away, some to their respective homes, and a few of them to the almshouse."[105] Many of the hired domestics were dismissed, and only 10 percent of charity patients were to be kept at Mount Hope on an ongoing basis. Rev. Deluol specifically forbade Sister Matilda as Sister Servant "to trespass on this regulation."[106] While Sister Matilda and the Sisters may have disagreed with Rev. Deluol's decision, they welcomed the challenges that ensued as a result of keeping the hospital open under the strained financial situation. Sister Matilda noted how she and the Sisters coped with the turn of events:

> All the Sisters with one heart and soul, entered into the views of the anxious Superior,[107] and tried to practise [sic] the most rigid economy. All was labor, privation, and hopeful endurance: and it is the opinion of many good, saintly Sisters who still survive, that the spirit of self-sacrificing then manifested, and the sufferings so cheerfully undergone by this first little colony of sisters drew upon Mt. Hope Institution the choicest blessings of Heaven. . . . At this period few of them enjoyed the luxury of a bed-stead, or comfortable bed: a husk-mattress, spread any where [sic] at night, & hidden early in the morning, was one among their many similar accommodations. Any thing would do. – No murmuring but the gayest and most playful acquiescence. The sisters were uniformly happy, and untiring in their efforts.[108]

Sister Matilda and the SC Nurses knew the power of charity to overcome any disturbances they felt about their mission. Mother Mary Xavier Clark had taught them: "We must wait on the sick to please God, and not to follow our miserable self-love, which often makes us go through painful labours, to please creatures, and draw a little breath of praise, to gratify our foolish self-love. Oh! This is real misery, & might indeed be called insanity."[109] Charity, she continued, "carries with it a soothing balm, something not earthly; and which never fails to produce happy results, if not on the body, at least on the mind."[110] Sister Matilda's charity towards the needy was immense; she treated them with the utmost respect and dignity. A Sister who accompanied her in her visits to the homes of the poor wrote that Sister Matilda "was so careful to speak to each one according to his state and capacity, being always so attentive not to wound the sensitiveness of the bashful poor, inquiring into their wants with such delicacy and charity, that it would seem she was receiving a favor rather than bestowing one."[111] Sister Matilda was also very practical. She, like leaders of other public asylums of the period, boldly faced the challenge of finding the balance between treatment ideologies and the daily realities of running a healthcare institution.

In addition to her ongoing financial challenges, Sister Matilda also dealt with the growing national civil liberties issues surrounding commitment[112] of an insane patient to an asylum such as Mount Hope. Influential physicians such as Samuel Woodward of Massachusetts, first president of the Association of Medical Superintendents of American Institutions for the Insane,[113] promoted early hospitalization of the insane as a means of achieving better outcomes.[114] Yet simultaneously, there was a growing public concern about the need for setting limits to protect the vulnerable insane, their civil liberties, and their dignity from families and physicians who would potentially misuse commitment power.[115]

The commitment of a person to an asylum in the early and mid-nineteenth century was usually the responsibility of the insane person's family and friends. Asylum care was typically sought for patients and families in crisis, when the behavior of the insane person grew beyond the capacity of the family or friends to manage. Sister Matilda's historical accounts and Dr. Stokes's *Annual Reports* frequently refer to the freedom of the patients within the confines of the asylum's secure environment, except in severe cases when restraint was necessary to keep the patient from hurting himself or others. Sister Matilda modeled the philosophy of voluntary commitment at the asylum. Wrongful confinement, about which the public was growing increasingly concerned, was against the SC tradition. The Sisters' goal was that patients and their families, who were intent on finding a solution to their mental health and lifestyle problems, find hope for healing and the possibility of a cure at Mount Hope [*see Case Study 3–2*]. Sister Matilda as Sister Servant was responsible for ensuring that each patient—whether he or she paid personally for care or was subsidized by the state, was Catholic or Protestant, or was acutely violent or convalescing—was best served by the care at Mount Hope and that his or her civil rights were never violated.

Charity Begins at Home ⌒

Sister Matilda's mental health nursing and leadership skills were also tested within her own religious Community. The SC were planning for the election of a new leader of the Community upon the completion of Mother Mary Xavier Clark's term. Sister Matilda was one of the two candidates in the Community election of July 1845. The majority of votes went to Sister Mary Etienne Hall (1806–1872), who won the election with sixty-nine votes, twenty more than Sister Matilda. The following year Mother Etienne sent Sister Matilda as an envoy of the council on a mission to New York City to handle a controversy that was spawning a separation of the New York Sisters from the Emmitsburg Community. According to the *Annals of the Community*, among the reasons for the New York Sisters' desire to separate were discontent with the election of Mother Etienne and the council's decision to give up the charge of boys' asylums and schools for the "welfare of their Community."[116] At the time Bishop John Hughes (1797–1864) had been trying to establish the SC under his jurisdiction in New York as an independent diocesan congregation. The conflict between Bishop Hughes and Rev. Deluol, his superior, became heated in their rapid-fire exchange of letters, which added to the controversy. The stress among the Sisters was great. Although thirty-three Emmitsburg Sisters remained in New York, approximately the same number of Sisters returned to Maryland after Sister Matilda's and others' interventions.[117]

It was a difficult time for the Community to experience a separation. Anti-Catholic sentiment was on the rise. The Protestant nativists, also known as "know-nothings," were gathering public support for their fears of "pope-ish" influence in American society and politics. Rapid industrialization and the rising numbers of poor immigrants in urban

CASE STUDY 3-2 **Come of Your Own Accord**

Patient Account at Mount Hope as Recorded by Sister Matilda

One day a fine carriage drove up to the gate, and the driver came to the house telling us that his Mistress wished to speak to a Sister at her carriage. A sister went to her; the lady asked: "Do you go to private houses to nurse the sick?" Answer. "No Madam, never: - we go to visit the sick poor, but never remain at their houses to serve them." "Would no circumstance or consideration move you to do so?" - "Circumstances might occur –" As the lady had her maid with her, she said "Good morning!" and drove off. The lady was middle-aged, of very fine appearance both in form & countenance, tho' sadness and [sic] were strongly expressed in her features. . . . We wondered who this might be, when a few days later the same carriage stopped at the gate, and the driver brought in a similar message. At this time the lady was alone, & entreated the Sister to enter the carriage & sit by her. She did so; and the lady thus accosted her: "I have a female friend, mentally afflicted, in whose welfare I am much concerned; what would you advise in her regard?" Sister replied; "It would be impossible to say, without knowing something of her previous to, and subsequent to the attack." – "Well"- she resumed; "she is distressingly sad; almost despairing; cannot eat, sleep or converse as before; - <u>cannot even read her Bible</u>." "Never mind the Bible," said Sister... "<u>What! not read the Bible</u>! - and can the mind come to that?" - "She is not able to read it now" said Sister, "And consequently she ought to omit it. Has she taken opiates; and to what extent or with what effect?" - "They no longer make impression, or else increase the excitement." - "Then use them no longer. – Has she any Physician?" - "Not at present; they do her no good. She is not willing to try them again." -- "Has she tried blistering or any other external irritations" -. "Yes, but all such remedies are equally useless." "What was formerly her disposition; what were her preferences, her state of health &c &c?" She was happy in her efforts to render others so. She was industrious in her household affairs; had the kindest husband and friends; with a mind & heart ready to enjoy all that friendship could desire: - but now, all is vacuum, disgust, fear, - apathy, and at times a violent eagerness to grasp again former enjoyments, especially those of the mental faculties. . . .

"O my God! if only I could pray again, and read my Bible!" – – She paused; then continued thus: "Could there be any hope for such a one?" "Oh yes!" said the Sister, "every hope." "<u>Can it be possible</u>!" Said the lady, emphatically; - "and <u>you will not go to her house to restore her</u>!" "We could not;" answered the Sister: "We have those around us who require our constant care, and I repeat, such is not our custom." The poor dear lady looked steadfastly on the Sister and then added; "What then shall her friends do for her?" – – The Sister responded; "Have patience, let her have change of air, without exciting senses; & as you say you have no physician

— continued next page

CASE STUDY 3-2 **Come of Your Own Accord**

for her, discontinue all opiates and medicines: – read pleasant books in her hearing; converse in her presence; relate sometimes cases similar to her own, but always with a happy termination of the incident. This is what physicians call, talking <u>at</u> the patient when persons would not venture to talk exactly <u>to</u> them." Then the lady, after a short silence, resumed thus: "And would you take <u>me</u> to be the patient in question?" The mind of the Sister darted over all she had heard, but fearing to make any remark that might prove injurious to the invalid, she composed herself and calmly answered: "No, Madame, I did not think it was yourself?"

"Yes, Sister," said she, "I am the miserable wretch that I have been describing; and all that the most loving kindness, all that expense could do, have been tried in vain for my cure! Oh! what an existence! at Midnight I quit my room and run, phrenzied into the street, through the vehemence of my tortured mind, longing for <u>peace</u>, or something to steady it.". . . The Sister said all she could to comfort and encourage the good lady, who answered her thus: "I will come to your Hospital, tho' my reason for not entering on these two occasions was the fear of meeting your lunatics; feeling myself so much like them." –

The Sister rejoined: "If you come of your own accord, you will also go away when you please, either from your own restlessness, or on account of our treatment, and then you will consider yourself worse than ever, saying, 'Well, I have tried the Hospital, and am no better.'– Wherefore do not come.". . . The lady left, and a few days after returned, accompanied by her husband & sister, who were evidently much dissatisfied at her resolution; for they being all [p22] of the first class in society, considered it a disgrace to have her at a Hospital. When the Sister entered the parlor, the lady advanced, and throwing herself in her arms she said, "Here I am, Sister, entirely in your hands!" The Sister replied; "My dear Madam, did I not tell you <u>not</u> to come?" "And why so?" "I gave you my reasons; your cure requires opposition; when you require a thing you must be denied, and what you would wish to have must be refused you; You must be in a manner remodelled. If you wish to do as you please, we will compel and restrain you into our views; and this treatment you will not endure; consequently you will leave and reasoning with yourself you will say: 'Alas! <u>I am no better; I have even tried a Hospital and am not improved</u>.' Then you will be more desponding than ever, imagining that your last chance had failed." The Lady exclaimed; "I will submit to any and every thing: - go home beloved husband & sister; these good ladies will cure me, for I <u>will</u> obey." Her friends were quite astonished, but seemed well satisfied with the candour of the Sister, for now they believed that the Lady had not [been] enticed to come. . . . She recovered under the above-named treatment; for often she was tied in her bed, being too restless to remain there otherwise. Her happy friends were delighted at her restoration; for she became <u>amiability itself</u>.[118]

Courtesy, Daughters of Charity Archives, Emmitsburg, Maryland

areas, especially Irish Catholics, were often cited as the cause of many peoples' concerns. While nativists sought to gather support for the deportation of the Irish, the Catholic Sisters were compassionate toward their plight. The Sisters' timing for the opening of their hospitals could not have been better, in that their success made them public figures in the Catholic community and in American society in general.

By the 1840s despite religious prejudice, the Catholic Church in America had grown exponentially. The SC Nurses contributed to that success. They exercised their religious freedom in a way that their counterparts in France had not been able to do. The SC, in addition to their nursing and educational work, assisted in the establishment of and ministry to the Catholic community in Emmitsburg and wherever they were missioned, including public hospitals. They continued their religious life and demonstrated it openly in the hospitals and infirmaries by wearing their religious dress, erecting altars[119] and chapels, praying for their patients, and reading scripture to those patients who wished it. However, unlike the male clergy and Sisters teaching in the schools who openly evangelized, the Sister-Nurses' ministry was more subtle. The SC Nurses modeled their religion in acts of faith, hope, and charity to the communities in which they nursed. Their mission and ministry were to nurse the sick, poor, and insane in body and spirit. The SC were committed to the health and comfort of their vulnerable patients, which took precedence over religious instruction and conversion.

The principle of *leaving God for God* permeated the Sisters' ministry from the beginning. In the case of urgent necessity, the Sisters were taught to prefer the service of the poor to saying prayers; however, if they planned well, they were able to find plenty of time for both. The apostolic women understood that if they left prayer and their Holy Mass (liturgical services) to respond to the urgent needs of poor persons they would not be losing. They knew that serving the poor was "to go to God," and they could see God in the persons they were serving.[120] For the Sisters charity was deeply rooted in their commitment to mission. Hence, they stood ready and available to serve the most urgent needs of those whom society was not serving. Their world view and mission were universal and inclusive, derived from the teachings of Vincent de Paul, who taught that "The Sister who has the spirit of a true Daughter of Charity is ready to go anywhere, prepared to leave everything to serve her neighbor."[121] Finding God everywhere—in the streets of the city, the wards of hospitals, on the battlefield, and in the asylums, the Sisters understood that there are the three "signs of charity: to love God and the poor, to make no distinction of persons, and to be indifferent to all places."[122]

The worldview of the Sisters toward the human family emanated from love, particularly for those who were suffering. This motivated the Sister-Nurses to view each of their patients with care, compassion, and a love meant to "wish him well."[123] Vincent understood the dynamism of human emotions, particularly love, which he described as "an ever-growing fire."[124] He believed that "if love of God is the fire, zeal is its flame."[125] He wanted the Sisters to be on fire with the love of God and neighbor. He saw them as mission-minded women whose passion for Christ impelled them to alleviate human suffering, especially among persons oppressed by poverty, disease, and illiteracy. This zeal of the Daughters of Charity in the seventeenth century passed through subsequent generations to nineteenth-century America and continues to animate Vincentian-Louisian sisters around the world today.

Sister Matilda and the SC's zealous approach to the care of the insane, some of the most marginalized individuals in society, stemmed from their religious fervor for charitable service to their fellow human beings. While the Sisters did not speak of Catholic doctrine to their patients unless requested, they often prayed for the safety and health of patients in their care. Despite their own deeply held attention upon their service to God in the nursing of the insane and their devotion to Catholicism as the "true religion," they were required to identify the proper boundaries between holistic, spiritual nursing care and proselytizing. They did not, according to Dr. Stokes, an Episcopalian, interfere with a patient's "religious profession," nor did they "make any distinction" between patients . . . and "the same self-sacrificing zeal, and the same absorption of their best energies, in the one great purpose of alleviating human suffering, are displayed to all."[126] Clergy as well as Sister-Nurses were expected to not interfere in a patient's religious belief and practice. This was discussed in the *Catholic Mirror* in 1849 in relation to the opening of the St. John's Infirmary in Milwaukee: "No minister, whether Protestant or Catholic, will be permitted to preach to, to pray aloud before, or interfere religiously, with such patients as do not ask for the exercise of his office. The rights of conscience must be held paramount to all others."[127]

The Sister-Nurses did not need to proselytize. Their works, as witnessed by others, were often sufficient to convey the nature of their Catholic beliefs and the Vincentian-Louisian-Setonian expression of their faith. Many patients who witnessed the Sisters' religious devotion did in fact ask for spiritual instruction, which Sister Matilda and the Sister-Nurses gave readily. Sister Matilda impressed upon the SC under her leadership the obligation to assess the needs of the souls of their patients. One Sister wrote, "To instruct the patients, to inspire them with a horror for sin, a great love for God; to soothe, comfort and encourage them was the constant employment of Sister Matilda."[128]

The success of the SC nursing ministry was demonstrated in the cholera hospitals, in the university infirmaries that served as clinical sites for medical residents' education, and in their own hospitals and was extended to all sick and insane persons. Although the Sisters were all Catholic and therefore a marginalized minority for that time, they were also all white women. In antebellum American society, crossing racial lines to provide any service to blacks or indigenous people would have been viewed by some as an act of courage. The Sisters provided social leadership by stating in their contract at the St. Louis Hospital (also known as Sisters' Hospital[129]), that they would, for example, "care for indigent sick free persons without respect to color, country, or religion."[130] The hospital, which opened in 1828, began as a two-room log cabin that housed eighteen patients, one of whom was insane. Slaves were cared for in the Sisters' Hospital, paid for by their masters.[131] For the Sisters providing care to any person in need was fulfillment of their mission.

The Sisters' missions also called for enthusiastic and generous response to emerging needs, despite the demands of time, energy, and personal sacrifice. Followers of Vincent and Louise learned early in their commitment that their vocation challenged them to love God both at times of prayer and hard work in ministry. In the words of Vincent: "Let us love God . . . but let it be with the strength of our arms and the sweat of our brows."[132] In other words the Vincentian-Louisian vocation called for a love that was both affective and effective. The foundation of their ministry was a vision of faith that saw Christ in the poor and the poor in Christ.

This belief enabled them to minister to Christ in suffering humanity for generations.

At times the fragility of the Sisters' own human nature required a courage recognized by Louise as necessary to the charitable ministry: "I beg all of you to renew your courage so that you may serve God and the poor with more fervor, humility, and charity than ever. Strive to acquire interior recollection in the midst of your occupations."[133] The love of Christ as described in the *Holy Bible*[134] impelled the Sisters in their mission and gave rise to the spiritual framework that shaped their nursing and other ministries: humility, simplicity, and charity. Two decades after entering the public sphere of American hospitals, regular physicians, and university medical colleges in Baltimore, the Sisters had established a reputation as expert nurses and ministers to the sick poor and insane, as well as devoted public servants.

Expanding the Reach of ⁓ Intercession and Inspiration ⁓

Sister Matilda left Mount Hope in 1847. The Sisters missioned at Mount Hope continued under the direction of Sister Mary Cephas Cook (1814–1855) who was Sister Servant until 1855, the year when the last note of the debt for Mount Hope was fully paid. There is no record that Sister Matilda's relocation was due to the financial difficulties at Mount Hope; it is evident that if she had suspected she was in any way responsible for the situation she would have asked to step aside. Her humility was often demonstrated in her writings: "We know that the work of God needs no individual instrument in order to its accomplishment."[135] Community records indicate that it was a mission that "called" Sister Matilda to expand the reach of her expertise in nursing and institutional administration beyond Mount Hope.

Sister Matilda first went to Emmitsburg for a few months of rest and then was sent to Rochester, New York. In 1845 the SC had assumed responsibility for the Saint Patrick's Asylum, an orphanage with an established board of managers and a staff of young women in residence. A plan for building expansion and fund-raising was required. Sister Matilda, now 48, had experience in both areas and left Emmitsburg for

Cᴀsᴇ Sᴛᴜᴅʏ 3-3 The Sisters' Daily Banquet

Patient Account at Mount Hope as Recorded by Sister Matilda

A shrewd, but insane old Lady was admitted into the Hospital. She had figures as a gay and fashionable belle when "Hail Columbia" was first sung as a National toast; and had excelled in singing it. Soon she found out that bad language was very disagreeable to us, wherefore whenever she felt unamiable, she would utter every bad & profane speech she could remember, in a loud voice; and when she had exhausted her store of such speeches, she would spell out slowly and emphatically, the words of each sentence. All this was at the top of her voice.

One day, being a little more lady-like than usual, she was busy in working some straws, strings &c. in company of some other lunatic ladies. One of these, while getting her dress fastened by Sister N. (Author's Note: Sister Matilda is Sister N) - suddenly turned upon her and spat in her face. A lunatic companion exclaimed; "If I were Sisters, I would slap you well for that, my lady--" . . . The Old Lady, without raising her eyes from her work, took up the word saying: "What is that you say, my dear, that you would slap the lady for spitting in Sister's face? Oh, no, no, that would be very wrong. Don't you know that these good Sisters have taken this house, and advertised to the public that now they are <u>ready for all kinds of abuse</u>? O my dear, you could not after that, resent any thing, O no, no, no."

In one of her quiet seasons, a company of travelling ladies & gentlemen called to see her, as being friends & acquaintances, but having no permission from her relatives, they were politely refused; Sister telling them that as she was now calm it wd be a pity to excite her, wh: would be the case, were she to speak with old friends; and not only <u>she</u> wd. be distressed but her paroxism [paroxysm] wd. affect others near her room. – The strangers listened, and were satisfied to abide by the refusal; but one of the ladies halting, said to Sr. . . . . "Madam, have you really embraced this state of life voluntarily?" – The Sister answered that it could not be entered into any other way. "Permit me then," said the visitor "to tell you that I think you have chosen the one least desirable on earth!" – "Well," said Sister, "you do not surprise me, but I think I can convince you to the contrary. Take history, hear-say or your own experience; ask all times and people, at what time of their lives they were most happy. and they will all answer you, that it was when they were mitigating the sorrows or wants of others. So, what <u>they</u> enjoy only occasionally, is our daily banquet."[136]

Rochester in November to replace Sister Ursula Mattingly (1808–1874) as Sister Servant. This was Sister Matilda's first mission north of her native Maryland, and very soon after her arrival, she began to do what she did well: she conducted a fair to raise money for construction of a new wing for the asylum, and she continued to expand the service to the sick poor.

During her fifteen years as a psychiatric nurse and asylum administrator, Sister Matilda had grown in her ability to inspire new SC Nurses, patients, and the Sister companions with whom she lived in Community. Her SC companions recorded stories about her that demonstrated her passion for religious life, often in the midst of great challenges. One Sister recalled that Sister Matilda's "fervent piety" had filled her with admiration when she was a young Sister.[137] Another wrote:

> When I cast a retrospective glance on those days, I marvel how it was, that any patient could be placed there (Mt Hope). The spirit of God, which filled the heart of our dear Sister Matilda, was the attraction. The world is very clear-sighted and rigid in its views of persons consecrated to God, and if it is scandalized at the imperfections it discovers in such persons, it also knows how to discern and reverence true virtue. We may very naturally ask, what was it that gave Sister Matilda such powerful influence over all classes of society? It was no doubt, because she had given herself unreservedly to God, and she had no other desire than to glorify Him, it was because she was animated by the spirit of our holy Founder, who, in his time could influence the greatest monarchs, that ruled France. This worthy imitator of Saint Vincent, took care to cultivate the virtues he bequeathed to his children, as their most precious inheritance, viz: humility, simplicity and charity.[138]

The Sisters did not aggrandize the exceptional qualities of Sister Matilda, however. They saw her as highly dedicated, sometimes to the point of being perceived as cold and austere by those who did not know her.[139] The Sisters knew that some physicians regarded her as an "oracle of wisdom," whom they consulted as if she were an "old professor"[140] and that patients often attributed their healing to her treatment and manner of acting toward them.[141] Yet the Sisters also witnessed their nurse leader "treated with the greatest contempt, her best actions misconstrued, her reputation blackened and her path at each step beset by trials of various kinds."[142] It seemed that Sister Matilda, an elder Sister in their midst, was simply a human being who faced life's challenges while aspiring to know God.

The Sisters noted a spiritual strength in Sister Matilda that allowed her to attract patients from the full gamut of Maryland society, from some of the most angry and violent to influential Protestants who put themselves in her care with great confidence. Though she was said to have been "sensitive," she built a spiritual practice that helped her to handle the "opprobrium hurled against her"[143] as Sister Servant at an insane asylum and as a Catholic religious woman. For example, one Sister recorded a "desperate case" of a male patient with mania a potu (delirium tremens) at the Maryland Hospital who admitted that he despised Catholics and the SC. He had healed, and while he was waiting for his friends to take him home from the hospital, Sister Matilda gave him lunch in the parlor. He "smiled with scorn and contempt on his countenance" and spoke insulting words to Sister Matilda. She abruptly left the room, and the Sisters supposed she went directly to the chapel to pray. When the man's friends came a few minutes later, the man was dead. The Sister wrote of the incident:

> Sister Matilda did not tell any one what had occurred. As soon however, as she saw the Rev. Superior she informed him of it. Not for years after, did she mention this to any one, and then only with a view to increase confidence in the protection of God over the whole Community and each member of it in particular.[144]

The records surrounding Sister Matilda's life include a number of references to the power of prayer, Providential protection and supernatural experiences such as this and what she perceived as divine intervention. In another story, a lady friend of Sister Matilda who had been visiting the Sisters' chapel to pray each day went on a trip. Before leaving she gave

Sister Matilda money for the altar and requested her to "light an extra lamp before our Lord, and let it burn one hour every day, the hour decided upon was from <u>ten till eleven o'clock</u>."[145] To clean and attend the sanctuary lamp was an office that Sister Matilda never delegated to anyone. She continued to light the lamp and pray for her friend during her absence:

> The lady had traveled two days, when one of the most fearful Rail-Road accidents, ever recorded happened. It was that of Norwalk, sixteen years ago. By some unaccountable neglect, the drawbridge was left up, and a long train of passenger cars with the Engine was precipitated into the river; nearly all were lost. By a special Providence, the lady in question was in the very last car, when the car preceding it, was going down, the connection suddenly snapped, leaving that in which the lady sat uninjured and on the very brink of the precipice. Sister Matilda on this fearful day, had been engaged with visitors, when they left, she went immediately to light the lamp, but discovered that it was one hour past the time; having placed it before our Lord, she knelt to make an act of atonement for her neglect of duty, and also offered an extra prayer for that good lady. Strange coincidence! At this very hour the car was saved.[146]

By the end of her mission at Mount Hope, patients and other Sisters were often seeking the intercession of Sister Matilda, who was a spiritual leader as well as a nursing leader in the SC Community.

The Catholic community greatly valued conversions of people to the "true religion." There are numerous accounts of conversions attributed to the care and ministry of Sister Matilda in particular. The SC Nurses' work positioned them in the lives of patients who were experiencing life-changing events. For this reason Sister Matilda and the SC Nurses often served as ministers to the sick and insane. Communities frequently regarded their work as similar in stature to that of a priest or minister, especially when they were caring for the dying. In providing pastoral care, they often dealt with the issues of baptism and confession with dying patients. The Sisters at one point had also acquired permission from the courts in Baltimore to see a former patient who was in jail on death row, a permission typically given only to clergymen and officers of the court.[147] In addition to patients, Sister Matilda provided spiritual instruction for the servants each night and prayed with them. In her role as Sister Servant, Sister Matilda also ministered and instructed the SC Nurses. The Sisters had a custom once a month of drawing for the names of those patients for whose salvation they "felt most uneasy." Each Sister said some special prayers for the one that fell to her in the drawing. One day Sister Zoé Gleeson impatiently and almost crying said to Sister Servant Matilda:

> "I will pray no longer for Mr. T. He is so obstinate that I am tired of praying for him." "Well!" replied Sr. N [Matilda], "if you give him up, he will be badly off, for you are more obliged to do it than any of us; and you are still doing all you can for his poor body; surely his soul ought not to be cast away before the flesh. Perhaps God will expect his salvation at your hands. Our perseverance in trying to save him, should at least equal that of the enemy [Satan] in trying to destroy him." The Sister renewed her fervor and prayed more anxiously than ever; for his time was now short.[148]

Sister Matilda was also known for her ability to save the lives as well as the souls of patients through her skilled nursing care and soothing demeanor. One account describes an insane patient who by some extraordinary maneuvering made his way to the roof of Mount Hope:

> He walked to the extreme edge, he was first seen from the yard, and all were terror-stricken; to call to him would have had a most disastrous result, to send men to seize him would have excited him and he would most certainly have precipitated himself to the ground. In this dilemma while all were considering the best means to be taken to save him, Sister Matilda walked quietly to the Cupola with two or three oranges in her hands and in a

cool, indifferent tone of voice said: 'John, come here and take an orange.' He walked to the window, received the oranges, got in and went down stairs to his room with Sister Matilda.[149]

Sister Matilda also had tremendous emergency nursing skills for a nurse of her time. On one occasion at Mount Hope, an attendant left a patient with a razor when he went to get water in the hall. The patient attempted to commit suicide by cutting his throat:

He had not been long in the house; appeared very sad as if some untold grief was killing him, yet no one suspected him of purposing suicide. The man was a Methodist; he was so frightened after having wounded himself that he ran the whole length of the hall before he fell. The jugular vein was cut through. The Sister [Matilda] sent at once for the Doctor. Then sitting by the bleeding patient, she turned him over on his side and laying his head upon her knee, she clapped her hand upon the gash, while the blood spouted up, smoking from his neck and hair, through her fingers, even into her face but soon it began to clot between the fingers, and after a while in the orifice; then it ceased flowing. The poor man, pale as death, looked up at Sister and said: "Will I die?" She said; "I cannot tell, but do you say: <u>O my God! how sorry I am for having offended you</u>!" In about 10 or 15 minutes the Dr. arrived, a Sister waiting at the front door showed him to the place, or rather she held his horse, bidding him hasten to the Gentlemen's Hall. . . . On seeing the blood he was terrified and asked where was the cut. The Sister answered: "Just under the palm of my hand, for seeing that the blood had stopped I would not remove it until you could arrive." – "Remove the hand," said he, and immediately the blood began to gush as before. "Stop it, stop it," he said hurriedly, and taking off his coat began to do something to save if possible the poor man's life.

> Two mattresses were fixed in a room near at hand, & the
> doctor assisted some other men in carrying the invalid to
> the bed, while the Sister kept along, still holding her hand
> on the wound. The Doctor succeeded in bandaging the
> wound, and in 48 hours the man was out of danger.[150]

As this account demonstrates, Sister Matilda's holistic focus in nursing situations included attendance to the soul of the patient as well as the body, even in emergency situations. Nursing service was the vehicle through which Sister Matilda and many other SC found expression for their charitable spirit wherever they were missioned.

Sister Matilda remained in Rochester, working untiringly along with five other Sisters of Charity to provide well for the care of the children in the asylum. It was during those two years in upstate New York that Amariah Brigham, the prominent superintendent physician from a state asylum in Utica two hours to the west of Rochester, decided to publicly challenge the institutional model of care at Mount Hope that Sister Matilda had established with the help of her physician-consultant, Dr. Stokes. The faith, hope, and charity of the Sisters as moral entrepreneurs would be put to the test again, this time by physicians who were rapidly rising in social status as they sought to establish dominance in setting national mental healthcare policies.

CHAPTER 4

The Doctor-Nurse Game: To Play or Not to Play

The same year that Sister Matilda left Mount Hope for upstate New York, Amariah Brigham, superintendent physician for the New York State Lunatic Asylum and founding member of the Association of Medical Superintendents of American Institutions for the Insane,[1] decided to pay a visit to Mount Hope. Shortly after his visit, an article by H. A. Buttolph, first assistant physician to Brigham, appeared in the *American Journal of Insanity*, the association's professional journal, of which Brigham also was the editor. Buttolph wrote on "Modern Asylums" after returning from his trip to Europe, where he had visited some of the prominent institutions for the insane. His article stressed the need for models of care that were hierarchical, with male physicians in leadership and residential positions. The required intellectual qualities of a chief resident officer, he wrote, should be like those of Dr. W. A. F. Browne of the Crichton Asylum in Dumfries, Scotland:

> The intellectual qualifications for such a trust are high and varied, but cannot be easily specified. They must comprehend a familiarity with the true and practical philosophy of the human mind, in order that its diseases may be understood, and controlled; as general an acquaintance as is practicable with the usages and workings of society, with the habits and pursuits, with the opinions and prejudices of different classes, with

literature and science so far as they contribute to the instruction, happiness, or amusement of these classes, with everything in short, which is or can be rendered influential in what may be called adult education, in the management or modification of character, in order that as great a number of moral means of cure, of restraining, persuading, engaging, teaching the dark and disordered mind may be created as possible. . . .[2] There must be benevolence. . . . But this gentleness must be controlled; it must be graduated. The purely benevolent physician can never be a good practitioner.[3]

Buttolph suggested that a woman be employed as matron to the institution. He defined the role of the matron based on that of Dr. James Macdonald of New York, formerly of the Bloomingdale Asylum:

The duties of the Matron, if well performed, are second in importance only to those of the Director. To appreciate her services, let us imagine a private family, consisting of young and helpless children, without the care and kindness, and sympathies of a woman. In the Matron of a Lunatic Asylum, should be found the highest qualities of the heart, directed by an intelligent and cultivated mind, and animated by that devotion and singleness of purpose, which Christianity [sic] alone can inspire...She will aid in carrying into effect the treatment ordered by the physician, direct the varied employments of the females, and administer to the unfortunate and afflicted in a thousand little things which no one else can suggest. But her duties should not be entirely limited to her sex; her spirit should in some degree pervade every portion of the institution...it is the more peculiar province and power of woman to enter into the feelings of the unfortunate.[4]

While Buttolph, MacDonald, and other physicians of the insane in America and in Europe voiced their support for women caring for the insane and lending patients their spiritual and emotional talents, that work had to be subservient at all times to the logical and learned (i.e., university-trained) physician. The physician of the institution had to properly oversee the care of the patients; therefore, they declared that he must live at the institution as did the matron, nurses, and attendants who worked with the patients around the clock.

When Brigham went with Buttolph on his "visit" to Mount Hope, he found the antithesis of the institutional model that he advocated. The SC Nurses, who were women, owned and administered Mount Hope. They had hired Dr. William Stokes to be their consultant physician, which meant that Stokes, who was quite happy with the arrangement, did not live at Mount Hope. Because of this, Brigham questioned whether Stokes could effectively serve as the director of the medical care of patients. He also questioned whether Stokes was "in control"[5] of the women who were administering that care.

⌒ The Game ⌒

The struggle for sociocultural authority and institutional power has defined the relationship between doctors and nurses for centuries. In fact, interprofessional rivalry existed between doctors and the DC Nurses in France in the seventeenth and eighteenth centuries. Doctors made many charges against the sisters' practice, such as that they overfed their patients. Physicians, who held power in the public sphere, believed that they knew best what patients needed. At one point they decided to bring semitrained personnel into the hospitals in Paris to do the work that the DC Nurses had always done.[6]

The DC's public reputation for excellent nursing care was not easily dismissed even by the physicians themselves. When physicians, under the inspiration of Enlightenment philosophy, became more interested in training their students at the bedside of hospitalized patients, they once again had to call upon the best, the DC Nurses. Physicians did not diminish the importance of the DC's nursing care simply because the DC were women; the physicians were threatened by the women nurses' renown for their enlightened and professional nursing and *medical* services. Medical power in earlier centuries was "at loggerheads with 'clerical power,' and the bitterness of the dispute was fuelled by similarities rather than contrasts in outlook."[7]

The sisters, in many cases, were just as successful in the care of the sick and insane as physicians, if not more so. The DC's determination to care properly for the sick poor and insane was grounded in a religious tradition in which God was "in control." While their *Common Rules* also clearly instructed the DC to value those in hierarchy and obey their superiors' directions, the sisters' direction from their own inner conscience and communion with God came first. If what physicians wanted was at odds in any way with what the sisters knew individually or collectively was best for the Christian care of patients or their own safety (physical and religious), they did not hesitate to challenge physician authority. Physicians wanted and needed the best nurses, those who were intelligent, educated in nursing, and, most importantly, completely devoted to a public service of physically and emotionally hard work that was out of keeping with the social instruction of middle- and upper-class women of the period. Physicians were in a bind, in that they really needed the skills and assistance of those women who could not and would not be under their complete control. Turf wars and what would later be called the "doctor-nurse game" were inevitable.

Three hundred years later, in 1967, a physician named Leonard Stein coined the term "doctor-nurse game." He described the game as

> clear agreement between doctors and nurses that their relationship was hierarchical and that physicians were superior. All interactions were carefully managed so as not to disturb the hierarchy. Nurses were to be bold, have initiative, and be responsible for making important recommendations, while seeming passive. Their recommendations had to appear to be initiated by the physician and physician requests for recommendations had to be covert.[8]

The cardinal rule of the game was that open disagreement was to be avoided at all costs. The rewards for playing the game well were that the doctor-nurse team functioned efficiently and the nurse gained self-esteem and professional satisfaction because the doctor used her as a "valuable" consultant, which in turn enabled the doctor to gain the respect, admiration, and support of the nurses.

In 1993 a study was published that compared approximately one hundred years of the doctor-nurse game from two physicians' perspectives.[9] The researchers compared two medical residents' journals, one from the 1990s and one from 1888. They concluded that there were many similarities. Twentieth-century doctors, like their predecessors, reacted to nurses' assertiveness on behalf of patients as "uncalled for" and "not tolerable." Yet the medical residents did not respond to what they perceived as the nurses' rudeness. While the nurse of the late nineteenth century was perceived by the physician as a "handmaiden" or "helpful machine" to the resident, the journals suggested that there was more collaboration in 1888 than in 1990.[10]

Twentieth-century studies have shown that collaboration between nurses and doctors improved both patient outcomes and nurse retention in hospitals.[11] Yet numerous studies describe physician abuse as a common consequence of nurses' not playing the game. One study for example, showed that 76 percent of a sample of 264 staff nurses in Honolulu, Hawaii, had been verbally abused by a physician at least once in their careers. Sixty-four percent of 500 nurses in a 1991 study in California said that they had been verbally abused by a physician at least once every two to three months, and 23 percent reported that they had been physically threatened by a doctor at least once. In 2001 questions about the doctor-nurse game still existed. One study of the doctor-nurse game in multidisciplinary health sciences research groups suggested that there was still a perception among some physicians that nurses were not their "intellectual equals."[12] The stereotyping of nurses and doctors and turf wars that has surrounded the care of patients at least since seventeenth-century France is still discussed today.

While educational opportunities in nursing—namely, the creation of doctoral degrees in nursing—have met and exceeded the education for the physician role, there is still an imbalance of power that prevails in the relationship. Social structures have delineated the legal authority of physicians as those who define patients and are responsible for their care. They were still in place in the twentieth century,[13] just as they were in the seventeenth century, breeding opportunities for the continuance of the doctor-nurse game, which, as will now be shown, also existed in the early and mid-nineteenth century during the years that Sister Matilda was fulfilling her vocation.

"Best" Practice and ⌒ Professional Culture Clash ⌒

In the 1840s, when Dorothea Dix first attempted to get the New York legislature to assign moneys for asylum reform, the average number of patients in state institutions was between 450 and 500. Amariah Brigham and H. A. Buttolph, who was also Dix's friend,[14] championed the best solution for improving the care of the insane in state hospitals, which they believed began with the establishment of the authority and residency of a physician for each and every asylum in the United States.

During the first years at Mount Hope, patient numbers were between sixty and one hundred; the institution was a manageable size. What bothered Brigham and Buttolph was not the fact that Dr. Stokes and the SC had implemented a moral therapy model of care for the insane based upon a law of humanity and kindness; they appreciated the contribution to the furthering of moral treatment. Instead, they questioned the credibility and effectiveness of an institution such as Mount Hope, in which care was administered by women nurses and medical needs were fulfilled by a consultant physician who did not live on site.

All the activities at Mount Hope were under the supervision of Sister Servant Matilda Coskery. She was also the person who paid Dr. Stokes. The establishment of Stokes's role in the 1840s as "consulting" physician rather than "resident" physician was a challenge to emerging physician dominance in American healthcare and asylum care in particular. Owning their own hospital for the insane was a highly unusual achievement for women of the period. In the early years of the Mount Hope mission, Dr. Stokes defended not only his right to serve as a consultant to Mount Hope but also the right of the Sisters to hold administrative and clinical control within their facility. He also supported their decision to collaborate in the leadership of the asylum and to reinvent the care of the institutionalized insane in America. By following their sense of the mission, Stokes, Sister

Matilda, and the SC Nurses bucked the doctor-nurse game in American psychiatry. They did not go unopposed.

In 1848 Amariah Brigham used his authority as editor of the *American Journal of Insanity* to openly challenge the working relationship of Dr. Stokes and the SC. He began what would be a years-long debate, writing of his concerns about the facilities at Mount Hope and about the quality of the care provided by his colleague, Dr. Stokes. Four months after Sister Matilda left for her new mission in Rochester, Brigham, in an editorial dated March 2, 1848, described the background for his forthcoming remarks. He stated that in February, two of the managers of the New York State Lunatic Asylum had accompanied him to New Orleans. He wrote that "the journey was mainly for recreation and pleasure and not for any specific object. Whenever it was convenient they visited Institutions for the Insane, though they did not vary their route for this purpose."[15] Yet Brigham felt he had the liberty and responsibility to record and publish the following observations of some of those institutions, in particular Mount Hope:

> We regret that Maryland has not a separate State Institu-
> tion for the Insane poor.... The Mount Hope hospital is but
> a short distance from Baltimore; it belongs to the "Sisters
> of Charity," and is wholly under their management. Dr.
> Stokes, of Baltimore, visits it daily. He was at the hospital
> when we called, and with one of the Sisters accompanied
> us through the entire establishment, which we found very
> neat and in good order. The number of insane was about
> sixty, three-fourths of whom were women. This hospital
> also receives cases of mania a potu.[16]

After reading this, anyone knowledgeable about issues in the care of the insane at the time might have begun to suspect that Brigham was about to render complaints against the institution. While he states that three-fourths of the sixty or more patients were women, what he does not say is that "the rest were men." It was not considered proper for women to care for men at that time. As stated previously, the Sisters, following the *Regulations* of their Community, were caring for men, although male attendants were hired to conduct more personal care under the direction of the Sisters.

In addition, Brigham's specific identification of mania a potu was a signal to his colleagues who read the journal. At the time there was a question as to whether or not mania a potu should be considered "insanity" at all and whether patients with the disorder should be included in patient statistics, especially those records that identified treatment cures. Because mania a potu was considered curable, institutions that treated these patients had better treatment statistics than those typically larger state institutions that treated idiots (those born with such mental illness as retardation) or the chronically mentally ill, such as those with psychoses.

Dr. Stokes had published a number of annual reports of the successful care of the insane at Mount Hope, a smaller private facility. Those successes posed challenges to the models of care provided in the larger state asylums. Brigham clearly sought to discredit Stokes, the Sisters and the Mount Hope retreat when he wrote:

> The institution is defective in many respects, especially as to proper means of heating and ventilation; in facilities for affording labor to patients and should also say in *Medical Supervision*. Dr. Stokes is well qualified, we believe, for the care of the insane, but he is, we understand, only hired to visit the institution daily and prescribe for such patients as the Sisters request. In his late Report he dwells at considerable length on the great importance of medical treatment in insanity, and apprehends Medical Officers of insane institutions have neglected too much the resources of medicine. This may be correct, but if so, how important is it that a household of insane persona should be under the supervision of a Resident Physician, who can vary the treatment according to the circumstances. . . . It must be difficult to establish a uniform and good *system* of moral treatment, unless the selection, instruction and discharge of the attendants on patients, are entirely in the hands of the Medical Officer. As we have said the Hospital as to neatness was in excellent order, and we

could not but admire the self-sacrificing spirit of the pious and benevolent females who have charge of it. They are we believe most faithful and excellent nurses; and we indulge hopes of seeing in our country an Institution for the instruction of such Protestant women as are willing to devote themselves to the care of the sick poor, and the relief of mental and bodily suffering.[17]

Brigham's motives for attacking Stokes, the Sisters, and Mount Hope publicly in the journal included his open concern for the care of the insane and establishing medical dominance as the best way of protecting insane patients from harm. It is also possible, as Stokes would imply in his retorts, that Brigham harbored prejudice toward the Sisters. Brigham was a religious skeptic who ultimately became agnostic after having been a Unitarian. Dorothea Dix was also a fervent Unitarian, as was Millard Fillmore, the 1856 presidential candidate for the American Party (which originated in New York), who championed the "know-nothing" agenda to curb immigration of Irish Catholics loyal to the pope in Rome.

In January of 1849 Brigham published a letter by Dr. Stokes that was his rebuttal of Brigham's remarks. Brigham republished Stokes's remarks on Mount Hope with the note,

It must be evident to every unprejudiced mind, that the foregoing remarks were dictated by kind and respectful feelings towards Dr. Stokes, and the proprietors of the Institution. But to our surprise Dr Stokes thinks differently; and in October last sent us the following letter which we cheerfully publish, and as early as possible.[18]

Stokes's letter to the editor, dated October 3, 1848, was published in the January 1849 issue. He wrote:

I must be permitted to express my deep regret, that you should have inspected the institution under the influence of feelings, which prevented your forming an unbiassed [sic] and correct judgment of its arrangements and

141

medical supervision. Otherwise, I am sure, you would not have given expression to statement so prejudicial to the establishment, and yet so wholly at variance with fact.[19]

Stokes then provided the facts of the heating and ventilation systems of the institution and positively compared Mount Hope to other successful institutions for the insane in America and Europe. He continued on to refute Brigham's claim that he was not providing adequate medical supervision:

> Every patient in the house is under my medical charge, and is seen and prescribed for by me. During the six years that I have presided over it in the capacity of the Physician, there has been no exception to this regulation, and it is not true that I prescribe for such patients only as the Sisters request. Contrary to your belief and expectation, I may be allowed to assure you that I have experienced no difficulty whatsoever in establishing a uniform and good *system* of moral treatment, and that too, "without having entirely the selection, instruction and discharge of the attendants on patients entirely in my own hands." The patients of Mount Hope are happy in possessing the priceless services of the Sisters of Charity. They constitute here the corps of attendants, and I presume you would hardly expect or desire the Physician to possess over them an appointing and expelling power. They are possessed of a degree of refinement and intelligence infinitely above the ordinary class of attendants, and impelled, as they are, to the performance of their duties by the highest and holiest of motives that can influence human action, I declare to you, that I experience no difficulty in establishing with their cooperation, a uniform and good *system* of moral treatment.[20]

He then referred Brigham to the published statistics on the percentage of recoveries at Mount Hope as one measure of the success of their treatment of the insane and concluded:

> Whatever may be your opinion of the subject, formed from a hurried inspection of the building, experience has demonstrated in the most satisfactory manner, that the institution is wanting in nothing that can contribute to the recovery, or promote the comfort of our patients. Your Obedient Servant Wm H Stokes Physician to Mount Hope.[21]

Brigham retorted that the "necessity for a Resident Medical Officer for such Institutions is everywhere acknowledged" in America and Europe.[22] He maintained his stand that the facilities were inadequate and that the Sisters should not be receiving medically ill patients with the insane in the same hospital—a practice that was falling out of favor. He all but accused Stokes of altering institutional records to suggest that the hospital was more successful than it was. For example, he suggested that patients were sent home to die so that the numbers of deaths documented in the hospital records were fewer. He also questioned Stokes's diagnosis of mania, basing his concerns on the fact that the patients were diagnosed with a type that persisted for only one to two weeks, which Brigham said he would not have classified as insanity. Brigham did ask if the Sisters were "attending upon the male patients" but did not pursue the issue further.

After Brigham's initial editorial was published, the Association of Asylum Superintendents held its third annual meeting. Stokes did not attend. Brigham continued to use the journal as a forum for his campaign and stated that based upon Stokes's assertion that Mount Hope was "wanting in nothing" he was "induced to look rather carefully" into Stokes's published reports. He felt it his "duty" to make the suggestions that he did for the welfare of present and potential patrons. He then proceeded to list the three major issues he had with Mount Hope and other institutions engaging in the same model of care:

> 1st Danger from private institutions for the insane not subject to legal inspection, nor under the control and supervision of a medical man.
> 2d The impropriety of treating the insane and personas affected with other diseases in the same building.

3d   The necessity of a Resident Medical Officer in an Institution for the cure of the insane.[23]

Citing precedent of the "evils" that resulted in England from letting asylums go uninspected, the "Mount Hope Institution," wrote Brigham,

> is an anomaly in this country, if not the world. It is a private Institution, and if we are correctly informed, not subject to legal visitation and regular inspection by the authorities of the State or city, and the proprietors of which manage it as they choose, without being required to give any account to the public of their proceedings. Hence, so far as we have been able to learn, they have never published their rules or regulations, their receipts or expenditures, the number of persons in their employ, or who have the care of patients, nor anything by which the public can judge from facts, how the Institution is managed, or what claim it has to be considered a *benevolent* one.[24]

He then unmasked himself completely in the final paragraphs of his editorial reply on Mount Hope:

> Its organization is objectionable, and establishments on a similar plan should at once be discouraged in this country. We do not, however, intend to condemn all private Institutions for the insane, especially those where an eminent member of the medical profession, who has devoted much attention to the study of insanity, and had good opportunities for studying it, takes a few patients under his charge. We have a few such in this country that are entitled to the greatest confidence. But very different are those established by individuals not belonging to the medical profession, and who have no knowledge of the treatment of insanity; who erect a building and advertise they will receive insane patients, and then hire a physician

who resides at a distance to visit it daily, but who has no
control of the Institution but what he derives from those
persons who own it. [25]

Brigham's primary reason for condemning Mount Hope was that Dr.
Stokes did not have "control" over the SC Nurses and that the Sisters, as
Dorothea Dix had suggested to Brigham and Buttolph, were successful as
nonmedical caregivers in administering a smaller institution for the care
of the insane. A number of negative claims and attempts to discredit the
success at Mount Hope would be laid against the Sisters and Dr. Stokes over
the years that ensued. They were accused not only of falsifying records but
of abusing patients. The most challenging allegation was one lawsuit they
endured much later in 1865 in which Dr. Stokes and the SC were indicted
for illegal imprisonment.[26] Stokes and the Sisters were acquitted.

Sister Matilda remained in Rochester during the flurry of Brigham's
editorials, in which he promoted his belief in the *resident* medical
superintendent model of care as the best system for American asylums.
Stokes, as well as at least one other member of the Association of
Superintendents, Dr. Joshua Worthington, resident physician of the
Friends' Asylum in Pennsylvania, stopped attending the meetings of the
Association of Superintendents during that time. Although Worthington
was a resident physician, the Friends' Asylum, like Mount Hope, had
been under lay management since its inception in 1817. Like the SC, the
founders of the Friends' Asylum modeled the York Retreat in England,
valued the therapeutic abilities of nonphysician staff in the implementation
and direction of the system of moral therapy. The lay management also
valued the diagnostic and treatment skills of consulting physicians for
the somatic concerns of patients.[27] It was not until 1850 that the Friends'
Asylum adopted a "medical superintendent" model of care under the
supervision of Dr. Charles Evans.

Dr. Stokes and the Sisters continued to support, as best they could,
their claims to successful treatment of the insane with statistics and
other evidence from their work. Amariah Brigham chose to present his
suspicions and innuendo based upon past experiences in Britain, but the
evidence from public and private records did not support his fears. Mount
Hope did not close its doors for another 130 years, and Dr. Stokes retired

at the end of a long life of service as consulting physician to the Sisters' Mount Hope mission in caring for the insane.

Amariah Brigham, on the other hand, died in 1849. Both he and his beloved son died of a disease contracted while Brigham served as resident physician at the New York State Lunatic Asylum. The death of his son was devastating to Brigham and weakened his already delicate constitution. He died of dysentery a few months before his fifty-first birthday. Brigham was described by a colleague in his obituary as "a philanthropist and a lover of his brother man in the strictest sense of the term; he no doubt was ambitious of fame and distinction."[28] He was described as holding a "high sense of justice, a strong feeling of self-reliance, a quickness of perception which enabled him to seize readily the views of others and use them for his own purpose; but above and before all an iron will and determination, which brooked no opposition, consequently in whatever situation he was placed, he must be absolute, or he was unhappy."[29]

There was no mention in Brigham's or Stokes's writings of the health risks encountered by physicians and nurses who lived in asylums, but Stokes's and his family's exposure to infectious disease would have been significantly less than Brigham's. Dr. John Galt, superintendent of the Eastern Lunatic Asylum of Virginia, presented a report the next year on the organization of asylums for the insane, in which he included commentary supporting the substitution of consulting physicians for resident superintendents in hopes of "prolonging their lives for the cause of the suffering insane." He said of the late Amariah Brigham, "If this eminent laborer in the field of benevolence, after establishing on a permanent basis, the important charity over which he so ably presided, had then acted in its behalf, under a less confining class of duties . . . we might still, perchance, have had the light of his intelligence among us."[30]

In 1850 the turf battle continued. The president of the association, Dr. William Awl of Ohio, invited Dr. J. M. Higgins to prepare a report to be published in the *American Journal of Insanity*, "on the necessity of a resident medical superintendent in an institution for the insane."[31] Although Higgins stated publicly that he had never managed an asylum, he concluded that the best practice in the asylum care of the insane required that a superintendent physician establish residency with his family in the facility.

In 1851 President Awl resigned on the first day of the association's annual meeting. It is not clear what transpired to cause the resignation, but Dr. Stokes, on the second day, "appeared and took his seat, as a member of the Association."[32] Dr. Charles Evans of the Friends' Asylum also returned. Although the debate continued in the *Journal* about the need for *resident* superintendents at American asylums, some became more tolerant of the notion of lay people and nurses taking the authority to administer care of the insane.

Initially, Stokes still did not attend the annual meetings of the association after Brigham's death. But in 1853, after the controversy died down, the association held its annual meeting in Baltimore. Not only did Stokes participate, he took the members on a tour of Mount Hope. A report of the event in the *Journal* proceedings stated that the "Association then returned to the Eutaw House much pleased with their visit, and with the kind and hospitable manner in which they had been received by the Sisters."[33] The association members seemed to have finally understood that Dr. Stokes's collegial partnership and shared leadership with the Sisters were not going to change. Stokes and the Sisters had successfully defended their right to opt out of the emerging doctor-nurse game in American asylum care. The doctor-nurse game was eclipsed by a powerful sense of mission and charitable intention.

What motivated two physicians—Brigham and Stokes, both educated, well-traveled, Protestant men—to have such diverse responses to the SC Nurses and their moral entrepreneurship? While this may never be fully understood, patterns in Brigham's writings clearly reflect his concern about the power and control that he thought the "medical officer" should hold, especially over nurses. He had little to no regard for the Sisters' expertise, their traditions, or their established relationship with physicians such as Dr. Stokes. His ambition and desire for medical authority seemed to blind him to the success of a system of treatment at Mount Hope that was contributing to the welfare of the insane, whom he claimed to love.

The Sisters' arrangement with Dr. Stokes was a new concept to American superintendents, many of whom sought to control matrons and nurses in their facilities, but it was not new to the Community of Sisters, and therefore it was not surprising that they were able to create a successful partnership with Dr. Stokes. Partnering with men and creating mutually beneficial working relationships was part of the tradition of which the Sisters were a part, as evidenced in the relationship between Vincent de Paul and Louise de Marillac and modeled by Elizabeth Ann Seton and Rev. Simon Bruté in America. Although Sister Matilda Coskery may not have consciously tied the decisions she made about nursing care at Mount Hope to her tradition, she had every reason to believe in the soundness and potential success of the design of a doctor-nurse relationship that, following the principles of the *Common Rules* and *Regulations* laid down by the French founders and then Mother Seton, mirrored the harmony of the others of her tradition.

⁓ *Sister Matilda's Middle Years, 1849–1855* ⁓

In 1850, as the controversy continued between the state asylum superintendants, Stokes, and the SC missioned at Mount Hope, Sister Matilda's years of pioneering nursing service began to take a toll. By July of 1849, at age fifty, she was in ill health, and her superiors decided that she should return to Emmitsburg for the sake of her health. Sister Romuald McGauran (1814–1884) replaced her in Rochester. Spending the summer of 1849 back in Saint Joseph's Valley improved her health, and toward the end of September, she was missioned to serve in Norfolk, Virginia, where the SC had begun St. Mary's Asylum and School the previous year. Sister Matilda replaced Sister Mary Aloysia Lilly (1808–1866) as the Sister Servant.

Sister Matilda and other Sisters were involved in a major Community transition being orchestrated by Rev. Deluol. He had returned to his native France to retire but before his departure had arranged that the Congregation of the Mission, the Vincentian priests, would assume governance and spiritual services to the Emmitsburg Sisters. As a result, the Sisters of Charity Community at Emmitsburg[34] formally joined the Company of the Daughters of Charity of St. Vincent de Paul of Paris on March 25, 1850. Sister Matilda and the SC based at Emmitsburg became Daughters of Charity. They exchanged their black dress, cape, and cap adopted by Mother Seton for the American SC for the blue-grey attire and large white cornette[35] of the French sisters.

That same year Mount Hope was challenged again. Neighbors who were concerned that the presence of the asylum would affect the sale of their lots attempted to have streets opened through the Mount Hope grounds and one to run directly through the building. Judge Frick, who heard the case, declined the American Daughters' (DC) appeal to stop the encroachment. He represented Mount Hope as a "public nuisance."[36] Fortunately for the DC, the judge died before finalizing the deliberations, but they still could make no further improvements to the buildings because of the "unsettled state of the streets."[37] The DC's need for more patient accommodations caused them to look for a new location, and in 1860 they moved into the new Mount Hope on a farm seat near Reisterstown, Maryland. This new facility was called Mount Hope Retreat until 1945, when a new title, The Seton Institute (1945–1973), was adopted. In her account of the Mount Hope mission, Sister Matilda reflected:

> But God will not permit his work to fail. Mount Hope is a standing monument of His Providence. It is an Institution that was commenced without one cent of capital; with few to sympathize with it and many to oppose it; even Catholic, who imagined that because it belonged to St. Joseph's it would be almost a sin to bestow an alms towards its foundation: for many persons erroneously supposed St. Joseph's House to be rich. Yet through all obstacles & prejudices, Mount Hope is still going on.[38]

Sister Matilda's work in Norfolk, of which little is known, was shortened by an urgent call to Detroit, Michigan, in October of 1850. Sister Matilda replaced Sister Servant Loyola Ritchie (1809–1850), who had died from cholera. Sister Loyola, with Sisters Felicia Fenwick (1808–1868), Rosaline Brown (1816–1885), and Rebecca Dellone (1801–1848) had left Emmitsburg in 1844 to open the SC mission in Detroit. Although she had not been well, Sister Loyola's death was nevertheless unexpected.

The Detroit Sisters started their mission in a cluster of old wooden buildings. In 1845 Sister Rebecca, who had helped to start the SC hospital in St. Louis, suggested that the Sisters convert the boys' school to a hospital. This became St. Vincent's Hospital, the first hospital in Michigan; it had a capacity of thirty patients. The first patient was an English Protestant named Robert Bridgeman, about whom the Sisters were told by a little girl in their school. The man recuperated from his "dreadfully sore" knee and then remained with the Sisters for "several years in the capacity of nurse."[39] The little hospital filled up quickly. In 1847 the Sisters began to receive support and donations from Protestants as well as Catholics to expand their hospital. In 1848 Sister Rebecca died at age 59, and in 1849 Sister Felicia left for another mission. In 1850, as the new hospital neared completion, another cholera epidemic broke out in the city, and the Sisters turned their schoolrooms into hospital wards for cholera victims. It was during this scourge that Sister Loyola contracted and subsequently died of cholera. Sister Chrysostom Fitzgerald (1808–1853) became the interim Sister Servant.

This was the situation into which Sister Matilda was missioned. Having had the experience of directing the expansion of the Mount Hope hospital mission, she was a logical choice for leading the Detroit Sisters through the period of transition. On November 1, 1850, just weeks after Sister Matilda's arrival, the nine Sisters transferred their patients from the old to the new hospital on Clinton Street. One of the first things Sister Matilda did as Sister Servant was to rename the new hospital St. Mary's House for Invalids.[40]

Sister Rosaline, who was the last of the original Sisters to remain, wrote a narrative of the Detroit mission during its first years. She described the new hospital as more "comfortable quarters"[41] for their patients, many of whom were sailors. In the summer of 1851, the Sisters treated men with ship fever, typhoid, and dysentery. Many of their patients were prisoners who had become ill. Forty-nine men who had been arrested simultaneously due to involvement in a railroad conspiracy took ill for various reasons and were transferred to the care of the Sisters. Many of the men were dying. Sister Rosaline described the men as "all grades of society. Ministers, Doctors, Lawyers, Farmers, Laborers and one Judge, charged as the leader of the band."[42] The Sisters ministered to the physical and spiritual needs of the dying prisoners as they would anyone else. Sister Rosaline's *Narrative* provided an objective observation of Sister Matilda's passion for nursing as a ministry of intercession for people's souls as well as their bodies.

Once of the Detroit Sisters was caring for a dying man who felt that he had been wrongly accused of a crime for which he had been serving time in jail. As he neared death, the Sister-Nurse asked the man if he "felt satisfied to die as he was."[43] The man expressed a desire to receive instruction in the Catholic faith if not too late. The Sister asked the patient if he believed in "all that the New Testament related of the teachings of our Savior" and that "our Lord's words are very expressive in regard to baptism."[44] Although his family was Episcopalian, the man had never been baptized. The nurse told Sister Matilda of the man's desire for baptism and asked the Sister Servant to pray for him. The Sisters knew that the man would probably not live another day. That evening after the Sisters had retired Sister Matilda went to the chapel:

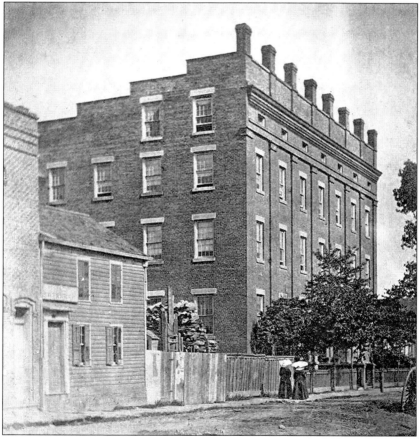

Fig. 4-1   *St. Mary's Hospital, Detroit, MI 1844*

Sister Matilda went into the chapel and prostrate before the Blessed Sacrament, implored our Lord not to let him die as he was. . . . The Sister opened the door and found her [Sister Matilda] kneeling before the altar with her arms stretched out in the shape of a cross. She followed the Sister out, and said: 'Now, Sister, don't let that good gentleman die without baptism.'[45]

Sister Matilda's and the DC Nurses' services often led to conversions. In a few cases their patients became Sisters and priests. One patient, John Finegan, entered the novitiate after his encounter with the Sisters in Detroit and took the name Brother Barbas. Finegan wrote a letter to the Detroit hospital Sisters in 1878, twenty-six years after being discharged from the Sisters' care, to express his gratitude. His "corporal infirmity" had been his "good fortune."[46] He wrote of the Sisters' care:

I remember especially Sister Jane Frances Chantal [Gartland], whom I used to call my mother. She was a mother to me, for besides her kindness in numberless other ways, she gave me her own old venerable beads, and so handed me over to our heavenly Mother. Sister Turebia [sic] [Turibius Donahoe] used to give me medicine; she also used to preside at evening prayer, and some devotions of that kind. Sister Stella was, I think, attending the chapel as sacristan. I forget the Mother Superior's name, but not herself; I think it was Matilda; also the Sister that attended to the medicines, who kept in fact an apothecary store on a small scale, - I had almost said the druggist Rosalia, [Rosaline Brown] if I mistake not. If you have an opportunity of seeing these, or any of the other Sisters that were then there, or any that knew me then, you will do me a great favor by remembering me to them in the most affectionate manner. . . . I almost forgot John, who worked around and prayed all the time.[47] I heard by a letter lately from Detroit that you still remembered me, and sometimes inquired of Mrs.

Finegan about me and it made me blush for shame that I
had never <u>testified</u> my gratitude by letter."[48]

Before her departure from Detroit in 1852, it seems that Sister Matilda
had instilled an enthusiasm and skill for hospital entrepreneurship and the
care of the insane in her companions. Sister Rebecca Dellone, who worked
with Sister Matilda in Detroit, also developed a passion for hospital fund-
raising. She was recorded by Sister Felicia Fenwick, who worked with her,
as being "a missionary of great experience and animated with the spirit of
holy vocation."[49] Sister Rebecca was raising funds for the new hospital when
she approached a merchant whose verbal abuses and accusations brought
Sister Felicia to tears. Sister Rebecca suggested to the man that he "no doubt
had had some disappointment" and that she would return to the shop in
thirty days to speak with him again about a donation for the hospital.[50] Sister
Felicia, with encouragement from Sister Rebecca, returned to the shop after
one month of daily prayers on behalf of the man. Sister Rebecca prompted
Sister Felicia's cooperation in the matter by telling her that her sacrifice to
once again bear the repugnance she felt for the man's abuse would certainly
"draw additional blessings on the mission."[51] Sister Rebecca's experience at
the beginning days of the St. Louis hospital mission was that the Sisters
were living in extreme poverty. She told the Detroit Sisters that she believed
that "poverty in the beginning guarantees success."[52]

Sister Mary Desales Tyler (1804–1899), who became Sister Servant
after Sister Matilda left, served in Detroit for thirty-five years. In 1853 she
led the DC in the purchase of a farm, where they expanded their nursing
services to include the care of the insane.[53] In 1855 the Detroit DC, much
like Sister Matilda and the Sisters in Baltimore, decided to build their own
asylum for the insane, which they would manage.

Sister Rosaline went to Buffalo, New York, in 1854 to the Buffalo Infant
Asylum. In 1860 Sister Rosaline exercised her entrepreneurial spirit and
spearheaded the acquisition and development of the Providence Retreat
in Buffalo, an insane asylum for the poor. An oral history recorded by
a sister who worked with Sister Rosaline beginning in 1868 described
how the DC came to the decision to open their own asylum. The mission
began during their daily excursions to town, when the sisters called at the
Erie County Poor House:

In going through, they found one portion of the building occupied exclusively by the poor insane, there being at that time no other place of refuge for those afflicted beings, in Buffalo, nor nearer than Utica. But the spectacle that met their gaze, in making the tour of the institution was not to be easily effaced from their memory. The condition of the insane department was truly appalling, there being a number of these poor unfortunates, strapped down to benches or chained to posts or anything to which they could be fastened, and most of them half naked, so that they appeared more like wild animals than anything human.[54]

Sister Rosaline is quoted as having said to their spiritual director, Rev. Francis Burlando, CM (1814–1873), that she "had not even one dollar to start an asylum," at which point he handed her a dollar and said, "Take this with my blessing and begin the work."[55] The DC received many inebriates at the asylum who paid $10 per week. Sister Rosaline "took quite an interest in them and made every effort possible to provide for their comfort," which was difficult at the beginning because the asylum accommodations were of the "poorest kind."[56] The sisters stored water at first in the bathtub, and when their supply ran out, they had to carry water in hogsheads for nearly a mile until they, with the help of Buffalo mayor Grover Cleveland,[57] received permission for the asylum to have access to city water. They made tallow candles to light the house. But while the house furnishings were sparse, food was not; the sisters ate well.

The Providence Retreat received many donations under Sister Rosaline's leadership. She instituted a subscription list of several business men and prominent citizens of Buffalo who donated from $5 to $50 dollars yearly. At one point, the asylum was bequeathed over $47,000, which Sister Rosaline attributed to the help of her first companion at the house, Sister Mary McGovern (1827–1887), who had died of typhoid and who, Sister Rosaline had assured the sisters, "would not forget them" in heaven.

Sister Rosaline died of cancer in 1885 at the age of sixty-nine. "Seldom was there a death so universally regretted as Sister Rosaline's, as she was widely known and highly respected by all classes and conditions."[58] Sister Rosaline had never been a Sister Servant, let alone an entrepreneur, before the Providence Retreat mission, but with the support of her superiors and companions and the experience of working with Sister Matilda in Detroit, who had a significant momentum in starting psychiatric hospitals, she was well equipped to pursue the mission. The Sisters treated the mentally ill at the retreat in Buffalo for eighty years.

After Detroit, Sister Matilda's doctor recommended a warmer climate, and she was missioned to the Baltimore Infirmary in April of 1852. Her flexibility, competence, and generosity made her able to be utilized on many missions of the province. Little is known about the brief time Sister Matilda spent as Sister Servant at the Baltimore Infirmary, but there is one record of her concern for the health of a young sister named Augusta Adams (1825–?), one of the companions at the infirmary. Sister Matilda proposed that Sister Augusta, who was suffering from dropsy (edema), be sent back to Detroit, where she had recently been a postulant. But the council decided that Sister Augusta should find proper medical care at the Baltimore Infirmary. Later, Sister Matilda and a priest advisor suggested that Sister Augusta leave the community, which she did on December 22, 1852.

In July of 1853 the council missioned Sister Matilda, as the Sister Servant of St. Peter's Asylum and school in Wilmington, Delaware. Established in 1830 by the SC, St. Peter's was the oldest childcare institution in the state of Delaware at the time. Little is known of Sister Matilda's Wilmington mission either. By early April of 1855, Sister Matilda's health had deteriorated again, necessitating another change in climate. An entry in the council minutes indicates that Sister Matilda was missioned to St. Vincent's Asylum, an orphanage located in the District of Columbia, on June 10, 1855, presumably a temporary assignment. Sister Matilda had limited responsibilities; however, she must have returned to the Baltimore Infirmary as either a convalescent or patient because late October records indicate that she had been recalled from Baltimore to Emmitsburg because someone was "needed to give instruction to the Children attending the Poor School and others employed at the wash-house."[59] Apparently, her health had improved.

⟿ *A Historical Privilege* ⟿

The Sisters of Charity Nurses, who had become Daughters of Charity in 1850, endured many personal, community, and professional hardships to engage in pioneer nursing and psychiatric care in early and mid-nineteenth-century America. They typically began their nursing missions in facilities that were physically well below the standards they required of healing environments for carrying out the holistic care for which their Community was known. Yet they, with the support of strong and compassionate leadership, carried the vision for their Community's ministry to care for the sick poor and insane from mission to mission.

Although the DC nursing missions were an extensive part of their Community's service, there was little documentation of the details of their work. There were many reasons for this, most notably that the sisters were too busy to stop to write down the details of their work when they were literally saving lives in healthcare facilities that needed their constant attention. Writing about one's work in a culture of religious service, especially in a sisterhood such as the DC, could also be viewed as an indulgence of the personal ego and a distraction from the focus of the mission, which was patient care. However, Sister Matilda Coskery did take the time to write down her thoughts on nursing the sick and insane. As will be discussed in greater detail in chapter 5, significant evidence suggests that Sister Matilda was the author of a nurses' instruction book archived in Emmitsburg entitled *Advices Concerning the Sick*.[60]

Advice books were a very important and popular genre in American literature in the nineteenth century. One of the most famous advice books for nurses, *Notes on Nursing*, was published by Florence Nightingale in Britain in 1859.[61] However, as Nightingale clearly states, her book was not written specifically for nurses but for all women whom she deemed capable of becoming nurses.[62] Sister Matilda's book, however, was written for the professional DC Nurse, who cared for some of the most sick, insane, and violent individuals in society.

The existing *Advices* document was not dated, so it is not completely clear when Sister Matilda wrote her book. It is most probable that she would have had to have achieved a certain level of leadership in her religious community before engaging in such a project. Internal evidence suggests that Sister Matilda wrote *Advices* when she was a Sister Servant, sometime after 1839 in Virginia. *Advices* includes extensive details on the care of the insane, suggesting that it was most likely written after she had established her special gift for the care of the insane at the Maryland Hospital and probably during the seven years that she was administrator and Sister Servant at Mount Hope.

Sister Matilda may have had a mentor in the project. The only other book on early nursing in the American DC Community was (as is noted in chapter 2) written by Sister Mary Xavier Clark, who had been Sister Matilda's Novice Mistress in the 1830s and became Mistress of Novices again in 1845 after years of service as Mother to the Community. Like Sister Mary Xavier, Sister Matilda had the responsibility of instructing new nurses in her role as Sister Servant and most likely wrote her advice book as part of that instruction. Mother Xavier, as was recorded in the Community's historical accounts, may have alluded to *Advices* when she told one sister who was being missioned to Mount Hope to serve with Sister Matilda, "My child, you are going to a saint, study her well, *she is a good book* for you to read daily."[63] Sister Mary Xavier, having just written her *Instruction on the Care of the Sick* in 1846, may have suggested that Sister Matilda document her *Advices* before leaving Mount Hope in 1847.

Additional evidence within the text of *Advices* suggests the date it was written. Sister Matilda refers to the hospital in which the Sister-Nurses worked as a "house," suggesting that the manual would have been written after she left the Maryland Hospital and most likely between 1840 and 1847, when she was Sister Servant at Mount Hope, which the sisters and patients referred to as a "house." The level of detail related to nursing the sick and insane that is present in *Advices* suggests that the book was written while Sister Matilda was still actively working with patients. If this was the case, it would have been written before the end of her Detroit mission in 1852 at the very latest. This was the time when she entered middle age, and poor health had started to preclude her performing patient care as she had in the past.

It was customary in the 1840s for every attendant[64] and nurse working in asylum care in Britain to receive a booklet with required duties described for each position by the author supervisor.[65] The nurses' details outlined in the instruction books at the Hanwell Asylum, for example, were cleaning, observing, and feeding their patients and accompanying their patients to social events such as chapel services and work. Based upon his experience in Britain, it is also possible that Dr. Stokes suggested that Matilda, as Sister Servant, write a manual of instruction for the nurses and attendants at Mount Hope. As the institution came under scrutiny by physicians and the public, it may have also become a professional necessity to have documentation of the training of the staff at the DC's asylums. Unfortunately, there is no existing reference to the date of any documentation of the use of the *Advices* manuscript by the DC in the education and training of nurses. There are, however, Community oral histories documented after Sister Matilda's death that stated that she did indeed mentor nurses for their missions when she was Sister Servant, as well as in her later years when she was living in Emmitsburg.[66]

Sister Matilda's book, *Advices Concerning the Sick,* provides an important understanding of the Daughters' early nursing practices and philosophies, especially during the period when moral therapy, the holistic care of the insane, centered on the notion of kindness as the "remedy of remedies." It also defines the roles of nurses in creating healing environments, believed by nurses, physicians, and the public to hold many keys to the humane treatment and curing of the insane.

In her choice of titles, Sister Matilda took yet another bold step. She used the word "advices" rather than "instruction" or "suggestions" or "notes." While "advice books" was a vernacular term used to describe publications on public self-care, the use of the word "advices" in a nursing instruction manual may have had a different connotation. "Advices" was the word often used by physicians to denote the "recommendations" or "orders" that they expected nurses and attendants to follow in the care of patients. For example, Sister Matilda wrote that in 1843 Dr. Stokes finished his regular visit to the patients at Mount Hope and "left his advices" for her and the staff.[67] Sister Matilda's *Advices* may have been equal to those of a physician in the eyes of some, perhaps even to Sister Matilda herself. The doctor-nurse game of defined order givers and order receivers was not fully established in the mid-nineteenth century, certainly not from Sister Matilda's perspective. Her *Advices* book, as will be presented in the next chapter, provides some insight into the nature of doctor-nurse relationships in the mid-nineteenth century from the view of a seasoned Daughter of Charity Nurse. It also provides a clearer picture of the role of the professional nurse of the period as it existed in juxtaposition and occasionally in opposition to the apostolic and charitable life of a Daughter of Charity.

CHAPTER 5

⁓ ♏ ⁓

Sister Matilda Coskery's
Advices Concerning the Sick

Vowing a life of humble service did not deny the Daughters of Charity
(DC) opportunity to be intelligent, creative, and expressive of
their God-given talents. Nursing was a skill as well as a ministry for the
Daughters. Sister Matilda Coskery's nursing is exemplary of the pioneering
work that the Daughters accomplished not only for their Church and
Community but also for the vocation of nursing. Sister Matilda's *Advices
Concerning the Sick* documents her nursing skill and ability to reason as
well as her ministry and caring spirit.

The enlightened DC, like other women of the period, valued rational
thought and intelligence in addition to compassion and benevolence.
Nursing, especially the care of the insane, was one social endeavor for
which intelligent nurses were actively sought. While it may have been
"written scores of times," according to Florence Nightingale,[1] that *every*
woman in the nineteenth-century culture made a "good nurse" and was
inspired to care for the sick and poor of society, nurses on both sides
of the Atlantic, Nightingale, and the DC realized that the contrary
was possibly truer. Not every woman was able to carry out the tasks
associated with professional nursing care, let alone the management
and leadership of healthcare institutions. Physicians like William Stokes
also knew the difference between caring women benevolently serving
in their communities and professional nurses. One physician from
Vermont wrote:

How often are the best directed efforts and the most
unremitted exertions of the scientific physician entirely
nullified, by the want of proper attention or the requisite
knowledge on the part of the nurse! The physician cannot
spare the time necessary to watch the varying phases
of the disease, or the minor but important wants and
annoyance it causes in the patient, and therefore must rely
on the nurse for information, as well as for carrying out
his plans and prescriptions for the relief of these as well as
the graver features of the malady; yet it is but seldom that
he can find a nurse on whose knowledge and judgment
he can rely with confidence. Kind-hearted and attentive
women are usually to be found in all communities, and in
most families, but the knowledge and judgment requisite
to constitute the *nurse* is a very rare endowment.[2]

The DC Nurses were particularly qualified by their ministerial and
nursing preparation for their professional role within the greater healthcare
culture. While every woman might have been expected to attain some level
of caregiving proficiency valued by society, not every woman was called to
nursing as a vocation. As discussed in chapter 2, the DC received formal
education in nursing care and ministry to prepare for their nursing missions.
The innate intelligence and character of a nurse was also taken into account,
especially when she was assigned to the nursing care of the insane.

Sister Matilda, as is demonstrated in her *Advices,* was a highly skilled
nurse. She was educated, literate, compassionate, and deeply devout. She
was not only a role model for DC Nurses but was also in many ways the
archetypal professional nurse of the period. Sister Matilda and the DC
Nurses laid the foundation for what the American public came to know as
professional nursing during the Civil War, through the 1860s, and into the
later part of the century, when the movement for secular reform of nursing
began in earnest in Britain and America under the banner of the Nightingale
training-school model. Secularization will be discussed in chapter 6.

In this chapter we provide our literary analysis and an explanation
for Sister Matilda's *Advices Concerning the Sick.* This seventy-six-page
text may have been a work in progress, one of the reasons it was not

published in the nineteenth century and lay dormant until now. Sister Matilda left a number of open spaces on some of the pages, possibly allowing for additional writing. Many "advice" books of the mid-nineteenth century were in essence working documents. Some of the most popular went through multiple editions.[3] Popular advice books, though they were often written by health professionals, were created for the public in an effort to employ people's abilities to "be their own doctors." Beecher[4] and Child,[5] popular mid-nineteenth-century advice-book writers on domestic medicine and nursing, were not nurses. And while their books included sections on sickroom management and the community caregiving practices of benevolent women, the books were not professional nursing texts. The purpose of sickroom-management content in advice books was to teach the individual woman in her home how to care for her family and friends. The purpose and intention of Sister Matilda's *Advices* was entirely different.

Advices imparts a holistic philosophy of nursing, addressing the corporal, mental, emotional, and spiritual needs of patients, which Sister Matilda advised that her DC Nurse companions employ in their nursing ministry. *Advices* was written for the professional nurse working in an institutional setting rather than for the woman engaged only in care of family and friends.

When assessing *Advices* from two historical perspectives—nursing and the Vincentian-Louisian-Setonian tradition, we find that Sister Matilda drew from her life as both a religious woman and a professional, hardworking nurse and public servant. Her lessons are often so simple that they are easy to miss at first glance. We have read and reread her text many times, each time finding more points of connection with the histories of the Daughters' nursing ministry, American healthcare, mid-nineteenth-century psychiatry, and nursing care. We have come to understand one of Sister Matilda's basic and yet profound teachings about the importance of simplicity. True to form, her text contains some of the most simple and yet elegant spiritual and practical *Advices* for nurses that we believe to be relevant for nurses and healthcare providers today, especially those working in healthcare institutions.

The content of *Advices Concerning the Sick* is presented here as Sister Matilda wrote it. There are no existing primary documents in which Sister

Matilda discusses her advice book or its meaning. Therefore, we rely upon her choices and the way she has ordered the content in her book, her language and writing style, to understand Sister Matilda's nursing skill and her intention or motivation as well to provide insight into the nature of the nursing care of the period. In this chapter we intersperse our editorial comments with the *Advices* content as it appears in the original text. The full text of *Advices* is also presented without commentary in Appendix B. A translation of the Douay-Rheims Bible, also known as the Rheims-Douai Bible or Douai Bible (abbreviated as D-R), the Roman Catholic version of the Bible used by Daughters of Charity during Matilda's lifetime,[6] was used to evaluate Sister Matilda's biblical references.

Advices Concerning the Sick is presented here in transcribed, type-written format so that the original loose-leaf pages written in ink would not have to be subjected to scanning technology. Our goal was that this transcription would represent the original document as closely as possible. Therefore the transcription preserves all of Sister Matilda's strikeouts and blank pages as well as headings, capitalization, and spelling. We made decisions about the presentation of the original text that we hope will aid the reading of it. There are some parts of the document, however, that needed some explanation. The notation "[*sic*]," typically used in references to historical documents to denote spelling errors that occur in the original document, is used here. There are also a few instances in which Sister Matilda included notes within parentheses to offer explanation to her readers. These notes are included as she wrote them. We have also added authors' notes to clarify that the material in the parentheses occurred in the original text.

⌒ *The Voice of an "Oracle"* ⌒

Sister Matilda was a nurse for nearly forty years. More than half of those years were spent in direct patient care, either as a Nurse companion or Sister Servant. Sister Servants during Sister Matilda's era were caregivers to patients as well as administrators. As will be discussed in chapter 6, Sister Matilda was a nurse during the Civil War and well into her later years in Emmitsburg, where she taught young sisters at the Central House and provided nursing care to her fellow sisters. Sister Matilda had achieved the respect of her Community for her accomplishments in the care of the insane and the establishment of hospitals. It was rare, given the nature of the DC Community, that a sister be singled out or recognized individually for her service—Louise de Marillac and Mother Seton had laid strong foundations for building a Community whose spiritual focus included the virtue of humility and equity among Community members.

Dr. Stokes's *Annual Reports* do not mention by name the Sister Servants or DC Nurses with whom he worked until later in the nineteenth century. At that time he listed the name of the Sister Servant on the *Report*'s cover page underneath the name of the consulting physician. When speaking of the DC Nurses' work, he always referred to the sisters' Community rather than any particular nurse. When W. G. Read wrote his report on the interview with Sister Matilda, he referred to her only as the "Sister who is charged with the direction of that establishment."[7] The Daughters' cultural beliefs precluded their drawing attention to themselves and away from the object of their mission, the patient. There are, however, two instances in which DC Nurses are named. One was the newspaper report of the two Sisters of Charity Nurses who died during the cholera epidemic in Baltimore; the second was the Catholic institutional records published in the *Catholic Almanac*[8] that named the Sister Servants of institutions in which they served in a leadership position. Sister Matilda was listed as the Sister Servant at the Mount Hope Retreat, for example. But for the most part, Sister Matilda and the DC strove for a life in which they would be recognized for their service by God rather than by people. It is not surprising that Sister Matilda did not sign either the *Cradle of Mount Hope* journal or *Advices Concerning the Sick*.

At this time there is no definitive evidence that the document in the archives at St. Joseph's Provincial House titled *Advices Concerning the Sick* was in fact penned by Sister Matilda Coskery. One expert we consulted who also works for the United States government compared the handwriting of two letters signed by Sister Matilda[9] *(See Fig. 5–1 on page 171)* and the existing *Advices* document *(See Fig. 5–2 on page 171)*. He stated that in his opinion the two letters were clearly written by the same person but the *Advices* book had unexplainable differences. From the handwriting evidence the *Advices* document in hand would not have been penned by Sister Matilda. There is, however, sufficient evidence, such as the oral tradition among the sisters attributing the advice book to Sister Matilda, to lead us to believe that the manuscript was written by Sister Matilda at some point and that Community secretaries or DC close to Sister Matilda made additional copies of her journal and *Advices*.

Although the handwriting in *Cradle*, as in *Advices*, is not Sister Matilda's, the "voice" can be attributed to Sister Matilda. The author speaks in the first person, saying such things as "We tried to get her on the bed . . ."[10] Sister Matilda, or "Sister N" as she is referred to in the *Cradle*, used the pronoun "we," meaning the sisters, when discussing historical events even though she was telling the story from her own perspective. For example, she wrote that "we told her (a patient's) husband that there was no hope of her recovery."[11] She most certainly did not mean here that all the nurses talked with the husband. That would have been inappropriate care, let alone unnecessary. Sister Matilda's use of "we" was an example of her way of not drawing attention to self and avoiding self-promotion. From the context it is also clear that a number of the patient issues discussed, such as patient prognosis, would have had to be dealt with by the Sister Servant, who was Sister Matilda. The amanuensis for the journal apparently took dictation from Sister Matilda or her notes for some of the content and then added her own accounts as well.

As noted previously, *Advices* and *Cradle* may have been written originally by Sister Matilda and then hand copied by another sister or sisters, a common practice by communities of women in the nineteenth century, who typically shared recipes and helpful advice. There were sisters in the DC Community whose assignment was to copy Community records and documents for posterity. Evidence for the possibility of multiple copies of *Cradle* is suggested in the theses written by two DC

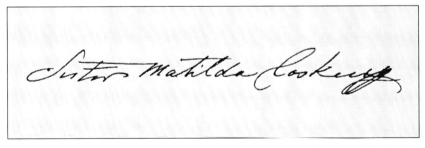

Fig. 5-1   *Signature of Sister Matilda Coskery*

in the mid-twentieth century, Sister Ambrose Byrne in 1950[12] and Sister Bernadette Armiger in 1947.[13] Both theses refer to the Mount Hope journal account by Sister Matilda. Sister Bernadette, in her history of the hospital work of the sisters cites, on page 54 of her thesis, Sister Matilda Coskery's "Account of the Beginning of Mt. Hope," "MS <u>Mount Hope Book</u>," held in the "Archives at Saint Joseph's Central House." This book is no longer in the Archives. On page 59 of her thesis, in footnote 29, Sister Bernadette references a document by Sister Thecla Murphy, which she titles "Notes drawn from Sister Matilda Coskery's <u>Account of the Beginning of Mt. Hope</u>," a manuscript in the Archives of The Seton Institute. Both were used to support content attributed to Sister Matilda that appears verbatim in the document presently held in the DC Archives at Emmitsburg. We distinguish the extant document from all other references to the journal by use of the title *Cradle of Mount Hope*. While the page numbers do not match and there are some references Sister Ambrose uses from "Mount Hope Book" that do not exist in *Cradle*,[14] the content in the *Cradle* document is identical to that which appears in the thesis.

Sister Thecla Murphy, identified in the theses as the copyist of some of the notes from Sister Matilda's journal, was a contemporary of Sister Matilda Coskery. Sister Thecla was born in 1809 and died ten years after Sister Matilda in 1880; she entered Emmitsburg in 1834 and was missioned to schools in Maryland, New York, Virginia, Pennsylvania, Massachusetts, and Delaware. She returned home in 1858 for her final mission at the Central House in Emmitsburg, where she lived in Community with Sister Matilda until Sister Matilda's death in 1870. Sister Thecla's notes on Sister Matilda's "Account of the Beginning of Mount Hope" that Sisters Ambrose and Bernadette used in their theses are not extant.

Sister Marie Louise Caulfield (1821-1905) was the First Secretary of the DC Community from 1844 to 1895, but there is no extant evidence suggesting that she took part in or knew about copies of the original manuscripts written by Sister Matilda. Sister Bernard Boyle (1803–1879), also a contemporary of Sister Matilda, shared the duties of Secretary in mid-1860. She fulfilled some of the duties of a historian for the Community, though she was not referred to as such. Sister Bernard ordered the documents that established a chronological history, referred to currently as the "Provincial Annals," for the Daughters from the earliest days under

Mother Seton until August of 1859. Sister Bernard entered the Community in 1820 before the death of Mother Seton. There is no record that she handled any of Sister Matilda's writings. Therefore, there is no definitive answer at this time as to who physically documented Sister Matilda's journal, but it is most probable, as some of the detailed excerpts of the journal presented in this book demonstrate, that the accounts are authored by Sister Matilda and others about her life as Sister Servant at Mount Hope.

Like Sister Bernadette, Sister Ambrose cites both the "Mount Hope Book" from the Archives at Saint Joseph's Central House and the Sister Thecla Murphy document. There is less evidence, however, surrounding the extant *Advices* document. Although she does discuss Sister Matilda and Mount Hope, Sister Bernadette does not refer to *Advices* in her thesis. She may not have known about *Advices* because the focus for her thesis was the Daughters' establishment of hospital institutions and not the specifics of the care provided. Sister Ambrose does not refer to *Advices* either. Her thesis, however, was on the history of The Seton Institute, the last name given to what was formerly Mount Hope. It seems very unlikely, had the Community secretaries known about *Advices*, that Sister Bernadette would have not included Sister Matilda's work in some way. It was only later, in 1989, that Sister Matilda's text was mentioned briefly in a publication about the American DC.[15] To date, the manuscript has not been shared with the wider nursing community.

The strongest evidence supporting Sister Matilda's authorship of the *Advices* text is the nature of the content and the record of Sister Matilda's contribution to DC nursing, especially of the insane. As will be described throughout this chapter, the author of *Advices* demonstrated a vast knowledge of nursing care and medical knowledge of the insane. Community records identify Sister Matilda as *the* expert in nursing and the care of the insane, as well as the author of *Advices*. Given our backgrounds in psychiatric nursing and social work, we wondered how anyone without extensive skill and experience in psychiatric nursing of the insane could have written an advice book with the level of detail displayed in *Advices*. It is our judgment that *Advices* was written by a Daughter of Charity; most probably, Sister Matilda Coskery.

To date, *Advices* has never been published. The Daughters' archival collection was organized into record groups and ordered, and finding aids were created beginning in 1979 under Sister Aloysia Dugan, the archivist, who previously had been the nursing educator at Saint Joseph College. Sister Aloysia recognized the inherent value of *Advices* but was also responsible for archival processing of the vast Seton collection and organizing the extensive SC/DC collection according to contemporary archival standards. The latter was the priority until the *Elizabeth Bayley Seton Collected Writings* (2000–2006) was published. Dr. Libster's first visit to the archives was in April 2002, and her work with the *Advices* book coincided with the completion of the Seton correspondence for publication. The decision to publish the book now was based upon two primary reasons, historical and clinical. First, there are patient-care situations, issues, and caregiving approaches that Sister Matilda addresses in her text that resonate with today's popular holistic- and integrative-care movements and the present demand for healthcare and hospital reform. The moral-treatment movement of the nineteenth century was one of the holistic, health-reform movements of that century. The call for healthcare reform and the humanization of healthcare in a fast-paced and changing technological world is not new to American culture. Hospital care, particularly of the insane, was reformed in antebellum America, and Sister Matilda and the DC Nurses were part of the solutions that emerged for that period. Sister Matilda's holistic approach to the care of the sick and insane as outlined in *Advices* may offer insight for present-day practice concerns and development of new models for institutionalized care.

Second, searches of the published literature in nursing have not produced any documentation of the textbooks used in the education of American nurses prior to the secularization movement in the later part of the nineteenth century after the Civil War. Present-day nursing texts, as will be discussed in the final chapter, do not include and often misrepresent the history of early professional nurses such as the DC. Sister Matilda's *Advices Concerning the Sick,* her journal, and the broader context of her nursing ministry provide American nurses an opportunity to read a history of early American nurses that suggests that the belief that professional nursing did not exist in America prior to the introduction of the Nightingale model is a myth. The perpetuation of this myth, which we will discuss further in the final chapter, has had a deep impact on American nursing identity and professional culture. This history of Sister

Matilda and the DC Nurses, especially as described in *Advices Concerning the Sick,* begins to fill a void in the understanding of America's history of *professional* nurses. The detailed actions and thoughts of Sister Matilda Coskery, nurse leader and educator of perhaps one of the most successful and certainly the largest nursing communities of the period in the United States, as are represented in *Advices,* provides considerable insight into the lived experience of the professional nurse of the mid-nineteenth century.

The "voice" of *Advices* is that of Sister Matilda, whose spiritual thoughts and intentions penetrated how she touched, spoke to, and attended patients. Though she cared for patients with many types of disease, her focus in *Advices* was clearly the *person* suffering from mental illness. Although cholera was the AIDS of Sister Matilda's time, she chose to include in her text two entire sections on what she knew best: the care of the patient with mania a potu (delirium tremens) and other types of insanity. She had developed an expertise in the care of patients with mental illness and also in the creation of healing environments in institutions that would support her caring mission.

Fig. 5-2   First Page of Handwritten *Advices Concerning the Sick*

Advices concerning the Sick.

1.

When a patient is brought to the house, place him according to sickness. If his condition would be disagreeable to others, put him by himself, or as far off in the ward as possible, without however letting him know why. If he is very sick or weak do not stop to question him about his sickness as the one at the door; the know his disease, and he may be questioned as to the treatment after he has rested. Then learn from him what has been done for him as to medicine, blistering, bleeding, dieting &c. Often the weakness of the Sick Poor is from hardship as to food, clothing or labor & exposure, so a little light broth &c be given to them soon after they come in. If he is faint-like give him a little wine, or toddy. Always keep a bed or two ready so that the poor sick may not be kept waiting. If he is able & needs a foot-wash, put a hand-full of common salt; or two table spoon of Mustard, or a pint of wood-ashes into a bucket of warm water, and only wash not bathe the feet before getting into bed, let them be dried well. If he has no clean linen, & needs one, loan him one, that his condition may be comfortable. If he is too weak to have the foot-wash, let him rest, and when he is more refreshed let his face, neck, hands, arms, feet & legs be wiped with whiskey, weak spirits of camphor or bay-rum. Whatever be his condition do not let him wait long for a drink if he is thirsty, but give him that, that suits his sickness. If he has fever & ague, he may have almost any thing, unless his bowels are too free, in this case, give him barley-water, rice water, toast-water, gum-water or water alone, and if he is not too feverish he may have pork

⁓ *Judicious Nurses Know the Curative Point* ⁓
(*Advices, Pages 1–7*)

Louise de Marillac, in the earliest days of the Community, prescribed a typical day for the DC Nurse. She based her recommendations upon the *Rules* being developed in a section called the "Order of the Day."[16] The order included such advice as what time to get out of bed in the morning (five-thirty) and the time for formal meditation (six o'clock). She also wrote specific guidelines for sisters missioned to a variety of locales. Appendix C contains a full account of the Order of the Day prescribed by Louise specifically for the DC working in hospitals. The sisters were to empty "night vessels" (i.e., bedpans) and make patients' beds when they arrived at the hospital at six in the morning. She instructed the nurses to have "a piece of bread and some wine" prior to going to the hospital in the morning except on days when they received Holy Communion. On these days, she wrote, "they shall content themselves with the scent of vinegar, putting some vinegar on their hands. This shall only be necessary until they become accustomed to the air in the rooms of the sick."[17] Although the guidelines were quite specific, she also suggested exceptions to the order, especially for those who were to care for the sick:

> Those who serve the sick keep a constant watch on their needs such as wood, linen, preserves, infusions[18] and other necessities[19] . . . A sister who cannot observe the Order of the Day as prescribed by Rule because of her work with the sick should unite herself to it in spirit from time to time.[20]

As demonstrated in this instruction to nurses about their Order of the Day, the early founders modeled flexibility as a way of being in religious community, which carried over into nursing service. The DC Nurses were encouraged to find ways to provide patient care without compromising their religious beliefs, obligations, their Community, and the spirit of the *Rules* that guided their lives. This flexibility in service appears also in Sister Matilda's *Advices*. The choice of the word "advices" was a softer approach, connoting a suggestion or consideration for the reader rather than implying that the instructions given were in some way an order, a requirement, or mandatory policy and procedure. Sister Matilda's *Advices* for nursing are exemplary of the wisdom gained through experience, a way of knowing that is often grounded in circumstance and context rather than in an ideal or dogma. She was a spiritual pragmatist who as Sister Servant of Mount Hope in Baltimore or St. Mary's House for Invalids in Detroit met all patients as they were when they appeared on the doorstep of the hospital or asylum, the sisters' house.

[Advices]   **[Pg 1] When a patient is brought to the house, place him according to sickness. If his condition would be disagreeable to others, put him by himself, or as far off in the ward as possible, without however letting him know why.**

This introduction suggests that *Advices* was written for the nurse in an institutional setting such as a hospital or asylum, which, as was mentioned previously, the sisters, their patients, and visitors often referred to as a "house." At the time Sister Matilda wrote this, the sisters were accepting both sick and insane patients. This caused some controversy with state asylum superintendents who thought that the mentally ill should be treated separately from those with physical illness. This is understandable in one respect because healthcare providers of the period were attempting to better understand the transmission of diseases such as cholera and typhoid fever.

The sisters often started their work at various locations in less than optimum conditions. Out of necessity, they may have learned through experience that some patients with physical or psychiatric illness actually improved in the presence of a patient with a different disease. Sister Matilda's *Advices* shows where she was in her scientific understanding of isolation and placement techniques. Regardless of the disease, each patient's suffering was the first issue to which Sister Matilda attended. Perhaps because of her tradition, she was particularly attuned to the immediate needs of the sick poor:

[Advices]   **If he is very sick or weak do not stop to question him about his sickness, as the one at the door [shd] know his**

> disease, & he may be questioned as to the treatment after
> he has rested. – Then learn from him what has been done
> for him as to medicine, blistering, bleeding, dieting, etc. –

Assessment is an important first step when admitting a patient. The patient assessment suggested by Sister Matilda in the mid-nineteenth century was similar to contemporary practice. The patient's previous history of treatment was critical information to obtain before implementing further treatment. All of the Mount Hope *Annual Reports* written by Dr. Stokes include the demographic data recorded by the nurses in the hospital "Register" that was part of their admission assessment. The data collected changed over time. The data that the sisters and Dr. Stokes collected represented what they believed was important for the record of the institution's work, particularly their treatment results. The table of information the nurses collected in the *First and Second Reports* included columns for date of admission, age, sex, civil condition (i.e., married or single), residence, occupation, date of discharge, and disease. The final two columns were labeled "results" and "remarks." Results could be "relieved," "cured," or "unimproved." Remarks were typically related to discharge status such as "discharged," "attended by another physician," "remains," "remains in house as an attendant," "left improved," or "died." The data on the insane patients was presented in a separate table from those with "general diseases," such as chronic catarrh, consumption (tuberculosis), fractures, and urinary tract "stricture."

Data collected on the insane patients was different.[21] The nurses recorded the admission date, age, marital status, and sex. They then recorded the "supposed cause" and whether the insanity was "recent" or "chronic" when the patient was admitted. The next columns were the "length of time in institution," presumably at Mount Hope; the "duration of disease"; "present condition"; and "remarks." Examples of patients that Sister Matilda, the Sister-Nurses, and Dr. Stokes cared for from 1840 to 1842 include:[22]

1. A seventeen-year-old female who for eight years had suffered moral insanity without mental delusion. She was cured after two years and seven months of treatment. The supposed cause of her problem was "indulgence in passion and pride."

2. A fifty-year-old male who had been chronically insane for four years and in treatment for two years and eleven months. He was not improved and was described as "morose, suspicious, paroxysms of dangerous violence, confined."

3. A fifty-year-old married female who was described as "melancholy, quiet, inoffensive" and improved after two years of treatment. She was admitted with a history of three years of chronic insanity related to "religious anxiety."

4. A thirty-four-year-old married male with recent intemperance and mania a potu who was cured in one week and discharged.

5. A thirty-eight-year-old married female who was recently insane, the cause listed as "puerperal." She was cured in two months and "removed by friends contrary to advice."[23]

In the *Second Report* the sisters and Dr. Stokes added a column of data called "apparent form." This is where they wrote the type of insanity that the patient was suffering, such as melancholia, senile insanity, dementia, mania, mania a potu, or monomania. They also included another column titled "prospect," where patients were deemed "favorable," "incurable," or "doubtful."

This admission data was used by Dr. Stokes for years as he defended the moral method of treatment employed at Mount Hope and the right of the DC to manage the asylum, with him as the physician consultant. Sister Matilda realized the importance of the admission assessment, but she demonstrated in the first paragraph of *Advices* that her nursing priority was to preserve the energy of the patient. She advised that the patient not be questioned if he was "very sick and weak." She then gave instruction for the interventions a nurse could consider to help raise the patients' energy level.

[*Advices*] **Often the weakness of the sick Poor, is from hardship as to food clothing or labor & exposure, so a little light broth shd be given to them soon after they come in.**

Giving broth, also called "bouillon," was a nursing tradition for the DC. Louise de Marillac had often "suggested" it for patients, the DC, and Vincent de Paul.[24] She included giving bouillon to the sick in her *Orders of the Day in the Hospital.* The nurses were to give bouillon or a fresh egg to the sickest patients in the hospital at seven o'clock in the morning.[25] On days when according to their religious beliefs the patients did not eat meat, Louise instructed the nurses to provide them two eggs and bouillon made with butter and egg whites with each meal.[26] Broth was viewed as an important treatment that strengthened the patient. It was made from meat, vegetables, and occasionally grain, such as barley. The nurses also used culinary and medicinal herbs in the preparation of their broths. The *Particular Rules* of the DC included the section title, "The Ordinary Diet to be Given to a Patient." The herbs that were considered best for a patient's broth were sorrel, lettuce, purslane, chicory, white beet, Chinese leaves or Chinese cabbage, and caraway. In winter, when herbs were not as available, the sisters used chicory, parsley root, and hulled barley.[27] Louise instructed the DC Nurses to remember that it was the "exactitude" by which she prepared the bouillon rather than "the quantity of meat" that made the bouillon "pleasing to patients."[28]

Prior to the later nineteenth century, nurses were considered experts in the prescription and preparation of "sick diet";[29] it was a vital part of women's domestic medicine skills. Because the DC were all women, they would have been skilled in sick diet including the preparation of broth; hence one possible reason that a recipe for broth is not included in the *Advices* text. One receipt book, *American Domestic Cookery* (1823),[30] belonged to Sister-Nurse Mary Felicitas Dellone (1799–1854), a contemporary of Sister Matilda and the elder sister of Sister-Nurse Rebecca Dellone, who worked with Sister Matilda in Detroit. The book is preserved at the Archives of the DC in Emmitsburg; it is a small manual, a size that could be carried in a sister's pocket. It includes a number of recipes for a variety of broths, including one for a clear broth made of beef, mutton, and veal that would "keep long" and one for a "nourishing veal broth"[31]; herbs such as thyme, onion, and parsley were used in the preparation of the broths. Sister Mary Felicitas may have shared these very recipes with her companions to be used in the preparation of sick diet for their patients.

Recipes for Healing ⌒

In the nineteenth century, recipe exchange was an important part of culture, particularly for women. Recipes, or "receipts" as they were often called at that time, were created for both culinary and medicinal purposes. A typical early and mid-nineteenth-century receipt book was recorded much like a diary or journal and used with the book cover opening from left to right. Culinary receipts were written from the beginning of the book. When documenting medicinal receipts, the owner turned the book upside down, opened the back cover, and recorded from right to left, thus differentiating the purpose of the recipe. Women often kept their more valuable recipes at the end of their receipt books.[32] Some ingredients, such as lemons, were used both in domestic and medicinal practices; as mentioned in Lydia Maria Child's *The Family Nurse*,[33] lemonade was taken as a refreshing drink in the summertime by those who were well and was also used in the care of those sick with fever. In both cases the purpose was to cool the body.

Knowledge of foods such as lemons and their growth and production patterns as recorded in receipt books provides the reader with clues to the history of the economy of the period. Receipt books documented local and acquired healing traditions, and they were also the record of the exchange of "intellectual property." Some recipes such as lemonade were so common that they might not even have been recorded. Child, however, did include a recipe for lemonade in her book under the heading "Food and Drink for Invalids." It is likely that the recommendation for using lemonade as a healing agent rather than the simple recipe for making lemonade was new information for the reader. Alternatively, recipes that were precious might be given only to those in a family, passing from generation to generation. Sister Matilda's *Advices* seems to have been treated as a book of special recipes because it was not shared outside of the Community.

Advices Concerning the Sick was a recipe book of sorts for the care of the sick poor and the insane. It is a historical record of Sister Matilda's knowledge, ingenuity, and beliefs. The influences on her work can be deciphered from her recipes for healing. Some of her *Advices*, such as the sections on mania a potu and insanity, required more detail than others and therefore were given more pages of descriptive instruction.

The knowledge of the care of the insane, including those suffering from alcoholism, was the key information that Sister Matilda offered her students. *Advices* was her intellectual property, based upon her clinical and ministerial experiences. Historian Janet Theophano writes that "the offering of a recipe book was a sign of affection, a tie binding together women of different generations."[34] Sister Matilda may have recorded the synthesis or essence of her nursing philosophy and practice in *Advices* as an inheritance for those who would follow her in the asylum ministry she helped to establish.

Although as Sister Servant she was the head of her "house," the hospital, Sister Matilda's *Advices* is different from many recipe books kept by the head of a household in the nineteenth century. First of all, she does not use the word "recipe," which comes from the Latin imperative "take" or "receive." Sister Matilda chose instead to write an "advice" book, a book that would counsel a member of her Community. Her counseling voice and the choice to write an "advice" book suggests a different relationship with her readers than if she had simply written a Community recipe book for nursing the sick and insane. Though it has some of the qualities of typical recipe books and popular advice books that included information on family nursing, the inclusion of medicinal receipts for the care of strangers, in particular the care of the insane, places the *Advices* text outside the realm of the common domestic receipt book and popular genre of American advice books. *Advices* was a professional textbook for the instruction and counsel of Daughters of Charity Nurses.

[*Advices*]   If he is faint-like, give him a little wine, or toddy.[35] Always keep a bed or two ready, so that the poor sick may not be kept waiting. If he is able & needs a foot wash,[36] put a handful of common salt, or two tablespoons of mustard, or a pint of wood-ashes, into a bucket of warm water, & only wash, not bathe, the feet before getting into bed, let them be dried well. If he has no clean linen, & needs one, loan him one, that his condition may be comfortable. If he is too weak to have the foot wash, let him rest, & when he is more refreshed, let his face, neck, hands, arms, feet & legs be wiped with whiskey, weak spirits of camphor[37] or bay rum.[38]

Whatever be his condition, do not let him wait long for a drink if he is thirsty, but give him that that suits his sickness.

There are numerous references in *Advices* to the beverages used in the care of the sick. The knowledge of what drinks to give, when to give them, and how much fluid to give a patient required that the DC Nurses have knowledge of anatomy, physiology, and pathophysiology. Fever was one of the most common illnesses treated by Sister Matilda and the nurses, but for nineteenth-century nurses it held a different meaning from today's definition of fever. Today's nurses define fever in terms of degrees of Celsius or Fahrenheit as measured with a thermometer placed in one of the body's orifices. Fever for Sister Matilda was a condition that emerged in many forms, each requiring a "general" as well as a "particular plan" of treatment. This is discussed further at the end of this chapter in the final section of *Advices* on fever.

Physicians in the 1840s and 1850s began to challenge the ability of nurses to prescribe beverages and sick diet for patients during acute conditions such as fever and during convalescence. As state medical societies formed to build professional momentum after losing licensure rights in the 1830s, American physicians, as their European colleagues had done since the 1700s, sought to gain control over nurses and midwives, who had been caring for patients autonomously in their communities for centuries.

Some physicians used their advice books to tout their own versions of what they considered the ideal nurse in the sickroom. One of the major issues they addressed was the errors nurses made in prescribing sick diet. Drs. Anthony Thomson and R. E. Griffith of Philadelphia called for the education of every "proper" sick nurse in a "public Hospital" to "certify her efficiency."[39] They wrote that any nurse trained in the manner they prescribed would not neglect cleanliness, ventilation, and temperature of the sickroom and would no longer present "obstinate and presumptuous opposition to the orders of the medical practitioner in reference to diet," which was so "prevalent."[40] The 1845 Thomson and Griffith book was a first American edition of a London edition written by Thomson, who was a Fellow of the Royal Academy of Physicians. The description of the "proper" nurse and the obstinacy to physicians, especially in regard to sick diet, was also published verbatim in an 1851 domestic medicine text by another Philadelphia physician named Francis Gurney Smith.[41] While some physicians may have viewed sick diet as their domain and expertise, Sister Matilda and Dr. Stokes demonstrated that sick diet was an important *interdisciplinary* concern because both physicians and nurses had made mistakes. Stokes wrote in 1852:

> No subject connected with the management of the insane has a more important bearing upon their restoration, comfort and general welfare that that of *diet*. In reference to this matter, very mistaken ideas have been entertained by medical men. The idea has too generally prevailed, that all the insane require is the mere nutrition of the body, and the satisfying the demands of the appetite, without regard being had to the quality, quantity, and preparation of the food. Hence, at no remote period from that we are not living in, the most flagrant injustice, inhumanity and privation have been practiced toward the insane. An ill-cooked, unwholesome and scanty diet has a pernicious tendency in various ways. Its effect is to impair vigor of the mind and body, and to induce a constant feeling of discomfort, uneasiness and fretfulness. On the contrary, food of good quality, well prepared and served up with the same care and particularity as for those of sane mind, exerts a salutary influence, and actually holds an important rank among remedial measures. By thus communicating pleasure and enjoyment with the act of partaking of food, we materially contribute to the restoration of mental quietude.... The Sisters always preside in person, and see that each one is properly provided for.[42]

Sister Matilda and the nurses made daily if not hourly prescriptions for the administration of sick diet, which included beverages. Advice about diet and nutrition remains a foundational part of nursing care. Many nursing-education programs require nutrition to be taught. Nutritional support skills are even more important in twenty-first-century American culture, where obesity in adults and children has reached epidemic levels. However, the nursing literature over the past ten to twenty years indicates that there is a decrease in nurses' nutrition knowledge at the baccalaureate, diploma, and graduate levels and at the same time an increased need for more clinical experience in the application of nutritional intervention skills.[43] In response, sickroom diet, now termed "nutritional assessment and intervention" is identified by some as an ethical responsibility of nurses.[44]

[Advices]   If he has fever & ague,[45] he may have almost anything, unless his bowels are too free, in this case, give him barley-water, rice-water, toast-water,[46] gum-water,[47] or water alone, and if he is not too feverish, he may have port [*Pg 2*] wine with a small piece of ice in it, but never much drink at a time, or the bowels become more free. If the bowels are in good state, he may have jelly-water,[48] lemonade, cream of tartar-water,[49] apple-water, or plain water.– Apple-water, or apple-tea, as it is called,[50] is made by slicing a few ripe apples thinly, pouring a pint of boiling water on them, and when cool, mix as much cold water with it as just leaves the pleasant taste.– If he seems in a sinking state, give him wine or brandy toddy, rub his temples with camphor[51] - put mustard plasters[52] on his ancles [*sic*] not the bones & wrists, & if there be pain of chest or bowels, put a plaster there also. If a patient has had bowel complaint for a long time, great care must be had to his food & drink. If allowed dry toast & tea, the tea shd be fresh & made palatable. – When he may have toast & tea, any of the following things are allowed too, & serve as a change for him, since all these watery things become distasteful to them when they are confined to them. They are as follows: thick rice, or barley water, seasoned with loaf sugar & milk – or arrow-root, sago, tapioca[53] – well cooked & seasoned as the others – Also thin pap,[54] which is made by boiling milk & water thickened with wheat flour, and, very well boiled, & with the sugar, & milk you may also add a few grains of salt for seasoning. When the

diet is of this kind, do not make too much at once, for it is
unpalatable if old; & the ſtomach sickens on it, which may
cause him to sink, as he is not allowed other food. If he is
very low & proſtrated, he may have a tableſpoonful about
every 15 or 20 minutes, but if not so low a teacup ful every
2 or 3 hours; or as beſt suits the ſtomach. . . . Tea shd be
made every few hours, or ſtand in an earthen vessel & kept
covered – given hot not warm. – [*Pg 3*] Toaſt sh [*should*] be
<u>browned</u> slowly, <u>not</u> burned, but prepared in a way to be
palatable. If they may have it, let it be what they <u>can</u> take,
or, as you wd [would] like it brought to yourself, to a sick
Parent, and, eſpecially as you shd prepare it for Jesus Chriſt,
who says: "What ye do to these ye do to me" – and: "<u>I</u> was
sick, hungry, thirſty, sad &c, and you consoled & miniſtered
to <u>me</u>."[55] When such kind of food is continued for some
time, you may give them a greater relish for it, by taking a
chicken bone, ſtrip the meat off it, and lay it on a <u>clean</u>, ~~gr~~
<u>hot</u> gridiron, till it schorches [*scorches*] or cooks, or if it had
been cooked til it gets hot – ſprinkle a few grains of fine salt
on it, & let him have it hot – At firſt he will be almoſt angry
that you wd bring him a bare bone, but after he has taſted
it, he will prefer the bare bone to all the other things he gets
– and the salty taſte of the juice gives him a better appetite
for the sloppy, watery things he is allowed[56] – Once or twice
a day he may have a bone if he wishes.– Sometimes a very
small thing ~~that~~ saves or deſtroys life.–

In fever, the face, hands, arms & feet shd be often wiped
with whiskey, bay- rum or weak ſpirits of camphor. If he
is in his senses & ſtrong enough to use a mouth-wash,
let it be by his bed, to rinse his mouth often with, and his
tongue may be scraped with a thin whale-bone to prevent
it from becoming coated. But if this is already so, & the
dark glue is around his teeth, it muſt be gently removed
by a soft mop, & the same for the tongue, as whalebone
cd [*could*] not be used on the sore tender tongue – neither
cd the brush then be used for the teeth in that condition.

> But, they must be cleaned little at a time, not at once. By
> keeping the mout[*h*] clean, there is less danger of the [*Pg
> 4*] disease spreading to others. In all contagious sickness,
> care shd be taken against receiving their breath into
> the lungs or stomach – This can easily be avoided, nor
> need the poor sick know it.– When there is tendency to
> contagion, let spirits of camphor be often sprinkled on his
> bed, dampen a towel with it also & leave it about his bed.

There was growing concern in the mid-nineteenth century among asylum superintendents that insane patients should be kept separate from those with general disease, especially those with contagious diseases. The DC and Dr. Stokes did not admit highly contagious patients such as cholera victims at Mount Hope; however, the sisters did admit medical patients with consumption and minor illnesses and injuries. Segregation of psychiatric and general medical patients was still an issue into the twentieth century. One factor in the decision for placement was the availability of resources; some cities with general and psychiatric hospitals may have been more inclined to argue for segregation to ensure the viability of both institutions. But psychiatric patients often had comorbid conditions. One twentieth-century study that ran from 1936 to 1983 showed that physical illness in psychiatric patients occurred at a rate of about 50 percent.[57] The argument of some physicians in the nineteenth century that the practice of general medicine and psychiatry be kept separate was accompanied by a motion in 1853 by some members of the Association of Asylum Superintendents to affiliate more closely with the American Medical Association, which had formed in 1847.[58] The motion was defeated.

Hospital and asylum admissions policies were not always determined by the mission and vision of the hospital administrators. Politics and economics were also part of the equation. Staff at a smaller private institution such as Mount Hope would have weighed the benefits and risks of declining to accept a patient simply because they had a medical disease. The DC at Mount Hope had *Rules* to guide them when making decisions, and they weighed any admission decisions against being able to sustain their hospital facility and mission. Sister Matilda's admission advice shows that she also carefully considered the health and safety of patients, was aware of infectious disease concerns, and knew the critical role nurses played in controlling disease, particularly by their attention to mouth care.

Sister Matilda advised the nurses to remove the excess tongue coating and glue around the teeth of the patient that formed during illness because its presence represented the potential for the spread of infection. She recommended the use of a brush or a whalebone for mouth care. The whalebone was stiff but still somewhat elastic and would have been a gentle way of scraping off the tongue fur.[59] Whale products were prevalent and popular because whaling was a large industry between the years of 1840 and 1860, considered the "Golden Age of Whaling" in America.[60] Sister Matilda also suggested the use of a "soft mop" for those with sore tongues.

Mouth care is still considered a standard in nursing care today. Just as Sister Matilda warned about the decreasing "danger" of disease with proper attention to mouth care, so too are American critical-care nurses concerned about documenting the effects of oral care in the intensive-care patient. One article on the state of the science published in 2004 stated that while the importance of oral care was noted in the literature, little research had been conducted on the various oral-care interventions used by nurses.[61] The authors identified two ways to remove "dental plaque and associated microbes: mechanical interventions such as tooth brushing and rinsing of the oral cavity and direct pharmacological intervention with antimicrobial agents."[62] While the study identified the oral cavity as a harbinger of organisms that can cause disease (in particular, pneumonia), it did not identify tongue brushing as an important deterrent. Tongue scraping is recognized in the current dentistry literature as a treatment for halitosis,[63] but scraping with a toothbrush was also shown to be more effective in reducing oral *Streptococcus mutans* than toothbrushing followed by a Listerine oral-care strip on the tongue or toothbrushing followed by an oral swish with a saline solution.[64] Twenty-first-century nursing research is validating what Sister Matilda taught in the nineteenth century before the discovery of antibiotics and the invention of plaque-removing toothpastes!

Nurses continue to prescribe the method of oral care for patients, a decision that has become more complicated by the presence of endotracheal tubes. Studies have shown that swabs do not remove plaque very well, especially in the intubated patient, and that toothbrushes are more effective. Nurses in their professional journals identify oral care as an important interdisciplinary issue in wellness and sick care[65] that can have physiological as well as psychological effects on and consequences for the patient's quality of life.[66]

[Advices] If he is allowed cold water, give it fresh & in a <u>clean</u> glass or cup. Not too full or in too large a cup, or he spills it. If he is allowed but little at a time, give him the right quantity only. If he is very weak & has constant thirst, it is handy for him to have his drink in a phial on his bed, as he prefers this to being served, especially as he can take it without fatiguing himself. When they cannot take much drink & the mouth is hot & dry, he may hold water in his mouth & then spit it in the basin.–

If ice, or cold cloths are ordered to the head, place a dry sheet about his neck, shoulders & pillow to prevent them from getting wet; or he may have lung disease by the time his fever is cured. Ice shd be in a bladder or silk-oil cloth bag,[67] which holds the water from running over him as it melts. If cold cloths are used, have two towels, fold them the size you want, & wring one out of the cold water dry enough to keep from dripping – spread it, or lay it in its folds over the forehead– and in 10 minutes or so - turn it over, laying the upper side next the head, presently changing it for the one that is in the basin, wringing it as the first one, but do not put the warm one in the basin in the fold, or it will soon make the water as warm as the head–but open it & fan it a little when it will be as cool as the water, & it need not be put in the water often, for this fanning makes it cold – keep changing the towels in turn till it is enough.[68] If he shudders from chilliness, stop the cold cloths immediately & [Pg 5] take the wet sheet from him, covering him up for the time, as this shivering is sometimes from some great change in his condition.–

If it shd continue long, give a little warm toddy, wine or
something to warm him, wipe the forehead dry as soon
as he shivers and rub camphor on the temples.– If the the
chilliness is only a few minutes & the head shd become hot
again, you may apply the cold again — The fanning of the
wet towels, often prevents the nurse from taking cold that
the dabbling so much in the ice water wd expose her to.–

One of the themes throughout *Advices* is that of caring for the caregiver.
Sister Matilda demonstrates concern for the nurse's health and well-being.
This is one way that she demonstrates her religious understanding of the
virtue of humility. Rather than inculcating in her writings a false sense
of humility that the nurse who serves God was somehow beyond human
and therefore impenetrable to illness, she acknowledged the humanity
and vulnerability of the nurse. This is an example of the grounded nature
of Sister Matilda's spirituality and ministry.

[Advices] The shivering, chilliness is apt to occur in Mania a Potu
cases, and must have prompt attention, and as often as it
comes on the same means of checking it must be used - and
when the heat returns, repeat the cloths. in some these
changes occur in 10 or 20 minutes of each other, give them
a teaspoon of brandy, or if they do not even occur so often
a table spoonful – however it may be, care must be had,
not to give too much brandy – you must judge of that. —

Giving a patient experiencing delirium tremens small amounts of
alcohol during detoxification as a sedative was part of care prior to the
creation of sedative drugs *(See Case Study 5–2 on page 210).* Sister Matilda
instructed nurses to exercise their judgment as to how much brandy to
administer when calming the patient. She demonstrated the same holistic,
thoughtful approach to implementing medical treatments recommended
by Louise de Marillac in the early days of the Community.

[Advices] Never let them sit up to have their sheets or linens changed
when they are very low or in a sweat[69] – But wait for

more ſtrength or till the Dr says it may be done safely –
Health & life is more than cleanliness[70] – At such times
avoid washing around his bed also.– A small thing near
the <u>crisis</u> of the patient, is very often the cause of death,
for being at its height, & on the point of changing for
better or worse, one little right matter neglecſed or one
little wrong thing done, takes from him his laſt chance
for recovery. This is what Drs call the curative point, and
moſtly reſts in the hands of the nurse & attendants. —

The term "curative point" is used in nineteenth-century medical
literature and often refers to a "point of view" in which the patient was
treated as if he would be cured, as opposed to given palliative care. The
way Sister Matilda used the phrase "curative point" in this context seems
a bit different, however. The term was not found in Dr. Stokes's *Annual
Reports*, but there is a section in the beginning of his *Reports* in which he
discussed the importance of the nurses' role at critical "points" during the
insane patient's convalescence. This has a similar tone to the notion of a
"curative point," which Sister Matilda mentions as resting in the hands of
the nurses and attendants. Stokes wrote in his *Sixth Annual Report*:

> It is at the period of convalescence, that the services of a
> judicious and skillful attendant are especially needed by
> the insane, in order rightly to lead the returning faculties
> into more healthy and rational channels. There is a certain
> dexterity and tact, which can alone be acquired by long
> familiarity with insanity in all its diversified shades and
> phases, and which enables their possessor to accomplish
> much good in controlling the morbid fancies of the
> patient, and in properly directing his thoughts, feelings,
> and affections. The judicious nurse and attendant will
> look with watchful eye for the earliest signs of recovery,
> and the moment the first glimmerings of right reason
> display themselves, will endeavor to promote the
> progress of improvement thus begun. . . . If neglected,
> they may pass away forever, and the patient speedily glide

into a darkness of mind of deeper gloom than before. Patients, therefore, at this critical period, require much delicate attention. . . . They are, at this time, particularly sensible to kind words, but easily disturbed by violent impressions or painful emotions; and it is now, when an indiscreet word, an unkind rebuke, may effectually retard recovery, that all the Physician's trust, and all his hope, rest on the judicious aid of a kind and gentle attendant. None can better appreciate than he the importance of the patient's having, at this critical moment, a nurse of intelligence and humanity. The happy manner in which the Sisters manage this interesting period, when the mind is beginning to release itself from the bondage of insane delusions, has been so often alluded to in former reports as to seem almost a useless repetition. Nevertheless as this is the distinguishing characteristic of the institution—the having the Sisters of Charity for nurses and attendants—a report of its system of management would be imperfect without a reference to the subject.[71]

The curative point was a turning point in the care of the insane patient and perhaps the patient with general disease as well. The nurses and attendants, who watched over their patients day and night, were in a particularly good position to observe for the curative point, the moment when the interventions would have their best effect. Stokes recognized that the sisters were particularly adept at identifying this moment and therefore were able to affect "cures" where other nurses, attendants, or superintendents might not, especially those who worked in larger asylums. The ability of assessing and intervening at the "curative point" was a major part of Dr. Stokes's explanation for the success at Mount Hope.

[*Advices*] **Avoid plaguing them with unnecessary attentions, these are hateful to God & man, but doubly so now, as life hangs on what is [*Pg 6*] what is [*sic*] right & proper; more, or less than this is injurious at this critical point.– The sick are weaker than we in body, but strong enough in mind, to see when we**

188

work for God, & when for Man. —

Others again who serve the sick, are so very neat, that the poor patient dare not turn in his bed, for fear of rumpling the bed clothes. —

Sister Matilda did not obsess over appearances in the sick room. She demonstrated in this entry her focus on patient comfort and what often was her more "home-like" rather than institutional focus to patient care.

[*Advices*] Do not raise a window or open a door too near them when sweating or in diseases that are increased by fresh air - & when smoothing the quilt do not fan or flirt it about their head, if sweating it checks it & if low takes the breath.[72]– If visitors see them in wet weather, do not permit them to loll, or reſt their wet arms on his bed. — If the illness has been long, it helps them to move to another room once or twice, ſtaying a week or two in each, but, shd they become house-sick for the room they had left, let them return to it, this indulgence will help them more then, than the ſtay there. Every reasonable gratification is an important means of recovery, because it excites to content of mind,[73] for the absence of which nothing supplies; and makes you more able to benefit soul & body.– Do not let them wait for their remedies, nourishment, drink or other comforts, for by this delay, besides the harm you may do the body, you irritate & discourage them — Where a disguſting dose is to be given, & the ſtomach is weak, you may put a <u>small</u> muſtard plaſter on the pit of the ſtomach 5 or 10 minutes before giving it, which will prevent their throwing it up again. Have something to give immediately after it, such as a bit of orange or its dried peel - apple - clove, allſpice &c— if salts is given, cold water, apple or lemonade is good – and salts may be mixed or dissolved in lemonade; and worked off with it or cold water - but all the other purgatives[74] require warm drinks to make them aćtive enough – but if there be Tendency to loose bowels, much drink shd not be given; and these ought to be one movement from the bowels before drink is taken, unless there be great thirst, then a [*Pg 7*] mouthful or two may occasionally be taken. or if the nature of the medicine does not prevent it, he may hold water in the mouth & then spit it out. When the convalescent take something for an action of the bowels only, he need not keep from drink or food unless he prefers it.– When medicine is too active it may be checked by a little port wine - or black coffe[*e*] without cream or sugar, & if it continues, give a few drops, 5 or 6 drops of laudanum occasionally – Or a mustard plaster over the bowels – if the sick is too weak for this, warm some whiskey, rum or brandy & dip a flannel several times folded & put it on as hot as he can bear it – have a second flannel to put on when the first cools.

The previous advices relate to the titration of remedies and the mitigation of known adverse effects to remedies. In contrast to the practice of medicine today, in which people seek a known outcome to drugs and treatments with supporting evidence from clinical trials whenever possible, mid-nineteenth-century nurses and physicians worked within a highly ambiguous climate regarding the treatments they were applying. In some ways that ambiguity forced the nurses to think critically before, during, and after administration of remedies and treatments and to make important choices about care related to treatments prescribed by physicians. The remedies they administered were meant not to disrupt the patient's energy level and were designed to help restore their mental, physical, and emotional balance.

Because each patient was viewed in the Vincentian-Louisian tradition as a unique person, individualizing care would have been particularly in keeping with the nurses' views. Dr. Stokes understood the level of ambiguity in patient care and, as quoted earlier, expected "intelligent, judicious" nurses to make decisions related to the treatments he prescribed. In the mid-nineteenth century and in the Vincentian-Louisian tradition, a nurse's work was not simply about administering treatments as ordered, no questions asked. The nurses and their patients implemented the treatments together, with the sisters managing the patients' responses to purgatives and plasters, foods and beverages, and the numerous cares provided each day during the patients' residency at the institution.

[*Advices*]   When they are weak from frequent sweatings, they may be sponged 2 or 3 times a day with warm spirits of camphor, but whilst sponging, keep the air from them by having them well covered at this time.

When pills are given have them of one size, or the smaller one will dissolve so long before the larger that no effect will be produced, and not allowing for this, stronger will be given which may do him harm; or be too much for him.

⌒ *Life and Death in the Hands of Nurses* ⌒
(Advices, Pages 7–16)

The importance of the DC Nurses' care was not only related to critical episodes in the lives of their patients, such as at the moment of the curative point; they also provided residential or custodial care for their patients. The ideal of moral therapy was that the patients create new lives within the asylum that they could then translate to life outside the asylum. They created new habits and thought patterns by interacting with the nurses throughout the day. They were also under the care of the sisters at night. The Daughters did not leave their night duties to paid attendants. They created a system of night watch, which Dr. Stokes described in one of his later reports:

> For many years we have had here a well organized system of night watch. It is composed of the Sisters themselves, and it is customary for them to go two together, making, at short periods, regular rounds through all the halls and through different parts of the building, all the night through. Thus we secured a watchful oversight over our patients at night, so that, should any one be taken suddenly ill, they can receive immediate care and atten-

tion; or, should anyone require medicine and nourishing drinks at regular periods, they continue under constant surveillance, and the treatment is carried on through the night with the same uniformity and regularity as during the day. The advantage and importance of this organized system during the silent watches of the night can be readily recognized and appreciated.[75]

Dr. Stokes and the Daughters worked closely together to establish systems of care. The DC Nurses' system of moral treatment encompassed engaging the patient physically and mentally during social interaction over meals and activities such as sewing parties and walking on the grounds. Nursing also included administering medical therapies, which they considered just as important to affecting a cure in some cases as the moral interventions. The treatments that were considered "medical" are discussed by Sister Matilda in the following sections. The nurse's role in medical treatments, according to Sister Matilda, was implementing the treatments ordered and monitoring and evaluating their effects.

Emetics ⌣

[*Advices*] When an emetic is given have two large basins, a bench or chair to put one on by the bed-side - place a chair, with the back against the bench for the sick to rest his hands or head on whilst vomiting. If he has no handkf [*handkerchief*], hand him a clean towel to wipe his mouth & face with. As soon as he has had one little vomiting or Severe gagging, give him a big drink of <u>warm</u> water, say about a pint & swallowed in big mouth-fuls, as this makes him vomit more easily & may prevent cramps. After each vomiting spell give <u>warm</u> water – if they do not seem easy to vomit you may make the water saltish with table-salt or put a little mustard in it. After he has puked 4 or 5 times freely, give no more water, let him rest if he can, but if the gagging continues put a small mustard plaster over [*Pg 8*] the pit of the stomach and give a few mouth fuls of strong black coffee, that is coffee without cream.– Two or three hours after, he may take a little light nourishment if he wishes.– As thirst usually follows vomiting, he shd not take right cold drinks even the same day unless the Dr allows it – he may have toast-water that has the cold air off a little at a time.

In the mid-nineteenth century, disease was thought to be the result of excess or deficiency of a "single biological property called excitability, the capacity to react to external stimuli."[76] Emetics, substances used to induce vomiting, were a common depletive remedy prescribed by physicians with the belief that they would purge the stomach of excess heat. Emetics, as well as other heroic treatments such as bloodletting, which were used by regular physicians were also commonly used in self-care, domestic medicine practices,[77] and in nursing care. Although there are records of the French DC and the early American sisters performing bloodletting, Sister Matilda does not mention it in *Advices* per se. She does refer to "wet cupping," which is a form of bloodletting. *(See cupping section on page 223.)* The nurses may have not performed bloodletting because they had consulting physicians who performed the task. They may also have not done bloodletting because it was believed by some asylum superintendents to be ineffective, providing only temporary relief of symptoms and at times even causing injury. Renowned physician Dr. Samuel B. Woodward of the State Lunatic Asylum in Worcester, Massachusetts, wrote in 1845 that general bleeding should not be used

> when blood-letting has been employed freely and frequently in active mania, the only form of insanity in which it is commonly used to excess, if the excitement, for a short period, an hour or two, and sometimes a day or two, abates, it is generally renewed with increased violence, and under circumstances far less favorable for the benefit of other remedies. The indications for active depletion are usually the *effect* and not the *cause* of excitement. . . . The effect of great loss of blood is often to produce pain in the head, a sense of stricture, as if a fillet were tied around it tightly, ringing in the ears, and noises

in the head which lead to false perceptions of sound and
illusions liable to result in permanent insanity.[78]

Woodward stated that he did not use emetics because they did not
relieve insanity.[79] The DC Nurses at the time of Matilda's writing of
Advices did apply emetics. Sister Matilda does not state here which
emetic the sisters were to use, but common emetics during the period
included tartarized antimony and also plant-based preparations of ipecac
(*Ipecacuanha hippo*), bloodroot (*Sanguinaria canadensis*), black cohosh
(*Actea racemosa*), and cayenne pepper (*Capsicum frutescens*), which was
popularly referred to as "pepper pukes." Woodward considered tartar
emetic "less safe" than the others.[80] Chamomile tea, one cup every few
minutes, was thought to "assist" other emetics.[81] Emetics were typically
given until they "operated"; i.e., the patient vomited.

Blistering ⌇

Topical applications such as cool compresses to the head were standard
sickroom care in the mid-nineteenth-century home, but blistering a patient
was not. It was an intervention that was typically reserved as "medical
treatment," to be employed by physicians and experienced nurses.[82] Dr.
Amariah Brigham wrote in 1847 that he tried blisters to the back of
the neck, but he "rarely witnessed any benefit from them, unless they
sometimes serve to direct the attention of the patient from his imaginary
sufferings and delusions."[83] Sister Matilda and the DC Nurses used blisters
as an "annoyance to engage the patient's attention and prevent their mind
from preying on itself."[84] Dr. Woodward occasionally used "insanity
blisters" for patients with melancholy and acute dementia.

Blisters were made by a physician or nurse by applying a substance
on the skin of the patient that caused irritation, discomfort, and then a
fluid-filled lesion. Sister Matilda described using "fly plaster," an ointment
rather than a plaster, as will be described in a subsequent section. The
wings of the Spanish fly, a green beetle also known as cantharides, were
ground up into a powder and placed on the skin to raise a blister. Even
used externally, cantharides can be very irritating to tissues and internal
organs.

Careful nursing was required to manage blistering treatment. One of the most common sequelae of blistering was strangury, or slow, painful urination. The size and placement of the blister was prescribed by the physician. The nurse placed the cantharides and after a period of time opened the blister and allowed it to drain. Salves were applied to the skin, with the purpose of continuing various levels of irritation, as is described below by Sister Matilda. When the blistering was to be discontinued, a healing salve was applied. Blistering treatment began to fall out of favor in the mid-1840s and 1850s,[85] which also suggests that Sister Matilda may have written *Advices*, or at least this part of the text, prior to the 1850s.

[Advices]   When a fly plaster is ordered, put it <u>on the place</u>, & <u>at the time</u> ordered for it. Have all things ready by the bed-side before his clothes are opened. If the Blister plaster is large & the weather very cold, warm it some before applying it. fix it comfortably tight to prevent its slipping about. If the plaster is for the abdomen, side or back, sprinkle a little powdered opium over it, or dampen it with laudanum[86] to prevent strangury. If this occurs, give him a tea-spoonful of sweet spirits of nitre[87] in a cup of warm flax seed tea,[88] or water once in 2 or 3 hours if continues so long.– When it has drawn enough, have all the dressings ready before openin[g] his blister. with sharp pointed scissors cut off the blistered skin – do not tear it off - warm the salve rag or the coldness of it on so hot a sore may cause congestion. twice a day will do for salve dressing. If it is to be kept running, let the morning dressing be of the drawing kind & the milder for the evening. or if it must have sharp salve every time, let the last or evening dressing be early enough to have the smarting gone before sleeping time. — When they take a distressing tormenting burning, they may be soothed by mopping them with a mixture of lime water & mild oil of equal parts–shaken well together to form a kind of cream. Never let the dregs or lumps of lime be [*Pg 9*] in the water. After this has quited it, the dressings may be

> put on again.– When cabbage leaves are the dressings, take
> the tender, small green ones. pare the coarse stems out of
> them, scald or crimp them on red hot coals & then squeeze
> them in a towel in yr. [*your*] hand, keeping them warm
> until the place is ready for them. they shd be laid on about
> 4 or 6 thick, or they will dry too soon, be very painful &
> do no good; & 3 times this dressing shd be made daily.—

Cabbage leaves (*Brassica oleracea*) were "highly praised" in the nineteenth century as a topical remedy for "indolent and fetid" ulcers.[89] See chapter 2 for an account of cabbage use by Sister Bridget (Ma Farrell) in dressing blisters. They relieve inflammation and therefore have also been used successfully on internal mucosa as a folk remedy for stomach ulcers. The anti-inflammatory action of the cabbage leaves is probably due to its sulfur compounds.

Crisippus, an ancient physician, wrote a whole volume on the virtues of cabbage applied to all parts of the body.[90] Nurses continue to use cabbage leaves today in the treatment of women with postpartum breast engorgement. Nurse Dr. Kathryn Roberts published research in the 1990s on the effects of chilled green cabbage leaves on breast engorgement. She found that cabbage leaves and cool gel paks were equally effective in relieving breast engorgement but that mothers preferred the cabbage leaves.[91] Lactation nurse-herbalist Sheila Humphrey suggests that the shape of cabbage leaves makes them ideal for their use in breast pain and swelling related to engorgement.[92]

Mustard, the plant used in the next remedy described by Sister Matilda, is in the same Brassicaceae plant family as cabbage. A plaster is an herbal topical application in which a paste, typically made from powdered plant material, is applied to a piece of cloth (linen or muslin) or leather and then is affixed to the skin for a period of time.[93] In traditional herbalism, mustard plasters are said to work by increasing circulation on the surface of the body, thereby relieving congestion of the organs and tissues below.[94] They are still used today by nurses in Russia, for example, but are used with caution.[95] Mustard should create redness, a counterirritant effect, but not blistering of the skin. Historically, mustard plasters typically have been used in the treatment of lung congestion and joint pain. They were also used on the abdomen following doses of an emetic to control the continued operation or action of the emetic.

Mustard Plasters ⌒

[*Advices*] Mix the mustard with <u>hot</u> <u>water</u> by the sick bed, as the hotter they are applied the quicker relief they give. For the instep, ancle [*sic*] or wrist one teaspoonful of the dry mustard flour is enough, but for the chest, abdomen or side a tablespoonful – let the paste, be thick so as not to run & wet the clothes, or have a large wet rag over the sick – have an old thin muslin or gauze rag to lay over the mustard to keep it from sticking to the skin, for when they make sores, they are hard to heal.– the time for leaving them on must be as circumstances call for.[96] Some can only bear them a few minutes, & if relief is soon given they may be removed – 15 or 20 minutes if they are not too painful, is not too long. for a tender, delicate skin this cd be too long if they burned much– A child cd not bear it long, & for a child a little corn-meal had better be mixed with the mustard-flour.– Never put them on the bony part of the ancle, [*sic*] that is the ancle [*sic*] bone or shin bone, but on the side of the ancle, [*sic*] on calf of the leg, or the instep.– When a mustard <u>poultice</u>[97] is ordered, make a stiff corn meal mush, & after it is spread 2 inches thick [*Pg 10*] on a rag, sprinkle mustard freely over it, if the pain be very great. but, if not, do not put on so much - but have the thin gauze over this. If mustard is not ordered, but only the hot mush, spread a little soft grease over the mush. A weak patient cd not bear so heavy a poultice – and as it must be thinner it must also be changed more frequently, as it cools quicker than a thick one.– Always make enough for 2 - so that one may be kept warm while one is on, & when warm poultices ar[e] needed, cold ones do harm – have a big dry cloth spread over the poultice to keep the clothes & bed-clothes dry & clean – When they are very important know whether they are to be kept on during the

night – if not, or at any time you are to leave them off, have
a large, folded flannel warmed, & lay it where the poultice
had been.– When poultices might serve, but the sick are
very weak & sick, it does well to warm whiskey, rum, ſpirits
of camphor or other such ſpirits, & apply it on a hot flannel
folded several times – keeping a warm one on all the time.

Try to prevent bed-sores,[98] for <u>no one is able</u> to tell the
violent, excruciating pain they cause, & when once formed
can hardly be cured.– When a delirious patient, after being
long in bed shows more reſtlessness, examine the back –
rather it shd be examined sooner & all means used to
prevent them.—

Teas, Tonics &c. ⌒

[*Advices*] Make them ſtrong, & in a clean vessel, have the water
boiling – keep them covered while boiling or ſteaming.
When done, ſtrain & cover it. In warm weather do not
make too much at a time, & keep it in a cool place. Nurses
are often careless in these things, thinking they are only
simple matters, thus, they prepare them negligently, [*Pg
11*] & are irregular in giving them – or give them after they
are sour & mouldy, and this makes the ſtomach sick, or
getting them irregular does no good. The Dr thinks it is
the fault of the tonic & changes it for something ſtronger,
perhaps, brandy or some other thing that does real harm–
He loses confidence in that tonic, names it to his ſtudents
and Medical friends, who likewise discontinue it, & in all
these cases that fall into their hands, some ſtronger thing is
given, when the thing itself was right, <u>in right hands</u>. How
often, these, <u>seemingly</u> small things, are the beginnings
of the death-bed & in many, many cases, Life & Death is
[*in*] the hands of the nurses, more than in the Physicians.

Sister Matilda refers here to the various herb teas that had been a
signature of the care of the nurses of the Vincentian-Louisian tradition

since its inception.[99] The role of prescribing, preparing, and administering teas, called tisanes or infusions in the French Daughters' history, fell to the Nurse-Infirmarian and Assistant Infirmarian.[100] She expanded upon Mother Mary Xavier's instructions about tisanes: "I have seen 'tisanes' and other drinks so thick, that it was a real task to take such, especially for a weak stomach."[101] But Sister Matilda adds a new twist on the importance of proper tea preparation that makes this section of *Advices* unique.

Sister Matilda offers an important realization of the impact of nurses' simple interventions precisely applied to development of medical treatment, as well as patient outcomes. She has observed that nurses' negligence in simple matters such as tea preparation are what led to the overtreatment of patients by physicians that Louise de Marillac warned against in her writings. Nurses, according to Sister Matilda, had to claim some responsibility for the phenomenon and in some cases patient death. She even goes one step further, stating that nurses may have an even bigger impact on patient outcomes than physicians. The example of tea preparation was a very poignant one for nurses of that period because it was a common task performed many times a day. Sister Matilda demonstrates her teaching style here in her role as a Community leader. Rather than telling the nurses about the heritage of tea making or commanding the nurses to make teas properly following a written mandate, Sister Matilda uses the tea-making example to drive home her point. She traces the result of choices while at the same time inspiring her readers as to the importance of their position as administrators of "simple" remedies.

Foot-Baths ⌒

[*Advices*] For a common foot-bath take hot, or right warm water, put into it one table spoonful of mustard, or a handful of coarse salt, or a pint of wood-ashes. Have it ready before the sick gets out of bed. Have cold water near, in case he says it is too hot, but, in pouring it in do not splash it on his feet. Let him sit comfortably, a blanket around his shoulders & something over his lap to keep him warm. 150 [*15*] or 20 minutes is long enough – have two towels to wipe them, either wipe both at once, or have one in the

> water while the first is getting dried – do this as quickly
> as possible & do not let him step on the floor, but get
> immediately into bed. If he becomes sick or faint-like,
> take him out of the water at once. Never let him take it if
> he be sweating, for, sweating is what you wish to gain by
> the bath, [Pg 12] and by rising at that time it is checked; &
> gives new cold, perhaps congestion.– A purgative medicine
> and a foot-bath ought not be given in the same night.

Footbaths are part of an ancient healing tradition called ablution or spiritual cleansing. They are known as *Wudu* or partial ablution in the Muslim faith and *Misogi* in the Shinto purification ritual. In the Christian tradition, foot washing was demonstrated by Jesus.[102] Jesus's act has been interpreted by some theological scholars as a lesson in humility and by others as a teaching that "service is the only guarantee of eternal life."[103] Still others have interpreted the ritual of the washing of the disciples' feet as a preparation for sharing in Jesus's death on the cross.

Sister Matilda, however, makes no religious reference here. She simply speaks to the physiological effects of the foot washing and the nursing management thereof. Louise de Marillac also did not reference Jesus's example[104] when she asked the Daughters, in particular the Sister Servant of the hospital, to wash each patient's feet upon admission. It is most probable that the sisters' absorption in religious life and familiarity with that the feet should be "washed" on admission, not "bathed." When the patient was admitted, the nurses were to "wash" the feet to prepare them for getting into bed. The footbath described above was the hydrotherapeutic intervention recommended by physicians and nurses.

The pores of the feet are the largest in the integument of the body, thereby providing a vehicle for the administration of the medicinal benefits of herbs. The pores of the feet take 15 to 20 minutes to open in a warm bath, as Sister Matilda indicated. She recommended adding mustard to the footbath as a common remedy for the sick and the insane. Dr. Woodward recommended mustard footbaths for those suffering from melancholy.[105] Dr. Brigham used warm footbaths for "cerebral excitement."[106] Lydia Maria Child recommended "dipping" the feet in cold water as soon as a person got out of bed in the morning, all year long, for complaints of cold feet or tendency of blood to go to the head.[107] The feet were to be dipped, removed immediately, and then rubbed vigorously with a coarse cloth or brush until they were "glowing." Thomas Jefferson attributed the fact that he had been free from catarrhs of the breast for eight to ten years and no fever for more than twenty-four hours except two to three times in his life to the practice of bathing his feet "in cold water every morning, for sixty years."[108]

There are many types of footbaths. The purpose of the footbath described by Sister Matilda was to produce sweating. Sweating the whole body, also referred to as "steaming," was an important therapy in nineteenth-century medicine and self-care practices, particularly among those who adhered to the philosophies of Thomsonian botanical medicine. Steaming had been considered health promoting in Roman and Greek times. Opening the pores with herbs and raising the body temperature in the sweat lodge is a healing ritual also practiced by First Nation people in North America. By performing footbaths, the DC Nurses contributed to the continuance of a healing tradition shared by many within and outside the Catholic faith and Christianity. Sister Matilda advised, however, that purgative medicine not be given on the same night as a footbath, demonstrating her understanding of the potential energetic interaction of remedies and therapeutics. Contemporary holistic nursing practice draws attention to the need for assessing the appropriate application of even some of the seemingly most simple complementary therapies in the care of patients.[109]

Injections[110] ⌣

[Advices] When only an action from the bowels is desired, warm water alone will do, or warm soap suds is better. A common injection for strong persons in slight sickness is: about a pint of warm water with one tablespoonful of table salt, the same quantity of molasses & lard. When a stronger one is necessary epsome [Epsom] salts may be used instead of table salt or castor oil instead of lard. let the salt be entirely melted. rinse the pipe with hot water, or its coldness will cool the mixture too much. Just before filling the pipe with

201

the mixture, draw the handle suddenly in & out of the pipe a few times to get all the air out of the tube. Then, put the small end into the mixture, holding it under the surface so as that the air cannot get into it. let the pipe fill, or as much as you need, by drawing the handle steadily & slowly. when you take it out, keep the finger on the small end of the tube until the patient is ready to help themselves – but if they are too weak for this, they must be previously fixed for it by having the hips raised by a pillow or something. If the hips are not raised the mixture will return when the pipe is withdrawn. When the pipe is placed, inject the mixture steadily & when the bowel has received it keep the pipe perfectly still for a minute or two, or if you take it suddenly away the contents follow it. Very soon the patient wishes to rise because the bowels seem disposed to act, but this feeling is only from the mix- [Pg 13] ture, and they must force themselves to wait half an hour or so, if possible, or, only the injection will pass & then it must be repeated, whereas by waiting a more natural action will be gained.– but if no good is derived, it must be repeated in about 2 hours – often the 2nd one is more successful.

When particular injections are required the Dr names the things that is to compose it, as in bad bowel complaint, starch & laudanum are used, and in some cases any injection wd be given after each movement of the bowels – You shd know from the Dr whether they shd be given cold or warm.

Opiates ⌒

[Advices] Usually in about half an hour after an opiate has been given, it shd compose or dispose to sleep. But if there be loud talking or other noise around him, the opiate cannot act favorably, & on the contrary, does harm & after a certain time, will not act however quiet things may be. care shd be taken therefore, to prevent their being disturbed at this time.

Opiates were considered a useful and successful medical adjuvant to moral therapy in the care of the insane. They were not used indiscriminately, however. Dr. Brigham warned that opiates were injurious in the patient with hot, dry skin and a "full hard pulse."[111] On page 21 of *Advices*, Sister Matilda provides insight into the nurse's role in the administration of opiates.

Cleanliness ⌒

The following section provides a picture of the sickroom in which the Daughters nursed their general medical patients. At Mount Hope many of the patients were ambulatory, and therefore the care provided was different. This section reminds us that the mid-nineteenth-century Daughters of Charity provided nursing care to patients who were often taking emetics, laxatives, and purgatives—without the benefits of modern plumbing. The DC Nurses had to be quite adept at handling body fluids safely.

[Advices] Keep the drinks that ſtand by their beds covered from duſt & flies – do not have it in heavy mugs, or so full that they ſpill it in taking it. wipe away slops & ſpills off the table or other things that serve to collect flies. do not let poultice or sore rags lay about or soiled clothes – empty the ſpit cup or basin frequently and return it quickly & clean. The chamber vessel should *[Pg 14]* [be] removed after each action from the bowels, unless the Dr is to examine it, in this case, have two vessels, setting one aside till the Dr sees it, & leaving the other by the bed. – When the bowels are too free, or if purgative medicine has been given, have two vessels with lids for their use. – In like manner, two basins when an emetic is given. – If mud or dirt is on the floor around the bed, do not have much of the floor wet at a time, & none at all if there be danger, or unless the Dr says it can be done without danger. Never let a love for cleanliness expose yr. poor patient, & thus endanger also, yr. conscience, for in some sicknesses a little damp air might

cause relapse & death.– There shd be changes of clothing
kept in the house for such as come in, in soiled clothes
and have no change, pay great attention to all clothing
sheets & bedding being perfectly dry before using them.

General Remarks ⌢

[*Advices*] Do not use any kind of metal spoons in medicine or sour
drink, but pewter or silver. if these cannot be had brittania[112]
[*sic*] is next best – neither let ~~such stand in this~~ medicine
or sour drinks or eatable stand in tin or metal cups. When
one is very weak, & wishes to wet his mouth often, he may
be relieved by leaving the drink in a phial on his bed. this
he can get without fatigue & he prefers this to being waited
on—

It is always in our power to render them many little
services by small attentions & little by little they help
towards recovery, and the charity that accompanies
[*Pg 15*] them does much for their content of mind.

This section on the type of metal to be used demonstrates the level of
detail that Sister Matilda paid to the creation of a healing environment for
her patients.

[*Advices*] In Summer, have large pieces of coarse bobinet lace or
cat-gut propped on a frame or sticks over their head &
shoulders & so as that their arms & hands will also be kept
from the flies – then they can use their hands inside of it –
even when they are not sleepy, they cannot rest, & fatigue
themselves by driving the flies off themselves. – There shd
be several of these for every ward, so that one might be
washed after a consumpted or fever patient, before giving
it to another. If you are ready to put their room in order,
but find the patient sleeping or nearly so, wait for awhile,
especially if they stand in need of sleep from having had but
little his rest will do him more good than a clean room or

all your other care might do: this is what we would do for a
sick friend or Parent, do not let the visit of friends cause him
to be awakened, if he has suffered for sleep, let friends wait;
when they are weak, all means for gaining ſtrength muſt be
afforded them, and in nervous complaints, it is so necessary
that they would die from this matter being neglecſted.

Let every phial or box of medicine have its name on it
and the quantity to be given, or serious miſtakes will be
the consequence: do not let dangerous medicines ſtand
about ~~unlockehed~~ unlocked, such as laudanum or others.

Not unlike nurses who work on busy hospital units today, Sister
Matilda took the responsibility for assuring that medicines, particularly
those that were addicting such as laudanum were controlled to protect
patients and staff.

[*Advices*] As the recovery and life itself often depends on the
suſtaining effecſts of nourishments and drinks the greateſt
care muſt be taken in these things, they muſt always
be properly and plateably [*sic*] prepared or their weak
ſtomachs not being able to keep or take them, they will
sink in ſpite of all the Dr can do; and when you see them
so proſtrate, it will probably, and moſt likely, be too late
to raise them or get back the ſtrength and little appetite
they had. What a misfortune to answer [*Pg 16*] answer
[*sic*] for!!. These things, if they had been prepared with St.
Vincent's ſpirit, that, is for his Jesus, such as the poor sick
could have taken, how much better the fruits would be for
them and the negligent nurses! let true pracſtical charity
season every thing they require, otherwise we are guilty of
injuſtice by with-holding from them their means of cure.

Charity as described here is practical, and yet it comes with deep
spiritual motive, to infuse their patient interventions with the spirit of St.
Vincent and St. Louise consumed with love for Jesus, whom he saw in the
sick poor.

[Advices] When spirits of camphor is used for sponging the skin, the diluted will do, that is, the gum camphor is dissolved in whiskey, some brandy, rum &c.–

When spirits of camphor is used inwardly, the gum is disolved [sic] in good Alcohol as long as it will disolve in it, and when the gum remains undissolved, it is strong enough. When a sudden distress finds you unprepared for the occasion, let this event & its anxiety teach you to be prepared for all things as much as possible; for instance, to be without adhesive plasters, bandages, lint, cups, injecting pipes, mustard, the medicines in common use, &c. &c. makes too much delay in urgent cases that would call for these.

Experience teaches in time, but too many are sacrificed by this method of teaching. A low tone of voice, with cheerful, kind manners must be strictly observed & practised [sic] by those who wait on the sick.

Sister Matilda may be providing a rationale for the writing of her *Advices*, that the process of learning through experience takes too long, and patients may suffer or die. The teacher provides the means for moving more quickly through the lessons of becoming a nurse. Sister Matilda followed this with the first lesson, the importance of communication and kind manners. She clearly did not ascribe to a trial-and-error method of learning. Sister Matilda provided formal vocational education through direct contact with students and indirectly through her writings.

⌒ *"Simple" Advice, Titration, and Regulation* ⌒
(*Advices, Pages 16–27*)

By agreeing to treat patients experiencing one of the greatest social ailments of the nineteenth century, intoxication and mania a potu, Sister Matilda, her DC Nurse companions, and Dr. Stokes placed themselves and their institution right in the center of some controversy among asylum superintendents. In the 1840s, mania a potu was classified as insanity, but some physicians questioned the practice. As with most types of insanity, it was thought that mania a potu was instigated by a person's lack of self-control and rational thought, hence its curability. In April 1845 the Association of Asylum Superintendents had British Reverend John Barlow's lecture, "On Man's Power over Himself to Prevent and Control Insanity," published in their journal.[113] Barlow spoke about the structure and function of the brain and the nerves. He then suggested that man had the ability to rise above the "vital power" of his animal nature by redirecting his "intellectual power," thus presenting an opportunity for preventing or curing "mental derangement," the term he preferred to insanity.[114] With the effect of the temperance movement of the early nineteenth century, excessive drinking was thought to be "bad" social behavior. Those who suffered from the disease were often judged by others. Nevertheless, the DC decided to treat those patients deemed morally and socially inferior because they could not control their desire for alcohol.

Statistical medicine was becoming very popular in the mid-nineteenth century. Dr. Stokes and the sisters reported data of their successful treatment of mania a potu in their annual reports. By 1849, Amariah Brigham, in his litany of concerns about Mount Hope, suggested that Dr. Stokes was "puffing"[115] the data of his successful cures of insane patients in his annual reports. Brigham had been raising the same concern with other institutions since 1846, and ultimately, Brigham and others established that "curable" forms of acute insanity such as mania a potu were not to be included in the statistical reports on other diseases. Although Stokes knew that Mount Hope was successful in its treatment of patients, he decided, after Brigham's accusations, to report the treatment-outcomes data for mania a potu separately. Dr. Brigham also criticized the DC for the impropriety of treating the insane and people afflicted with other diseases in the same building. He condemned them for exposing their milder chronically insane and quiet, physically ill patients to "so many drunkards" who were "noisy and violent" and stated that "no one with proper feelings of humanity"[116] would "attempt to justify" the action. Sister Matilda often saw the humanity in partnering unlikely patients together, as described in the account of the young patient with spinal disease who became the roommate of a forty-year-old woman with extreme melancholy *(See Case Study 5–1)*.

CASE STUDY 5-1 **Partnering Patients**

Patient Account at Mount Hope as Recorded by Sister Matilda

A young lady was admitted for spinal disease. She was beautiful, full of life & love of the world, tho' not able to stand straight, and only able to move around the room in a doubled up form; hopping about the house from chair to chair. She was extremely passionate and profane in speech and manner. No religion, and without baptism.

She was placed as a room-mate with a single lady of about 37 or 40 years of age. This one was of a most amiable and self-sacrificing turn; a great lover of silence, unless when charity or reason called for conversation. She was considerable improved from an extreme melancholy, yet liable to brain-fever, from too great sensibility, exercised by domestic disappointments, having lavished her fortune on a bank-rupt brother, who failing a second time, reduced her almost to beggary. She was of no religion, without baptism; but a perfect lady, ever occupied, & willing to oblige any one less happy or comfortable than herself. The crippled young girl was for turning every thing, even misery itself into cruel merriment, whenever she was in a playful mood. She was a great novel-reader. . . . These two persons being constantly together could not fail of being an annoyance to each other, or else of feeling some interest in each other's concerns. Gradually the morality and refined deportment of the grave lady, together with her unalterable patience and gentleness, medicated somewhat the savage manners of the other; and little by little, the routing of the Hospital discipline, together with hourly associations among the Sisters, became for them channels of faith and grace.

The young profligate became upright in soul and body, was baptized, became a faithful, edifying Catholic and went home an altered being. The spirit of the world had yielded its empire and given way to Religion. She was, if we may say so, the first ray of Christianity that ever shone under her father's roof. After spreading around her large circle of relatives & friends, the good odour of Christ, she fell into consumption, and died most piously.

[T]he other was reading also; they were receiving instructions at the same time. The solace of religion seemed to be the only remedy necessary for our melancholy patient. She seemed to have put on a new existence; and became an ornament to society & an exemplary Christian. ------[117]

Courtesy, Daughters of Charity Archives, Emmitsburg, Maryland

The care of the mania a potu patient focused first on the acute phase of the disease, the detoxification and management of potentially life-threatening physiological and psychological symptoms, such as seizures and extreme paranoia with hallucinations. It was common at Mount Hope and other institutions for patients with delirium tremens, once they were out of danger, to be discharged. The detoxification phase often took many days to complete. See Case Study 5-2 for an example of the medical treatment of a patient at the Baltimore Almshouse in the 1830s written by the attending physician, Dr. James Miller (1788–1853).

Patients who had regained their sanity often demanded to leave the asylum. Brigham insisted in his response to Dr. Stokes's rebuttal of his accusations about Mount Hope that those with delirium tremens be kept longer than the one-week period typically employed by Dr. Stokes and the sisters, with the "praise-worthy purpose of curing them of their propensity of intoxicating drinks."[118] Those who stayed in asylum treatment beyond the acute phase would have the benefit of longer periods of controlled abstinence. Many of the patients with mania a potu, according to Dr. Stokes, had three or four bouts of the disease every year, causing him to state that the patients might do better if placed under legal restraint.[119]

By mid-century physicians had begun to assign the concept of disease to alcoholism so that they could have a rationale for involuntary treatment and imposing abstinence.[120] Later in the nineteenth century, the role of inebriety specialists emerged in American society. Histories have marked the evolution of physician treatment of alcoholism and identified that little was offered the patient in antebellum America. The following section by Sister Matilda on the early and mid-nineteenth-century nursing care associated with mania a potu demonstrates the opposite: that nurses played an important role in the management of this public health issue. It seems that Sister Matilda and the DC Nurses were some of the early "inebriate specialists."

CASE STUDY 5-2 **Detoxification**

Josiah Manty --- was admitted into the Alms House labouring under confirmed Delerium Tremens of five or six days existence. His whole frame was in constant & violent tremor when left alone he appeared deranged. Fancying himself annoyed [sic] by Devils & Gosts [sic] etc. but more particularly by individuals who he imagined intended to murder & rob him. When interrogated on any subject his answer was always rational. If by constant conversations his thoughts ware [sic] diverted from the disgusting and fearful objects that tormented him continually when left alone he have evidence of a sane mind and was conscious of the disease under which he laboured.

During the interval of delirium I learned from him that he had been drinking to excess for 4 or 5 weeks that he had not enjoyed a moments sleep for 4 or 5 nights and partook of no food for three days previous to his admission –I have since learned that his statement is perfectly correct having sufficient evidence to sanction the presumption that the stomach & bowels in the case after a protracted course of intemperance must of necessity be surcharged with morbid secretions. I administered an emetic which operated freely and likewise produced an evacuation of the bowels. By the combined effects of the medicine and warm bath he became more tranquil for a short time. But in a few hours the disease assumed its most violent form and in less than twenty four hours he became raving mad. And had to be confined to his bed by use of straps to prevent his injuring himself. Opiates were freely given until the morning of the third day but without producing any effect. The stomach was now again evacuated by an emetic & the warm bath repeated. Finding that sleep could not be induced. The opiates ware [sic] resumed and continued until the morning of the forth [sic] day. When he obstinately refused to take any medicine declaring they ware [were] mixed with poison – and their only object was to destroy him. Finding that persuasion and threats ware alik [sic] ineffectual to the accomplishment of our object – we from Necessity abandoned him to his fate. On the fifth and sixth day he partook of nothing except a few drinks of cold water. By this time the tremor had in a great measure subsided but the delirium had terminated imperfect mania on the seventh day. The straps with which he had been confined ware taken off—The debility which was induced by this time prevented him from making any effort by which he might injure himself. He was now prevailed on to take a cup of strong coffee, which he did frequently during the day. But never without a ___ of being poisoned. On the 3rd and 9th days he drank coffee freely & eat a small quantity of bread and ham, and occasionally drank a small quantity of brandy & water, still refraining from taking medicine, on the tenth day perceiving that he was more sane than usual he was removed from the cells to the Hospital. During all this time he was never observed to sleep a single moment though regularly attended to.[121]

Mania a Potu or Delirium Tremens ⁓

[*Advices*] Delirium Tremens, which is the lighter stage of this malady is produced by intoxication. The trembling stage should be attended to in time for fear of the worst condition. As soon as such a patient is brought in take him to his room, having learned from [*Pg 17*] from [*sic*] his friends as to the violence or otherwise state of his mind, & if necessary have all things, that he would be disposed to break or throw at you removed from the room such as bowls, pitchers, looking-glasses, tables, &c. have a trusty person to undress them, handing each piece as he takes them off: the patient usually objects to stay or undress &c., but the attendant says, it is necessary that he gets some sleep and therefore she entreats and insists very politely & helping off with coat, vest, &c. and leaving the hired man to finish the remains out-side the door to take the clothes from him, for fear the patient hides something he should not keep; it is better to put the clothes on a chair until all is there,[122] and then hand the chair out-side saying, they will be put away, or they will get dusty &c. as they sometimes hide things in a belt under the shirt, have a night shirt ready for him, that he may be more comfortable; thus you may be satisfied whether you have left any thing about him. When they object strongly to taking off their cravat, boots &c. you may fear they have a special reason: in some cases you must not insist then, but stay in the room as though through politeness &c. until you may ask him again that he takes them off, and saying always that you know that they cannot be [*e*]asy with them on: sometimes they only have money that they are trying to keep from their friends, but you should try by all means to satisfy yourself that they have no intention to hurt themselves, yet this fear you have must not enter into their thoughts, or you would do them more harm by this than you could ever repair.

Sister Matilda's concerns about the patient's and staff's safety were very congruent with the treatment of patients hospitalized for mental illness even to the present day. What is unique perhaps about this section is Sister Matilda's instruction that a nurse should not in any way convey to the patient her concern about risk of suicide. Suicide prevention, as discussed throughout this section by Sister Matilda, was important to the proper care of the mania a potu patient. Suicide, though not talked about as openly as it is today, was quite prevalent in the mid-nineteenth century. Asylum superintendents knew that it was a critical social problem and had started to track it statistically in their states. In 1845 Dr. E. K. Hunt of Connecticut reported to the association that 184 persons in the United States had been reported in weekly newspapers to have committed suicide. Sixty-four people hung themselves. Drowning, shooting with a pistol or gun, cutting the throat, and taking overdoses of opiates all claimed about twenty-five people each.[123] Hunt stated that he knew the newspaper statistics were most likely inaccurate. Editor Brigham followed up the Hunt report with suicide statistics from New York State that were the same number in some years as were reported by Hunt to represent the entire country. In 1846 the association established a Committee on Suicide, and all asylums' medical superintendents were asked to collect suicide data for a formal national report.

[*Advices*] **All insane or delirious persons should [have] the same examination upon coming in; and even if friends assure you that they have nothing of dangerous matters about them, do not fail going through this precaution: experience teaches the necessity; after this provision for destroying themselves comes into their mind as soon as they find the [*Pg 18*] the [*sic*] friends are determined to take them from home and though they give no reason for the friends thinking of it, they prepare themselves now, and will try to secret razors or pen=knives [*sic*] &c. under pretence [*sic*] of pairing their nails &c.=, pocket=comb with nail=pail=[*sic*] in it, thumb=lance, opium=phials, powders, small=ropes &c. &c, Sometimes a favorite pocket=hkf [*handkerchief*] will be kept unknown to the friends on purpose for hanging himself, or his suspenders may do. With the insane the thing they first** thought of using for this is the <u>one</u> thing they try to secure and this should be a great point of information to gain, for this one thing may be kept from them, they may in time lose the intention: but in the minia [*sic*]a potu, if the thought or desire to destroy himself exists, he will do it by any manner, even to beat his brains out against the wall if left alone.

If the mania=a=potu[*sic*] patient wishes he were dead you may be on the watch, for the next thing to effect it: the greatest prudence is necessary; if you saw that they had kept something, but do not know what, you must judge of the propriety of insisting on seeing it, for this would let him know what you feared and would make him more determined, fearing let he would be watched &c, and so lose the chance, or if he had no thought of killing himself before he is now put in the mind of it by your suspicion and thinks he ought to do it since you thought of it: so the better way is to stop a while longer and not leave him alone until you are certain about it; but by providing the night shirt you have the best way of knowing whether he hides any thing or not. Never reproach those suffering from intoxication, for their own thoughts are often more than they can bear, even when you may feel nothing: in most cases it is better to [*Pg 19*] to [*sic*] console them saying that others have reformed from this vice or habit and became the joy & credit of their family and that they must now make strong resolutions and imitate them in their last state since they had fallen into their first state &c. &c.

Sister Matilda had experiences of patients being cured of intoxication, one of which she described in her journal *(See Case Study 3-1 in Chapter 3)*. In *Advices* Sister Matilda provided a sample script for her students who were learning how to best communicate with patients when they were potentially suicidal, a problem that had much assigned social stigma and was identified as a "vice" rather than a disease. Learning how to care for the intoxicated patient continues to be a challenging assignment for many nurses, nurse-educators, and nursing students today.[124]

[*Advices*] As they get more out of their senses they think they see enemies going to kill their parents, wives, children &c, or that some one is aiming a gun or bow at them, this makes him dodge about & try to hide and often he tries to kill himself, rather than let one who was once his friend, kill him &c. these excessive fears excites and heats the already injured brain until it can bear no more, and his fright makes him sweat so much that if he is confined in a strict way, or held down, he will surely die. At times they think hell-flames are all around them, then they reproach themselves & deplore the shame, disgrace they bring their friends to, and the loss of their soul. Reason comes & goes almost in the same moment, their terror, horror & torment are not to be expressed.– Now in this misery and despair, it is plain to be seen that the kindest, mildest, persuasion is the only course to pursue. You cannot have greater objects for your charity.

Let every attendant see in this poor creature a beloved Father or Brother, and act accordingly.

Sister Matilda showed in the care of the inebriate the perfect object of the DC Nurses' charity and the opportunity for Vincentian-Louisian holistic nursing care that would comfort the soul and the body.

[*Advices*] They should not be left alone even when they are calm, for often self-reproach is keenest then, & remorse like a fiend is more fiercely at work, – remembering past joys, respect, honor, dear friends &c., and now the horrid future he is about to enter, all all [*sic*] rack his mind so that he seems to see only one thing to do which is to destroy himself!

For God's sake do not laugh at them or suffer others to treat them with contempt, [*Pg 20*] though this shd be the hundredth time he has been brought to yr. care, you may save the soul the last time, and this done, all is right. Perhaps, crushed by frowns at home, he hopes to find pity from the Daughters of Charity[125] as channels of mercy from Jesus & pity from Mary, & cheered & sustained by you, he

may, like Magdelaine rise to fall no more, instead of leaving
this life Judas, saying: only hell remains for me.– Tell them
to take courage, that this will pass off, and they must now
resolve to serve God and pray for grace to avoid falling
again.– that they must now do as the Dr & Srs. [*Sisters*] tell
them and all will soon be right, that they will then go home
and give their dear friends great happiness by showing them
how well they will do the remainder of their lives.

    These seem like simple advices, but only experience can
tell their value. —

Sister Matilda demonstrated the values of many who practiced moral
therapy in the nineteenth century. It was believed that demonstrating
charity and mercy in simple acts of kindness, such as providing comforting
words of encouragement, were seemingly simple but powerful healing
interventions. In this paragraph Sister Matilda gives specific advice on the
care of what is referred to in contemporary vernacular as the "frequent
flyer" patients. Frequent flyers return over and over to hospitals for care
because it may be the only place that they receive care and understanding.
They rely heavily on the staff and the healthcare institution to provide the
structure in their lives that they have not been able to create or sustain
for themselves. Caregivers can experience these patients as frustrating
when they make little progress because the philosophy and ethic of the
caregivers and the hospital is not to turn away any person requesting
care. Sister Matilda provided spiritual advice in this section; the nurses
would never stand in contempt of any patient even if they were coming to
the hospital for the "hundredth time." The nurse was to look toward the
prospect of "saving the soul" and acknowledge that it could occur at any
time in the care of the patient, perhaps even on the hundredth visit. She
then provided instruction as to the specific ways nurses and staff were to
handle the insane patient within the moral therapy framework.

[*Advices*]   When they have not sense enough for such things, but
        violent in trying to get away, have two strong, but <u>kind</u> men,
        and a Sister present to direct them. Let them pick up the
        patient & put him on the bed, or he may sit in an easy chair,

comfortably, but not held rudely – Some hired men kneel on the patients chest or abdomen to hold him down, or holding his hands in theirs clenched & pressed down hard on the bowels or chest of the poor patient so as to cause his death, even after the delirium has passed off. This hard usage causes the patient to say hard things to the men & then there is no limits to their cruelty.

Our good Savior did not break the bruised reed.[126] We shd imitate Him.[127] [*Pg 21*] After the Dr has named the kind, quantity & frequency of the opiates & stimulants, there is still much depending on the attendants, as in many cases these remedies increase excitement & shd therefore be discontinued until the Dr comes again, & telling why these were not given– Hop tea is a good substitute as opiate & tonic; & often serves better than opiates or spirits. Chicken soup is a good remedy, also, because it strengthens them.

This is an example of titration and regulation of remedies that the judicious nurse was expected to exercise in the early and mid-nineteenth century. In this case Sister Matilda demonstrated her knowledge of the medical theory of excitement, of the action of crude opiate medications, and her role as the one to decide if an opiate should be given or held. Holding a medication "until the doctor comes again" does not challenge the status quo, but offering a substitute, hop tea, as potentially better than opiates or spirits prescribed to the insane by a physician suggests that Sister Matilda and the nurses she instructed practiced with a certain level of therapeutic autonomy. Sister Matilda's guidelines for following doctors' orders will be discussed again in the content on nursing, page 45 of *Advices*.

In the early and mid-nineteenth century, "nurses" were always women in the establishments where the Daughters of Charity provided their ministry. Male caregivers were referred to as "attendants." While nurses for the insane were expected to be intelligent and judicious, there were different expectations for male attendants. In 1852 an article on the qualifications and duties of attendants on the insane was published in the *American Journal of Insanity*. The attendant was to be sober, discreet, and virtuous, said Dr. Francis Stribling of Virginia. "He should possess a cheerful, accommodating disposition, an amiable, kind, sympathizing nature, and his manner should be pleasing and conciliatory. His temper should have been properly trained, and fully subject to his control, under all circumstances of disappointment, or provocation, and he should be eminently endowed with the virtues of patience and perseverance. . . . It is not important, that the intellect be highly cultivated, not indeed, if desirable, would it be practicable, within the limited means at command of most of our asylums to obtain for such as post, the services of those who have devoted much time to literary, or scientific pursuits."[128] They were, however, to have common sense and a basic school education. The male attendants were expected to use their intellect to devise amusements and occupation as part of the moral therapy of the patients in the asylum.

By 1854, however, the same year that the Royal College and American physicians published their concerns about nurses' management of sick diet, the Association of Medical Superintendents published a translation of an article by a French physician, Dr. Henri Falret, "On the Construction and Organization of Establishments for the Insane." In the article Falret stated that in France the nurses of the insane needed the "best qualities of mind and heart." He said that the DC Nurses and nurses in other religious orders were hired as hospital personnel because the people of the "class of society" that the physicians and hospitals wanted to hire for the nursing work had not "received the benefits of education" that the DC Nurses had. He wrote:

> This system has great advantages; the Sisters have more patience, greater discernment and love of their duties than personals ordinarily employed; they are better instructed and educated, and they can fulfill their duties equally well towards women and men, and render even greater services in the last division, where the difference of sex gives always a more extensive influence. The only objection that can be made against the introduction of Sisters of Charity into an establishment for the insane, is the fear so often realized, that their mode of organization disposes them rather to follow their own plans and desires, than those of the physician.[129]

Although it is unclear in this article by Falret that the "Sisters of Charity" he refers to are indeed of the same Community as the Vincentian-Louisian Daughters in Paris, he says quite plainly that there was a "fear" among physicians in France of the power of the religious nurse. This fear existed on both sides of the Atlantic and seemed to reach a crescendo in the mid-1850s. The Daughters' *Common Rules* had not changed, however. They still followed the admonishment of Vincent de Paul that "the principal aim of your obedience, dear Sisters, should be to please God"[130] and that their obedience to their superiors, their *Rules*, and Divine Providence would ensure that they went "straight to God."[131] The Daughters' understanding of obedience to their superiors (priests, hospital administrators, physicians, and Sister Servants) in the United States developed from Article III of the *Regulations* of the Sisters of Charity, which stated that they were to first and foremost follow their rules.[132] And the first rule of the Community was the "principle end for which God has called and assembled the Sisters of Charity"—to "honor Jesus Christ as the source and model of all Charity by rendering to him every temporal and spiritual service in their power to persons of the poor, either sick, invalid, children, prisoners, even the insane or others."[133]

It was in the day-to-day practical application of her spiritual life and ministry that Sister Matilda worked out how to be obedient to her superiors so as to please God *and* also follow the dictates of her own heart as to how best to minister to and nurse the sick poor and insane. She had witnessed the process of withdrawal at the Maryland Hospital before and after she left for Richmond and had led the reconstruction of the sisters' ministry to the insane, with the blessing of clergy and her Community, when they had established their own institution at Mount Hope. Sister Matilda knew through experience that there was a limit to obedience to physicians when it came to patient care. She demonstrated her thoughts on the subject in *Advices*. For example, it was known that opiates could have an adverse effect on insane patients, exciting rather than calming and sedating the patient. Sister Matilda not only declined to administer the doctor's prescribed treatment if it was not appropriate for a person, she also made decisions to give a remedy she prescribed herself, which in this case was hop tea.

Hops (*Humulus lupulus*) is a climbing perennial plant with heart-shaped leaves and bundles of flowers known as "strobiles." While hops is more commonly known today as the plant that lends its flavor to beer, its strobiles have been used medicinally for centuries. Hops is best known for its hypnotic and sedative effects, and nurses used hops poultices (topically) in practice well into the twentieth century. In the 1920s Bertha Harmer suggested using them on the abdomen to relieve postoperative distension and on the lungs during pneumonia. Hops poultices were also applied to wounds that were infected, painful, or inflamed.[134] Hops-distilled water was used in the Colonial period for "cleansing the blood and opening an obstructed liver and spleen."[135] It was used in the nineteenth century for delirium tremens to allay "morbid excitement and vigilance."[136] Later in the nineteenth century, a tincture (an alcohol extract) of the constituent lupulin was more commonly used for delirium tremens than was an infusion or decoction.

Sister Matilda continued her instructions on the management of the mania a potu patient. She described the specific ways the nurse could use herself as a therapeutic instrument; her "simple" techniques for using her voice to soothe and de-escalate the patient . . . and possibly to "save a soul" from demon possession. Insanity was viewed in the Catholic tradition during Sister Matilda's time as pathology and also as besiegement by inner demons. The DC acknowledged the reality of evil in the world and were vigilant to prevent its dominance.[137] Daughters of Charity to the present day recognize that Divine Providence permits diabolical activity in the world, and yet they believe that it is possible for them to have an impact on evil in that "all things work for good for those who love God, who are called according to his purpose."[138] Like Jesus who had "driven out demons, anointed with oil many who were sick and cured them,"[139] Sister Matilda and the DC sought to help patients overcome their inner demons with assistance from the nursing interventions described in detail in *Advices*, through prayer on behalf of patients, and by sending for a priest to bring the sacraments to the repentant who wished to be reconciled with God. Sister Matilda's ministry as a Vincentian-Louisian disciple of Jesus Christ gave her an outlook on sick persons, illness, and insanity that was filled with compassion for the soul and spirit as well as the body.

[Advices] An old, worn-out drinker will not be able to digest his fill of water, but a stronger one may drink as much cold water as he craves, unless it causes too much vomiting or pain.—

If he will be still enough, or even when he is jumping & dodgeing [sic] about, you may begin to ask him the most familiar questions, speaking in a mild, moderate tone, but with earnestness, as though you wished very much to know, & do not smile, or allow others present to do so, or you will do no good. Let yr. questions be short & such as wd give his understanding no trouble to answer. Such as: What is yr. christian name? What was yr Father's? Are you married? What is yr. wife's name? how many brothers have you? how many Sisters? What is yr oldest brother named? then the next & so on with the Sisters. Then have you children? how many? What the oldest's name? And so with the others. Then, what street is yr house in? Is it brick? What no? how many stories high &c. &c. &c. [Pg 22] At first he will give no attention to you, but, the questions being so short & easy to answer, he answers at last in hopes you, will then let him be. But as soon as he has answered the first one, then, with the same calm but earnest manner, ask him another, keeping to <u>that</u> one until he speaks in reply. If you were to speak loud or hurriedly, he would confound yr voice with those he imagines he hears, and therefore you wd not gain his understanding. —

But if often asking him, he seems too busy to hear you, having to dodge to avoid that gun, axe &c, say quietly: All is right, dont fear &c – Then begin the questions again.

Immediately after he has answered one question, you will see some improvement, and if he is not a worn-out drinker, or in danger of congestion, he will be cured by these questions, for soon, your voice has more influence over his senses than his fancied terrors; & he, who to all appearance had but an hour to live, is, if he is carefully spoken to, entirely out of danger in an hour after he begins to answer the questions. –

If he shd show sleepiness, of course you wd stop
speaking & give him every chance for sleep.– Do not grow
weary of this simple method, for the demon is not weary in
trying to put some new folly on the poor brain, in order to
prevent your success, so the good Samaritan[140] must not give
up first; for while life is in the body the soul & body may
both be saved.

~ --------

If he is a Catholic, the presence of a Priest may
help to bring him to his senses, as often happens, even
though he may have been [*Pg 23*] negligent in christian
duties when sober, for the horror he has now of hell,
makes a hope Spring up in his mind on seeing a Priest,
and often the[y] are able to make a confession– In
many, intemperance is their only fault or vice, and
God, seeing their hearts and human weakness, does not
reprobate them as readily as men do who see neither.

While local prohibition laws went into effect and the physicians of the
early and mid-nineteenth century were debating the "disease" nature of
inebriation, Sister Matilda focused on the psychological and soul aspects
of the "vice."

[*Advices*] Some patients will remain all the night kneeling by a hat or
coat on a chair, thinking he is making confession to a Priest.
A Priest shd be sent for, for them although some Priests,
not knowing much about the state of delirium, say they can
do nothing for them, and almost wonder at being sent for,
but, having sent, begin then to question yr poor patient so
as to have him calmer by the time he arrives, but conjure
the Priest to stay with him awhile, even if he is yet very
wild and excited. Your questions in this occasion may be
of confession, as: When was you at Confession? do you not
wish to go now? Who did you go to? But, quiet him in any
manner, so that composure be gained. Do all you can, and
if you fail as regards yr.[*your*] patient, you will have at least

did all you cd for his soul & so avoided sin by neglect.

Do not put restraints[141] on them unless obliged to do so to prevent their killing themselves or others[142] – but if you must do so, and they get angry at it, say to them kindly: My dear friend you oblige us to do so, for, you need composure & you will not take it, but as soon as your fever is off, we will set you free &c. Say too: If you were my Father or Brother, I wd do the same – we do this for your benefit, not to irritate or trouble you. &c [*Pg 24*] Let us indeed bear in mind how we wd do our very best for a dear Father or Brother, and wd not suffer them to be badly treated or laughed at.– Our Vocation is Charity, we must, as St. Paul says: put on the bowels of Jesus Christ[143] wherewith to serve His suffering members; our fallen Brethren.– Always speak to yr patients in a kind, sympathising [*sic*] manner, you thus excite their courage & confidence and lessen their wretchedness. What a blessed duty![144]

If such patients are determined to kill themselves, they will pretend to sleep, thinking the attendants will then leave him, & thus leave them to their opportunity. In one instance a man did so for th two or three days & nights, after which the man attendant went to his breakfast, without being replaced by another, and the Patient rose immediately, but his hands being confined some, he commenced beating his head against the door case; a Sr. passing heard the blood falling on the floor & went in. The Dr was called to sew up & dress the cut, but, the Patient did all he cd to prevent the Dr from doing him a Service.– But time & care restored him & every such case as was brought to the Hospital while he staid there, he wd stand by their bed to give himself a new fear of ever falling again, and as far as we were informed several years after, he never did.

The word suicide or self-destruction must never be used in their [*presence*], or any other weak-minded patient.– When opiates excites when given internally, sleep may be gained by rubbing laudanum in the hair & eyebrows, laying

also a little lint or rag wet with [*it*] near enough for him to
smell it.– [*Pg 25*] If you have not a Physician's prescription
to treat him, you may, with great advantage, perhaps, give
the following, as it has often produced ſpeedy cure.–

The principle of titration and regulation Sister Matilda teaches in the
case example of the suicidal patient is the difference in the action of a
remedy administered topically versus orally. She advises the nurses to
apply laudanum topically if the patient is excited by the internal use of the
narcotic. Sister Matilda provides another personal prescription for use in
the absence of a physician.

[*Advices*]   Take, Caſtor oil – 2 ounces
           " Spirits of Turpentine ½ ounce
           " Elm emulsion 4 ounces
           " Laudanum 1½ ounces

           Mix and give him one tea-ſpoonful
           every two hours until he sleeps.

Cupping ⁓

[*Advices*]   When cups are to be applied on the head, temples or any
           other place near the bone, the lancets muſt be set very
           shallow, or the griſtle that covers the bone will be injured. It
           is better for the Dr to apply them when done on the temples.
           If it cannot be set shallow, beare very little on the scarificator
           whilſt cutting.
               Have near the bed, a table with a lighted candle, two
           basins, one holding hot water, the other empty for the blood.
           the cups in the hot water – about 20 or 30 pieces of soft
           paper, tissue or news paper in size of a silver dollar, a ſponge
           in the water – a soft towel on the table to pass the cups
           quickly over when [*Pg 26*] taking it from the water. When
           the place to be cupped is ready, dampen the parts with a hot
           ſponge squeezed out of the hot water – then take a cup in

one hand, one of the little papers lit & blazing in the other, throw it in the cup & place it quickly on the ſpot – then another in the same manner until all are on, or as many as you intend to use. Have the scarificator ready while these are drawing, and when the cups have drawn the flesh pretty well into them, begin taking them off, taking off the one you put on firſt. You may take all of[f] before you begin to cut them, or you can cut one at a time, putting on the cup again before you take another off.–

As soon as you cut the place, light a paper as in the firſt inſtance & put it over the bleeding ſpot. If you take all the cups off before you cut any, cut all before you put on any; or the raised flesh will flatten down too much & thus too the bone wd be in danger.

When the cup is filled, or even half full, or that you see the blood is not coming any more, squeeze your ſponge again & remove the cups carefully, holding the ſponge near so as to catch the blood if it shd run – And, wetting the ſpot again, with the hot ſponge, put the cup on again, unless you have as much as was required. – If you do not know well how to cup, do not be ashamed to ask one who does know, for you may not get as much blood as wd benefit the patient. If you did not take the quantity ordered, let the Dr know it that he may know what else to do. Always have a large, dry cloth to prevent the clothes of the sick or the beg [bed] from getting wet or bloody. [Pg 27] Dry the scarificater [sic] & ſtrike it into a <u>mutton</u> tallow to prevent ruſt. Dry the moiſture from the skin of the patient with a soft towel & then lay a soft rag over it if necessary.

When cupping is ordered for the back, <u>avoid</u> the ſpine (back-bone),[145] but cup each side of it. <u>Avoid</u> also the shoulder blade. <u>Do</u> <u>not</u> cup on the side of the neck or the front, (the throat) and even for the temples, it is better to have the Dr, as some times it is hard to ſtop the Blood, there being so many veins and so little flesh there.

When <u>Dry</u> cupping is ordered, the cups are used as in

**the other, but the scarificator (the lancets) are not used
consequently no blood is to be taken, as a better circulation
is all that is wanting in this case, & often gives great relief.–**

After the air in the glass cups or bulbs is heated, they are placed on
specific points on the back. As the air in the cups cools, suction is produced,
drawing the skin into the cup and the blood with it. Many ethnic groups
practice the ancient remedy of cupping; it is used for varying reasons
depending upon each group's cultural beliefs. In traditional Chinese
medicine, cupping is practiced to move *qi* (energy). Dry cupping, as
Sister Matilda mentioned, was used in her nursing practice to promote
circulation. The stimulation of the skin with the intent to bring blood to
the surface, known as counterirritation, was popular in nursing care in the
nineteenth and twentieth centuries. An increase in the local circulation
caused the dilation of blood vessels. Herbal applications such as cayenne
pepper (*Capsicum frutescens*) poultices and liniments and the mustard
plasters discussed earlier also created counterirritant effects. Wet cupping,
which Sister Matilda also taught, was a type of bloodletting technique. The
presence of cupping in *Advices* suggests that the document was written
prior to 1850, when bloodletting, like blistering, was falling out of favor in
the care of the insane.

This passage in *Advices* also represents a significant change in
professional relationships between physicians and the Daughters since
the founding of the Community in France. In the seventeenth century the
Common Rules for the motherhouse clarifying the sisters' roles stated that
the DC Pharmacist was to make sure that no patient was bled who had
the means to go to a surgeon. She stated that there were two exceptions:
if the patient who "needed" to be bled was "well-known by the Sister-
Pharmacist or at least, not without the advice of a doctor."[146] At the time
of the writing of *Advices*, it appears from Sister Matilda's description that
the nurses, or at least the Sister Servant, had a standing order of sorts to
cup and bleed a patient as needed.

~ *Kindness, the Remedy of Remedies* ~
(Advices, Pages 28–44)

Advices was divided into sections: The first section contained general instruction on the care of the sick. It was followed by detailed explanations of therapeutic interventions, such as emetics, footbaths, and teas. Then Sister Matilda discussed cleanliness and her "General Remarks" on patient care. The next sections focus on the care of the person suffering from mania a potu and the insane in a section that she subtitled "A Few Remarks on Insanity." These two sections contain unique nursing-care content when compared with early, mid- and late nineteenth-century advice books and domestic medicine books written by physicians, reformers, and lay authors that typically focused on the management of the sickroom, implementing therapeutics, and how to follow physician instructions. Sister Matilda included her advice on all of these nursing skills in her text prior to and subsequent to these two sections on the care of the insane person. While a glimmer of the author's presence is sensed in the first sections, it is in the two sections on mania a potu and insanity that Sister Matilda's person, her voice, beliefs, and motivations are most clearly encapsulated. Here we find the expression of her deeply religious nature and her expertise as a seasoned nurse in the care of the insane.

Expertise in nursing care in the early and mid-nineteenth century has been defined throughout this book from the traditional perspectives of the Vincentian-Louisian Daughters, the physicians with whom the DC Nurses worked, and the patients. Sister Matilda and the DC Nurses' skills were described by the public, health reformers such as Dorothea Dix, and representatives for medical associations and the State of Maryland such as W. G Read, who took tours of Mount Hope. The sisters' nursing was described as judicious, intelligent, and enlightened. The content in *Advices* points to the particular tasks that were the demonstration of those expert qualities. Sister Matilda also included the way in which DC Nurses went about their nursing ministry; they were to cultivate an awareness of the importance of the simple details of their work.

Would Sister Matilda and the nineteenth-century DC Nurses be considered experts today? Certainly not, if expertise were measured by nurses, their colleagues, and society only in terms of the mastery of certain tasks, such as flushing a central line or extubating a patient. Although examinations of the expertise of people are typically done within the context of the time period in which those people live, we decided to make a comparison between contemporary and mid-nineteenth-century definitions of expertise. We found that there are some poignant similarities between the definitions of expertise in the two centuries. Researchers of at least one study of nurses in the twenty-first century, The Expertise in Practice Project,[147] for example, found that expertise among British nurses was not measured in terms of the mastery of tasks. It was described in a much broader sense, as it also was in the nineteenth century. The five attributes of expert nursing identified in the recent study are holistic-practice knowledge, saliency, knowing the patient, skilled know-how, and moral agency.[148]

Holistic-practice knowledge is described as "drawing from the range of knowledge bases to assess situations and inform appropriate action with consideration of consequences."[149] Saliency includes observing nonverbal cues, understanding the patient's individual situation, listening to the patient's verbal cues, and regarding the patient as a whole person to inform treatment process. Knowing the patient means respecting people and their views and perspective on illness or their particular situation. It also means promoting ways to relinquish efforts to control the patient. Skilled know-how refers to the ability to enable others by mobilizing all available resources and a willingness to share knowledge and skills. Lastly, moral agency is promoting another person's dignity and individuality and living one's values and beliefs without enforcing them on others.[150]

Given this contemporary definition of expertise, Sister Matilda might well be considered an expert today. She taught nurses how to demonstrate respect for their patients: the suicidal, the insane, the inebriates, and criminals, including homicidal patients.[151] The focus of the sisters' care was always to elevate their patients' self-esteem. They treated the insane as "rational beings," as far as safety allowed.[152]

Sister Matilda drew upon all the resources available to her and always sought more in constructing hospitals that would not only comfort patients but also convey the values of her ministry. She crossed gender and professional boundaries to create programs of care that were innovative for her time and timely, given the war that was looming, when women would be called to care for men on the battlefields as well as in the hospitals. She shared her nursing and health-related knowledge with her DC Nurse companions, her medical colleagues, and her patients. Sister Matilda and the Daughters practiced an early form of theory-based (moral therapy) nursing that valued kindness and nonrestraint.[153] She was an expert in the implementation of moral therapy and its philosophy and was an innovator in associated nursing practices. While the specific therapeutic agents in the hands of the nurse have changed over time, the expertise identified in the nineteenth century and in the study published in 2006 may be closer to defining the essence of nursing, which has been elusive.[154]

The next section of *Advices* demonstrates Sister Matilda's unique way of weaving her spiritual and professional knowledge and skill in the service of the insane.

A Few Remarks on Insanity

[Advices] [Pg 28] When an Insane or Melancholy Patient is proposed for admission into the Hospital,[155] gain all the information you can concerning previous health, disposition, temper, whether quick & angry- minded or the contrary, natural character, habits, business, &c. – Request also the friends to make you acquainted with any thing that the[y] noticed as being different from what the patient used to be – telling them that a very small matter as they think, may help very much to restore him provided the Dr or Sisters were to know it. – Ask them especially, what he did or said that first made them think that his mind was getting wrong. – This information is so necessary that, Some Institutions have printed forms to be used by those who receive them.

The following are some of them in addition to those above named:

What is his age? How long since you first saw a change in him? What was it that made you fear that something was wrong with him? What did he do or say that made you think so? Was he ever this way before this time? How long ago & how long did it last? how old was he then? What did

228

you think caused it then? had he had trouble of any kind,
or sickness, & what sickness & of how long standing. Is
he married? is his wife living or how long dead? did other
deaths occur that distressed him greatly? had he difference
with members of his own family or neighbours? how did he
behave during this disagreement? Is he kind in his family?
had he loss of property or injustices done him, or spiteful
enemies that talked hard of him? [Pg 29] how did he bear
these things? Was he disappointed in his affections?[156] What
was his general health before this strangeness came on? Are
any of his Relations in this way? Was he much with them, &
how did it affect him? What was his appetite before this, &
how is it now? how much did he use to sleep, & how much
now? Was he often from home? Was he a drinking man, &
how long & what was his usual condition? how long since he
quit it? has he smoked, chewed or snuffed Tobacco greatly?
& how long since he quit it, or is he a great snuffer yet?
did, or does he chew opium, or has he used laudanum or
Paregoric often? has he quit these & how long ago? and is
there a change in him Since? Was he free & pleasant among
his friends, or Sad & gloomy before this? Does he desire to
be alone now? what seems to be his greatest desire? desire
to wander from home? Seem to fear friends?[157] Does he
hate or love some one particularly? who is that one? how
long has he had a Drs care & what was done for him? Was
he bled, cupped, blistered, leeched &c? how often or has he
lost much blood in any way? has he been dieted, how long
& what was the kind of food & how much was he allowed
& how much did he take, or did or does he still desire more
food than the Dr allowed him? Was he freely purged? What
used to be the State of the bowels & what are they now? did
the Dr order opiates, such as Morphine, Laudanum, or what
kind of opiates, how much & how did they seem to affect
him & how long did he use them, and how long since he quit
them? how was he different in taking, or not taking them?[158]
Does he [Pg 30] or has he at any time since he is so, wished

he were dead? has he tried to hurt others? or himself? and how? for usually, the way they first tried to kill themselves, will be the one they will think of most, & perhaps if the thing or kind of thing were kept out of their way, they might forget their intention entirely. this has been told after their recovery. But in some this desire to kill themselves is so fixed that it seems to be itself the derangement – these will use any means in their power & no Sane person cd think of their inventions.

A gentleman so disposed was brought to the Hospital. His friends told us that he had expressed the wish to kill himself, because he thought he was a disgrace to the family &c., but that they had no fears of it, since a very emminent [*sic*] Dr them that such as intended to do so, never told their wish or intention – As friends seemed easy, we hoped for the best, at the same time kept it in mind to use what care we cd prudently, for if the Patient suspects that you fear it, he is sure to do it, thinking then that he must since you have thought of it. – the means this unfortunate man had intended was to hang himself with a Silk pockt [*sic*] hdf. [*handkerchief*] he had about him & which he never sent to the wash with his soiled linen. this we were ignorant of, but, with this, seeing it daily & pondering over it he succeeded – had this been told us by friends, we knowing the importance of taking it from him, wd have managed some way of getting it, without exciting his suspicion, and we have cause to believe he wd have [*Pg 31*] given up the idea, as he seemed to be improving in mind[159] _____ __ __ __

When the Patient is a Female their age and condition of general health must be particularly enquired into.

While Sister Matilda alludes here to her belief in some of the differences in the needs of females versus males, she does not imply in *Advices* that women are particularly susceptible to mental disease because of their gender nor does she represent women as "Natural Invalids," the picture of Victorian womanhood prevalent in white women's culture during the mid-nineteenth century. Sister Matilda may simply be referring to assessing for the possibility of menopause.[160]

[Advices]   The best writers on Insanity;[161] say: that kindness is the main remedy, because this method treats them as if they were Sane: this excites to self-respect, for the poor patient feels there is something wrong with him, but seeing he is treated like others – his remarks and wishes attended to, he begins to think he is not out of his mind, or that if he has been so, he must be better now, since he is considered & respected like others. This bright hope makes him try to deport himself in the best manner, he suppresses rising emotions. Even Idiots[162] love kindness, and may be improved by it.

Kindness in paroxisms [*sic*] of great excitement is of the best results,[163] and in their rage and fury, no harsh word or treatment should be used with them. but whatever may be the force or restraint you may be obliged to use with them, let it be done as to a loved parent or Brother – Saying to them kindly! My dear Friend, do not be angry with us for this, you are so out of humour, that we are obliged to do this. When you are better, all will be right again. You have fever, makes you do as you do, and when it passes off, you will be comfortable again – Why, the thing you wish to do, would not be for your good, or we would be too glad to gratify you – We like to see you happy. If you were my own dear Brother, I could not grant it – It is because we love and respect you, that we [*Pg 32*] refuse you now, &c.&c — Such mild remarks as these, calm their feelings, though they may rave on – And when these paroxisms occur they do not injure them, if they are treated kindly during them, for, it is harshness in their treatment that does them harm. They forever remember what bitter things were said to them and by whom – An excitement you can always explain to them, by calling it fever, and this raises their broken spirits, but they know they must have been very bad to have brought such things as they remember was said or done to them.

This debases them so in their own mind, that they say:
I know I am crazy, as they treated me as such, I can destroy
myself at any rate – Even though it may not go so far,
they are always depressed at remembering the contempt
or hard things said to them – O break not, the bruised
reed![164] But if you are kind, gentle, patient under all their
violence and abuse, they love and respect you as Angels of
consolation,[165] and each paroxism will be lighter, as they
recollect your tender compassion for them. thus too, they
lose their dread of these attacks, and improve rapidly. _____

Sister Matilda described how the DC Nurses could become instruments
of healing to the insane by the use of their words and their tone of voice.
The previous section also represents Sister Matilda's in-depth analysis of
the psychology of the patient in response to kindness versus harshness.
Kindness, in her estimation, raised the spirit of the patient above self-
condemnation, allowing the patient to take responsibility for his or her
behavior and life. Caregivers' harshness justified and further incited the
insane person's "debasement" or humiliation and potentially made his
illness worse, causing the "bruised" person to actually "break" under the
weight of his or her illness.

[Advices]   We should bear in mind that God leaves us our reason,
whilst He takes it from our patient, but shall we outrage this
God of Charity by making a cruel use of ours over His poor
Servant, who, without sense, is put under our care by Him?

Sister Matilda is instructing nurses to resist using rationality and sanity
as a means to control those who are irrational and insane. Instruction
on the proper use of power and patient empowerment is still given to
prelicensure nursing students today.

[Advices]   Or will we by anger, add our own violence to theirs?
Their attacks of excitement hurt their constitution,
whilst your harshness, hurts their mind! [Pg 33] Even
those who are subject to greatest violence, have a

232

sense of self-reſpect, on which you may ſtill rebuild
their tottering mind, but, your contempt by hard
treatment & manners towards them deſtroys this, and
ſtrength of scattered reason cannot be rallied again.

Sister Matilda places much responsibility for the spiritual and corporal
welfare of the insane squarely on the shoulders of the nurses and attendants.

[Advices] Could we push back in to the deep, a ſtruggling, drowning,
fellow creature, a Brother? – Too often the attendant thinks
they ~~they~~ are not capable of feeling while in this ſtate of
rage, thu[s] what is the use of rudness [*sic*], but to exercise
your own vexation? You have not kept your reason calm,
and they would gladly be able to give you no trouble! Ah let
us not love a cruel authority! It is better by far to be without
reason, than abuse it by a bad or uncharitable use of it!

——————

An angry man feels & remembers all hard things
said to him, because, the hard ones, or hard things, pain
us. this is why these are longer on the mind than other
things. On the contrary, gentle, mild, pity &c, is so sweet
to the poor chained brain, that it soothes and binds
the wounds they endure. His power of thinking, feels
muffled, or as groping about in the dark, confusedly.
Your mild tone of voice, is like a ray of light, or taking the
hand of a blind man, saying: this way, my friend. Thus
you loan them your reason, till their's [*sic*] returns.

Sister Matilda makes an exquisite analogy between the nurse who
takes the hand of a blind man and the nurse "loaning their reason" to a
patient, thus further solidifying the belief in the mind-body connection.
Sister Matilda was able to translate her early medical nursing training into
practical instructions for those nurses who had never cared for the insane.
No comparable description of nursing care of the insane has been found
in any other nineteenth-, twentieth-, or twenty-first-century nursing literature at this time.

233

[Advices] like the strong friend gives his arm to his sick, or weak friend. [166] – This is a glorious application of our faculties – His is the part of the good Samaritan.–

We should never show that their bad speeches or manners towards us had pained us – especially as they sometimes [*Pg 34*] say such horrible things that it would be a great mercy to help them forget them –

The Daughters did endure great physical and verbal abuses as a result of nursing the insane. Physicians such as Dr. Stokes were aware of the women's abilities to continue in their charitable work. As shown in previous chapters, younger nurses had to be helped by more experienced nurses to learn how to protect themselves physically and emotionally from remarks made by the insane and how to endure their mission with joy.

[Advices] They seeing you are always the same kind friend towards them, begin to think, those hateful things were only dreams.___ But should they make an apology for improprieties of speech or manner, say pleasantly: O if I had had your fever, I might have done far worse, do not think of it. I do not care for what my dear Brother said to me last month in his ship-fever &c.

This is another example of scripting for the novice nurse to follow. Sister Matilda demonstrates a psychotherapeutic communication technique here known as "normalizing." Her choice of words may also be her adapted version of the Vincentian teaching: "Meekness makes us not only excuse the affronts and injustices we receive, but even inclines us to treat with gentleness those from whom we receive them, by means of kind words, . . . it makes us endure all for God."[167]

[Advices] These precious words are registered in Heaven, as they are on the grateful heart of your poor patient. How then does the Heart of your Jesus view them! ___ And if in the course of time, they, or their grateful Friends[168] may come to know & embrace the true Religion, it will be because its

truths were written in honey. But a hasty, self-opinioned, or negligent & unfeeling attendant, prevents good from being done. She serves him as a Swine-herd, without respect to him, or merit to herself, and by one short word or remark, makes quick work of the Slender chance that had been carefully Studied in better hands – This chance gone, all future care, perhaps, may be useless – like the tender plant in taking root, must have time, tender care, and preserved from the boisterous winds, or it withers, never to be restored.– The diseased mind is like an Infant trying to walk – if another child leads him, he will be injured by falling and vexation, but if one capable of directing his crooked steps is with him, all will soon be right.

Sister Matilda's voice softens even more here and becomes more poetic with her use of metaphor.

[Advices]   Happy, happy lot of the Sister of Charity, whose duty is, Service to the Insane!

Duty in the Vincentian-Louisian tradition refers to one's ministry to which a sister is assigned or missioned.

[Advices]   [*Pg 35*] Conversation is a matter on which much depends for the Insane. What they say should not be abruptly contradicted, or turned into ridicule, contempt &c, as though at first thought we saw it wrong – but seem to be pleased with their remark, or considering it, even to add your own to it, and then presently, as if you took another view of it, propose that which might be better . . .

This communication technique is redirection and possibly confrontation, which is explaining the patient's behavioral discrepancies to him.

[Advices]   that is if this is necessary, for if the thing is trifling, let it remain as they first said, for this respect for

235

their opinion is very useful to them – it is another
stone in your building, especially as being picked
from among the ruins of what once stood higher.

Sister Matilda reminds the reader about the fundamental Vincentian-Louisian value of respect for the patient and his or her opinion, even when it seems inconsequential, because the very act of verbal affirmation and validation has therapeutic value. The analogy which Sister Matilda uses, comparing respectful communication to rebuilding an edifice, stone by stone, may be predicated upon the biblical teaching, "Do you not know that you are the temple of God?"[169]

[*Advices*]   But if the thing is bad & would lead to ill consequences,
Seem to be thinking about it. and then as though you just
saw it right, propose the contrary quietly.
          When first little remarks of theirs meet with our
attention & respect they begin little by little to speak
more freely to us of themselves or of other patients.

As discussed in previous chapters, Sister Matilda and the DC Nurses encouraged patient interactions as a means of promoting healing. They did, however, monitor those interactions and as shown here also learned much about their patients from hearing of the content of patient interactions.

[*Advices*]   – thus you gain their confidence, and, becoming better
acquainted with them & those of whom they speak, (for
often they know each other better than we yet know them)
[*Note: Parenthesis and enclosed words in original document*]
and this information becomes very profitable to them if
we make a right use of it – but we must not show much
eagerness to know from one patient of another, or they
will become Suspicious and guarded on these things. –
They often become the confidents of each other, for the
Dr and Srs are looked on as instrumental in keeping
them there, &c. and so they are slow in trusting them.

As kind and compassionate as the DC Nurses and Dr. Stokes may have been, the mentally ill patient, especially the psychotic patient, could have still viewed their hospitalization as incarceration.

[*Advices*]   once [*sic*] they receive always from you [*Pg 36*] a kind, respectful bearing, seeing you so towards all, also (For they are quick sighted in partialities, indeed, in all our weak points) [*Note: Parenthesis and enclosed words in original document*] they lose their distrust and begin to view you as their best, often their only friend – In a word, we only succeed with them by taking God's way with them, that is: Justice, Charity, clemency, or in His own words: "Do to others, as you would have them do to you."[170]

　　　　　The tendrils of the plant will run wild without support, and so do the thoughts of the insane when they converse only with each other.

The nurses and attendants are considered as much of the scaffolding for the emotional and mental support of the insane patient as was the physical milieu.

[*Advices*]   But should the attendant be an improper prop, they are badly off.– But by prudence we may gain a timely knowledge of the strange things they had planned among themselves, and thus prevent terrible consequences.

　　　　　It require [*sic*] great prudence also, for selecting right topics for conversation, as you must avoid what excites or exasperates them. One thing or subject is odius [*sic*] to one & indifferent to another, you must be like an able Pilot on dangerous waters – often a little misplaced word or sentence tears open a closing wound that had taken much time & care; or excites another to violence.

The counseling technique Sister Matilda is referring to here is called "pacing" today. In this technique the nurse or counselor establishes rapport with the client by being flexible and using the same information processes as the client. For example, if the client speaks in terms of his or her feelings (kinesthetic reference), then the nurse also references feelings during the interaction to match the primary representational system of the client.[171]

[Advices] **With the Melancholy or desponding patient, it is well to advise them never to speak of their troubles to the other patients, who believing what they say, are apt to confirm them in their sad impressions.**

This is a very astute example of the redirection that was used by the nurses in the milieu during patient interactions.

[Advices] **And if they wish to speak of them constantly to you, you would do better to say to them: "Now [Pg 37] my dear friend, I believe you distress yourself too much by speaking always of your troubles, so I cannot let you do so, but if you cannot join in other subjects of conversation, at least try to entertain yourself on what others are talking about." Do not grow weary of giving this advice, for a little gained, is a great thing.**

In this, Sister Matilda instructed the nurses in what is today called "inviting"—a technique in which the nurse or counselor asks the client questions and politely engages them in a search for new meaning.[172]

[Advices] **After they have refrained from speaking of it or from warning it a couple of days or so, do you, yourself say to them kindly: "Well how is your poor heart now? don't you think you can bear your troubles now better than when it first came to you? I think you will soon be better – I know what sadness is, and bitter as it is, it is only a sickness of the mind, as fever is of the body, and like fever too may be cured, but we must have patience – It will pass away.**

This technique of offering encouragement is often referred to as "cheerleading." Nurse and counselors use their emotions to support changes in patient behaviors, even small steps forward. Sister Matilda included normalizing with cheerleading in this example. Cheerleading can also go awry. If Sister Matilda was to say what she does here to the highly depressed and suicidal patient on their first interaction, her words might be perceived as invalidating. This may be why Sister Matilda advised to "wait a few days" before offering encouragement (i.e., cheerleading).

[Advices]   Our Heavenly Father can heal us when all others fail, but He knows the best time for healing our poor wounded hearts – You have had bodily sickness, and you got well again & so you will of this – take courage – many have been like you, and are well and happy now – when you get well and go home to your people, you will be so brave, that if any of your dear friends should be in trouble, you will be their comfort & encouragement, for the mind is like other things it becomes stronger by having been seasoned by keen trials and afflictions. I can bear much more now, having had trials of the mind.

Believe me, a sickness like this, wonderfully fortifies the mind for coming troubles, or common occurrences of life." *[Pg 38]* Such things said kindly to them occasionally help them so much, that you might call them the means of their restoration.

The sisters modeled new ways of thinking and being for their insane patients. This is known today as cognitive behavioral therapy and is particularly helpful for the depressed or melancholy client, as Sister Matilda notes here. The technique is also called "reframing."

[Advices]   – Consequently, when these assistances of consolation are omitted, the Melancholy becomes derangement & fixed. The diseased or the troubled mind is like a fractured limb, which does not often heal without help – So too much pains cannot be taken to become a proper aid to the fractured or shattered mind._____

By creating the analogy between physical and mental illness, Sister Matilda attempted to raise the spirit of her patient by normalizing and challenging the social stigma and associated self-condemnation surrounding insanity that could threaten the patient's healing and cure.

[Advices] Be careful that the gloomy or sad patient is not made the ſport and derision, of the rough, jolly wit of the unthinking class of Patients, for the very being associated with such, they consider a degradation & painful to their too sensitive feelings.

Some attendants, for want of experience, think it well to turn them into ridicule, but it is injurious, and to such as were diſposed to deſtroy themselves, it would increase the desire to do so, and thus shew their abhorrence of such low jeſting and gross annoyance as they now deem it. "Break not, the bruised reed."

It is often advantageous to permit one low-ſpirited patient to talk to you of her troubles in the presence, or hearing of another like her without your seeming to know she is there. The one who hears the other ſpeak of herself as the worſt off in the world, and also hears your replies, thinks juſt as you do in her case – She becomes for the time entirely occupied in liſtening to her, and is surprised that anyone can be so miſtaken, since she herself is the only one so truly wretched. She continues to liſten to her woes, so as moſt to forget her own for a moment – She [Pg 39] thinks about it, believes her entirely miſtaken, & that your advices to her were perfectly right, and in a day or two, she will begin to tell you of the reality of her own case, but the other she heard ſpeaking, was only imaginary, &c.

Slowly and gently, draw the comparison & gradually you will weaken the ſtrength of her opinion on such & such points, she used to be positive on. – She, who before this would not ſpeak to any one, now seeks the company of her fellow-sufferer, and if they are not left too long together at a time, will very much improve each other without their knowing it. _____ ___

Associations of males and females is not of advantage to either side, and should be carefully avoided.

_____ _____ _____

The word: suicide or self-destruction should never [*be*] used in their hearing.

The word: punish for every slight fault or mischief they do, will make your government odius [*sic*] to them, and threats exasperate them. When shower baths are necessary, do not let them think they are given as a punishment, but only as a remedy & for their benifit [*sic*] or health &c.

Sister Matilda specifically rejects the use of the word "punishment." She advocated that the DC Nurses take a sisterly rather than parental role in the care of the insane. Showers had been used as punishments in asylums even during the era of moral therapy.

[*Advices*] – If they resist so far as to get in a great heat, they should not be put in, or the consequence may be death, as has happened. Or if you might fear, that other reasons, (with females) [*Note: Parenthesis and enclosed words in original document*] should prohibit it – Do not fear that giving up to their objections, will make them more outrageous another time, thinking, that they conquered you, &c.

Sister Matilda may be referring to the power struggles that occur between nurses and attendants and the patients in hospitals.

[*Advices*] no, no, if you show [*Pg 40*] no impatience in mood or manner, they will think you give up, because you pity & feel for them, and this supposition will make them love you, and this may bring about the beginning of their good deportment, and again we see the fruits of kindness, for [*it*] is, and forever will be, the remedy of remedies, whereas, showering, or such things, are in most cases only a power of subduing the body, but often hurts the poor head by giving

some new aversion for you & any who have any control over
them, as also it is often too great a shock to the Brain.

Only time, daily associations and experience can teach
us of how much we can help, or injure them. According
as a thing is precious or valuable, so does it call for care
and attention. Now what price would we take for our
Reason? Then let us pray and labor, & labor and pray for
light and charity, by which we may be able to help our
dear fellow creatures in this blessed work of Mercy.

This closing paragraph is a summary of Sister Matilda's philosophy and
spirituality of care for the insane and perhaps therefore the statement of the
"inner compass" that ultimately determined her expertise. She then offered
a witness to one of her spiritual guides, St. Francis de Sales.

[Advices]   **The great St. Francis de Sales cured the moſt**
violent, by, patience, kindness and prayer.

Sister Matilda's voice changed again, almost as if she wrote the next
page in a separate sitting. In the next section she provided the reader with
a very didactic account of some of the most common medical terminology
of her day. As mentioned in chapter 2, the DC Nurses studied medicine
and sciences such as chemistry with their physician colleagues and with
Rev. Bruté, who had been a physician. Because of Sister Matilda's pragmatic
nature, it is most probable that she would have only included this content
if it had been something that the nurses needed to know for their nursing
work. As in previous sections, Sister Matilda included lay language in
parentheses when she deemed it necessary. The remedies used by the
sisters were often botanical in origin, and examples of botanical remedies
were included.

[Advices]   **[Pg 41] General Remedies include 1ſt Arterial Stimulants;[173]**
sometimes called: Incitants, which, while they raise the
actions of the Syſtem above the ſtandard of health, shew
their influence chiefly upon the heart & arteries: 2nd
Narcotics,[174] which eſþecially affect the cerebral (brain)

[*Note: Parenthesis and enclosed words in original document*]
functions, & are either stimulant or sedative according as
they increase or diminish action; 3d Antispasmodics,[175]
which, with a general stimulant power, exert a peculiar
influence over the nervous system, by the relaxation of
spasms, the calming of nervous irritation &c., without any
special & decided tendency to the Brain; 4th Tonics,[176] which
moderately and permanently exalt the energies of all parts
of the frame, without necessarily producing any apparent
increase of the healthy actions; 5thly Astringents,[177] which
have the property of producing contraction in the living
tissues with which they may come in contact.

Local Remedies may be divided into four sections:
those affecting the function of a part; namely, 1st
Emetics,[178] which act on the stomach, producing vomiting;
2nd Cathartics,[179] which act on the bowels, producing a
purgative effect; 3rd Diuretics,[180] which act on the kidneys,
producing an increased flow of urine; 4th Antilithics,[181]
which act on the same organs, preventing the formation of
calculous (gritty or stony) [*Note: Parenthesis and enclosed
words in original document*] matter; 5th Diaphoretics,[182]
which increase the cutaneous discharge; 6th Expectorants,[183]
which augment the secretions from the pulmonary
mucous membrane, or promote the discharge of the
Secreted Matter. [*Pg 42*] [*Nothing written on this page.*]

Of Measurement ⌒

[*Advices*] [*Pg 43*] For the sake of convenience, in the absence of
proper instruments, we often make use of means of
measurement, which, tho' not precise, afford results
sufficiently accurate for ordinary purposes –

The difference between "ordinary" purposes and nonordinary purposes
is not fully explained but it would seem that Sister Matilda was making a
distinction here between domestic medicine and that which they did when

carrying out physician's orders. American nurses of the mid-nineteenth century, such as those in the Daughters of Charity, Shakers, and Latter-day Saints communities were "cultural diplomats," in that they applied many ways of knowing in their care.[184] The DC Nurses drew knowledge from the "professional" medical culture, such as what they learned from Dr. Stokes and from community and household medicine practices that they learned while growing up and from living in the DC Community. Their nursing knowledge and practice was the representation of an integrated approach to caring for others.

[Advices]   There are certain household implements, corresponding to a certain extent with the regular standard measures.

Custom has attached a fixed value to these implements, that is well to be familiar with.

A tea cup is about 4 fluid ounces or a gill.

A wineglass holds 2 fluid ounces.

A good sized table spoon, ½ a fluid ounce.

A tea spoon (60 drops) [*Note: Parenthesis and enclosed words in original document*] holds a fluid drachm.

One drop is called a minim, or sixtieth part of a fluid drachm – but, as some liquids form larger drops than others, the safer method is, to use the minim measure in important cases.

As the abbreviations are mostly from the Latin, we give them here in english, as also the signs of the weights.

℞	stands for, take	Collyr.	Means, an eye water
āā	" of each	Cong.	" a gallon
lb.	" a pound	Decoct	" a decoction
℥	" an ounce	Ft.	" make
ʒ	" a drachm	Garg.	" a gargle
℈	" a scruple	Gr.	" a grain
O	" a pint	Gtt.	" a drop
f ℥	" fluid ounce	Haust	" a draught
f ʒ	" fluid [d]rachm	Infus.	" An infusion
℩	" Minim	M.	" Mix
chart	" a small paper	Mass.	" A Mass
coch.	" a spoonful	Mist.	" A Mixture
qs.	" sufficient	Pil.	" A pill

[Pg 44]   **Pulv. means a powder**

S.	"	write
Sf[?]	"	a half

245

⌒ *Nursing Science in the Mid-Nineteenth Century* ⌒
(Advices, Pages 45–76)

The organization of the next section follows a typical layout of mid-nineteenth-century advice books on the subject of sickroom management. The sickroom was the domain of the mid-nineteenth-century nurse, lay and professional. It was the place where innovations in care were tested. The sickroom was and continues to be the laboratory of the nurse. Developing expertise in creating a space for the promotion of health and healing was not only an art, it was the nursing "science" of the nineteenth century. As mentioned before, every woman was expected to have some knowledge of sickroom management and therefore it was a common topic, and often a chapter, in household-advice and domestic-medicine books.

Nineteenth-century nurses like Sister Matilda, however, had more than "ordinary" knowledge of sickroom management.[185] Sister Matilda and other professional nurses of the period were innovators of care and educators. They researched and developed the knowledge base for the best practices in sickroom management and in the creation of a healing environment. One of the core beliefs underpinning medical and nursing knowledge in the mid-nineteenth century was the notion of the importance of nature in the care and cure of the sick.

"Nature cure" philosophy appeared in advice books and medical literature. In 1835 Dr. Jacob Bigelow read his essay on self-limited diseases before the Massachusetts Medical Society. He stated that some diseases were "controlled by nature alone" and that the physician was but the "minister and servant of nature" who was to "aid nature in her salutary intentions, or to remove obstacles out of her path."[186] Dr. Wooster Beach, a regular and botanical physician, wrote in 1843:

> In reality we can cure nothing. We can only remove the offending cause, while nature performs a cure; and, therefore, lay it down as a fundamental maxim in medicine, that all the physician can do is, to act as a servant or handmaid to nature.[187]

Lydia Maria Child wrote in *The Family Nurse* that "both doctors and nurses, as they grow older and wiser, use as little medicine as possible, and simply content themselves with recommending fasting, or light diet as will best assist the kindly efforts of nature."[188]

While physicians demonstrated their belief in nature cure by adjusting their treatment regimens, nurses expressed the belief by creating healing environments for their patients. They utilized the elements of nature— fire, air, water, and earth[189]—to design a space that would nurture and comfort. In 1859 Florence Nightingale published her own advice book on sickroom management for all women who had "personal charge of others," in which she wrote that "nature alone cures . . . and what nursing has to do in either case, is to put the patient in the best condition for nature to act upon him."[190] Physicians, nurses, and the public who were being their own doctors and their families' nurses were often interested in nature's healing powers.

Environment was a key health issue in the mid-nineteenth century: Americans had experienced a number of cholera outbreaks and were beginning to feel the effects of rapid industrialization on health and family life. They had begun to assume more individual responsibility for creating the health of the newly formed democracy. Popular physician authors such as Englishman William Buchan[191] and American John Gunn[192] encouraged people to use the remedies found in their own kitchens and gardens.

Sister Matilda did all of this and more. She exemplified the role of the nurse scientist of her day as an expert in sickroom management when she created an entire healing environment for the insane, the asylum named the Mount Hope Retreat. She implemented a program in moral therapy in which nature was utilized in activities and occupations that would bring a patient back to a rational state. The *Advices* text, in its totality, is an account of the work of a professional nurse in the mid-nineteenth century whose focus was creating and "being" the healing environment of the patient.

The next section of the text follows the typical mid-nineteenth-century sickroom-management-book format. It is a similar structure to that which was used by Lydia Maria Child in *The Family Nurse* and by Nightingale in *Notes on Nursing*. Nightingale's *Notes* begins with a prologue of general comments followed by instructions on the management of such things as ventilation, warmth, noise, cleanliness, and bed making. The next section of *Advices* on sickroom management also includes these headings. Comparing *Advices* with the mid-nineteenth-century advice and domestic-medicine literature, it is apparent that sickroom management advice books or chapters in books typically included the same subjects found in *Notes on Nursing* and the following section in *Advices*. However, when first analyzing the overall layout and tone of the next section of *Advices* in the context of the whole manuscript, the section appeared to have been written not only during a different sitting from the previous section but also in a different voice. The explanation for this change appeared a few years ago when this section of *Advices* was found verbatim in *A Practice of Physic* published in the 1830s by a Dr. William Dewees (1768–1841). Dr. Dewees was an American-born physician of some renown, having studied with Dr. Benjamin Rush. He was best known for his work in establishing obstetrics as a practice of medicine as opposed to midwifery. Dr. Dewees wrote numerous books, including *A Practice of Physic*, which the *London Medical and Surgical Journal* in 1830 dubbed "one of the best systems of medicine extant."[193]

Sister Matilda was an *editor* and *commentator* rather than the author of the following sections on nursing (i.e., sickroom management) and fever. Her inclusion of large excerpts from Dewees' book was not uncommon practice in the nineteenth century. Some advice-book authors lifted entire books and placed them in their own. For example, Dr. John Milton Scudder, who published domestic-medicine books for families later in the nineteenth century, acknowledged the nursing work of Florence Nightingale by putting the entire content of *Notes on Nursing* in his book.[194] Sister Matilda did not do what Scudder did, however. She did not reproduce each and every word of Dewees' chapters on nursing and fever in her *Advices*; she cleverly edited selected sections of the work for the nurses and students who read her text. Sister Matilda's choices about what to include and perhaps more importantly what to exclude from Dewees' work imply much about her thoughts on professional nursing. Her choices also suggest what her relationship was to Dewees' views of nursing in terms of the values and beliefs associated with the Vincentian-Louisian ministry of the DC Nurses. These final two sections of Sister Matilda's edited copy of the chapter on sickroom management from

Dewees' *A Practice of Physic* are provided now with editorial comments and a literary comparison of the original Dewees text and that which Sister Matilda chose to reproduce in her *Advices*.

A Professional's Exceptions ⌢

The first excerpt of *Advices* is taken from Dewees' book, page 21.

[*Advices*]   [*Pg 45*] The office of "Nurse" is one of awful responsibility if its duties be properly considered; for on the faithful discharge of them, will the Life of a fellow being, in very many instances, almost exclusively depend.

How much intelligence, good sense and fidelity are therefore required, that the patient may profit by her attentions; or that [s]he may not be injured by her self-willedness or neglect! Where there is a Medical Attendant, the duties of a Nurse are reduced to two simple, but highly important rules; the observance of which Should be most rigidly insisted upon. First, to do every thing that the Physician orders to be done, and this in the strict letter of the commands. Second, to do nothing herself, nor permit any one else to do, that which he has not ordered; for it is fairly to be presumed, that the Physician will direct to the best of his knowledge, whatever he may think is essential to the welfare of his patient. —

Sister Matilda left out the remainder of Dewees' sentence here and a number of paragraphs on the "mistaken notions" of "disingenuous and ignorant nurses" who challenge the authority of a physician and who engage the assistance of the patient's family to do so.[195] Dewees wrote, "therefore, for a nurse to put her judgment in opposition to that of the physician, is arrogant and dangerous."[196] From all accounts of the work of the sisters at the Maryland Hospital, the Baltimore Infirmary and Mount Hope, not to mention the other DC hospital missions across the United States, there is no evidence that the sisters believed that their challenges to physicians were centered in arrogance or that they were dangerous.

Instead, when they exercised their own judgment to intervene on behalf of patients, it was often on behalf of patient safety or their own. Dewees based the justification for his commentary ridiculing nurses on their lack of education and the fact that they had not researched disease the way physicians had. "Now can it be for a moment supposed, that an ignorant uneducated woman, (be her experience what it may), shall be as well qualified to judge of the condition of a patient, as the man who has devoted the better portion of his life to the investigation of diseases?"[197]

Women, however, were socially excluded from participating as men did in the investigation of diseases, and it was rare for women in the mid-nineteenth century to study medicine at universities or even apprentice with physicians. Harriot K. Hunt (1805–1875) was the first woman to apply to Harvard Medical School, which did not admit women until 1946. She was allowed in 1850 to sit in on lectures, after twelve years of practicing as a physician trained in Boston under British naturalist physicians Dr. Richard and Mrs. Elizabeth Mott.[198] In 1949 Dr. Elizabeth Blackwell was the first American woman to obtain a medical degree.[199] Dewees devalues the education that professional nurses of the period received and criticized their abilities because they did not have the opportunities extended to them that men did. It is understandable that the sisters would have explored every possible avenue for receiving medical education, as did men in the society, and engaged the help of the physicians with whom they worked to aid in the process. It is neither surprising that Sister Matilda disregarded Dewees' comments nor that she added her own at this point:

[Advices] There are however, exceptions to these remarks, that
the Medical faculty admit of, that is; when the nurse is
experienced and faithful, and has also shewen herself equal
to her duty, she may, and should, withhold medicines,
drinks &c, which she observes acts contrary to the designs
or wishes of the Phyn, but, this liberty is only to be exercised
between his visits, and she should relate to him as soon as
he comes of what she had done, & why.– The injury usually
done in nursing is, by being in the advance of the Phyn
when improvement appears, for then, She, of her own
accord, allows him more nourishing drinks, food &c, or tests

his strength too fast by having him [*Pg 46*] rise too soon, often &c.– Could all the consequences of ill timed omissions or commissions, as regards nursing, be laid down, or sufficiently remembered, the remedy would be gained – It is believed that a majority of relapses in acute diseases is owing to the injudicious employment of what is considered a very innocent indulgence of something, "more palatable": as in one case, three table spoonfuls of chicken water, created so much fever, and so severe a renewal of the pain of Pleurisy, that severe bleedings were required to subdue them; tho' when it was given, even the Phyn thought the patient convalescent – Therefore, it is in the injudicious use of animal substances, either entire or in solution, that Nurses most frequently effect the mischief complained of above – In the same way they venture on seasoning their nourishment with, "a little dash of Wine or Brandy", tho' contrary to the positive orders of the Phyn — Is it then surprising that fever should have so many Victims, when the force of the disease is <u>aided</u> by the attendants on their recovery?

The previous paragraph is an edited version of Dewees' book, pages 25–26. The references to chicken water as a detriment to patient progress come from Dewees; however, what Sister Matilda leaves out is Dewees' commentary that the nurses' "injudicious employment of the 'innocent chicken water,'" which he reported was an everyday occurrence, was more harmful to patients than the occasional "mischief" reported from problems with bloodletting and mercury.[200] This was a serious charge against nurses and those practicing domestic medicine. Sister Matilda believed that chicken broth was "strengthening" to patients, but she also clearly knew when to withhold broth and substitute the chicken bone instead *(See page 3 of Advices)*. Dewees knew that he was on shaky ground. He wrote that the "prejudices" in favor of using chicken water were so "common and inveterate" that he felt that his directions would "rarely be believed."[201]

Sickroom Management ⁓

[Advices] [Pg 47] Hitherto we have spoken only of the Patient, let us now pay some attention to the Sick <u>Room</u>. If "good nursing is half the cure", let us see in what it consists.

Dewees did say that it was "universally admitted" that good nursing was half the cure.[202] The following paragraph is taken almost verbatim from Dewees.

[Advices] The Phyn acknowledges that his attentions upon the sick would be altogether unavailing, were his directions not obeyed by the Nurse, and this, in the most faithful manner, for the Phyn sometimes rests his hopes on what may seem small in the mind of the nurse, she must therefore follow his directions most implicitly; except as in circumstances before alluded to- On the nurse depends most important responsibilities; the faithful administration of the medicines, in <u>time</u> and manner; the giving drinks and nourishments; attention to comfort and cleanliness; keeping the room quiet; procuring its proper ventilation; preserving a proper temperature of the air of the room; regulating the warmth of the Patient; the examination and preservation of his excretions; her management of his sitting up; making of the bed; the proper attention to the utensils for the evacuations; the mode of giving him drinks; the application & dressing of blisters; the administration of enemata; & management of the patient during Convalescence.

The only part that Sister Matilda left out in the previous paragraph is "the rule to be followed by the nurse must therefore be obvious; namely to follow them, most implicitly."[203] While there is no explicit note as to why Sister Matilda leaves out this sentence, it is plausible that she left it out because the Daughters of Charity had their own *Common Rules*, which they followed implicitly in practice rather than the physician's rules. The first State Nurse Practice Acts in America were not established until the early twentieth century. Prior to that time, the sisters' *Regulations* served the purpose: *The*

Rule of 1812: Regulations for the Society of Sisters of Charity in the United States of America[204] was the document of rules under which Sister Matilda and her students initially performed their ministry and nursing services.

The next sections in Dewees' book that Sister Matilda also excluded explicated his definition of the moral qualities of a nurse. He stated that

> she should possess moral honesty, that she may completely understand her situation as regards those, whose orders from the nature of her office, she has voluntarily bound herself to obey. Her duty consists in passive obedience; and when she refuses this, she breaks a contract; and if she follow her own promptings in the management of the patient, she betrays a trust, by which, she may counteract the best devised plan of treatment.[205]

The Daughters' rule on obedience from the inception of the Community in France never suggested "passive" obedience. Hence it is apparent from Sister Matilda's edits of this renowned physician's beliefs about nursing that she was aware of the physician rhetoric and struggle for greater sociocultural authority in healthcare. Sister Matilda, in the fashion of a cultural diplomat, read and utilized what she agreed with in the famous author's book and left the rest.

[Advices] **The nurse shd be cleanly in person, apparel & habits. She shd after each meal rinse her mouth, that the breath, or flavor of what she had taken disturb the weak stomach of her patient –**
Her hands must be always clean –

This brief hygiene section was adapted by Sister Matilda. The next section was taken nearly verbatim from Dewees:

[Advices] <u>too</u> **much duty must not be given her, or she may fail at a moment, when of all others, her services may be most necessary. [*Pg 48*] To prevent this, ~~her~~ her health, strength & constitution shd be consulted, that no more**

be put upon her than she will be able to bear – In cases
of long protracted illness therefore, other assistance
shd be added, so as to give her occasional rest.

The following paragraphs are Sister Matilda's voice:

[Advices] This is better than to withdraw her entirely, for she having
become acquainted with his strengths, habits & disposition,
is, during his sickness, almost necessary for him, as also,
any matter of pain or annoyance wd now cause him to feel,
that it is from the change of nurses. This interfering with his
quiet & content, interrupts improvement, besides the reality
of very frequently being seriously important to the patient –
When the disease is acute, no or very little talking
or conversation shd be allowed in his room – If some
conversation may be, let it always be of a cheerful nature,
in a tone of voice that the patient may hear it distinctly
without straining his attention – and never relate a thing of
fatal or sad termination – whispering must never be used in
the sick room – The nurse must speak to her sick in a low,
kind, gentle and respectful manner – just loud enough to
be heard without the patient being obliged to ask her what
she said – Therefore she shd speak plainly, simply and in
proper terms – She shd never be "talkative"- Sickness may
become supportable by a nurse of kind, willing & amiable
deportment, & the obligation of gratitude is long felt by
the object of her affectionate care – So important is this,
that it is often necessary for recovery, & the contrary has
destroyed the nervous, sensitive or debilitated sufferer ⏝

Sister Matilda provided one paragraph of instruction on the topic of
quiet in the sickroom. Dewees spent two pages giving instructions point
by point as to when the nurse could and could not speak in the sickroom
and how to control noises such as "creaking" shoes and doors.[206] Sister
Matilda may have considered Dewees' level of detail too ordinary to
include in her text.

Of the Faithful Administration of Medicines

[*Advices*] [*Pg 49*] The power of medicine over disease, is owing to its proper selection. This belongs to the Phyn, but it depends too often upon the nurse, whether it be efficacious or otherwise – In many cases, life itself is at the mercy of the nurse, as she may faithfully or negligently perform her duty.[207] How necessary is it then, that this important personage, shd feel the responsibility attatched to her situation; & be influenced by a conscientious regard, for the proper fulfilment of the duties, her position has imposed upon her.

In insisting on the entire conformity of the Nurse to the directions of the Phyn however, we repeat, there are exceptions to this rule –

The previous sentence is Sister Matilda's voice. She then included Dewees' words:

[*Advices*] The patient as well as the Phyn are occasionally indebted to the nurse, for a judicious, or weltimed [*sic*] suspension, or perseverence [*sic*] in remedies, beyond the strict letter of her orders; and especially, when such departures have proceeded from a genuine exercise of judgement [*sic*]; and not from a preference for her own method, carelessness &c.–

Dewees' words at the end of the previous section were somewhat different from those recorded by Sister Matilda. He wrote, "such departures have proceeded, from a genuine exercise of judgment; and not from a wayward determination to disobey."[208] Sister Matilda substituted other reasons for not following orders to the letter that might be in keeping with what might occur in the work of a professional nurse: "preference for her own method and carelessness." The next section, another synthesis of Dewees, continued:

[*Advices*] Variety of constitutions may deceive or escape the

expectation of the Phyn, no one can be certain that his
remedy will act up to his desires; consequently were the
medicine not suspended, or sometimes urged, beyond the
common direction, much injury might follow.

In such instances, the judicious interference of the
nurse, may be highly valuable & fortunate. But she shd
not presume on a frequency of these, as they are rare.

The following section was added by Sister Matilda:

[Advices] Much depends on the mode of giving the medicine – A
cheerful, persuasive manner on the part of the nurse, with
disposition to lessen its nauseating effect, by having some
little thing [*Pg 50*] of pleasant taste to present immediately
after swallowing the disgusting dose. good sense must
prevent her from insisting on his taking it at a moment
when he discloses he cannot retain it, as in case he had
just vomited, or been greatly disposed towards it, wait,
in this case, even 10 or 15 minutes over time appointed

Of Giving Drinks and Nourishments

[Advices] [*Pg 51*] Greater errors are committed in the use of
drinks and nourishments, than in the neglect, or mal-
administration of medicine. A nurse may suppose
that thirst must be allayed whenever it is great & then
allow free drinks unmindful of quantity or quality –

This paragraph is very close to what Dewees wrote.

[Advices] This is sometimes of very serious moment, as it either
overloads the weak stomach, or causes it to be vomited,[209]
much to the inconvenience or injury of the patient. An
over <u>quantity</u> causes oppression; an improper <u>quality</u> may
seriously injure him.

> **The nurse, therefore, shd never depart from the**
> **quantity or quality of the drinks prescribed.**

Sister Matilda left out a number of specific instructions that Dewees included in his section on nourishments. He wrote, for example, that "from a vulgar belief, that all the 'herb teas' as they are called, are perfectly innocent, we find nurses in the constant habit of employing them, without the sanction of the physician, by which the most serious evils oftentimes arise."[210] Historical research has shown that nurses in the early and mid-nineteenth century, when Dewees' book was written, did indeed use herbal teas in their practice.[211] In Sister Matilda's tradition the practice also extended back to the time of the first Daughters of Charity, as noted in many of Louise de Marillac's writings,[212] and Sister Matilda seemed to have been perfectly at liberty to recommend hops tea for the patient who had adverse reactions to opiates. She, like many other nurses and physicians,[213] had great success with herbal teas, which they often believed to be "gentler" medicine than the medicines Dewees advocated. Dewees continued on in his book to say that "nurses should never be permitted to prescribe drinks, any more than medicine."[214] Sister Matilda also excluded that statement.

[Advices] The same care is necessary in point of food or nourishment – too much of the right kind wd be as bad as to give what had been objected to – If the over quantity remains undigested, he suffers much pain, and if it digest[s], it may afford too much nutriment to the system at a time when it requires less – Nothing shd be thought small in the mind of the Nurse, where the benefit or injury of her patient is in question –

Of Cleanliness in the Sick Room

[Advices] [Pg 52] Pure air is so necessary for the sick room, that every means must be used to preserve it.

Dewees wrote that "no single agent is of more importance in the sick chamber, than pure air."[215] Sister Matilda modified the language:

[Advices] On the nurse, this duty almost entirely depends. Every thing disgusting smell or sight must be removed as soon as possible – The evacuations removed immediately from the room; the body, & the bed clothes shd be as frequently changed as circumstances will allow. Fresh air shd be admitted as freely as the condition of the sick will allow of; no filth to remain on the floor, tables, bed, hearth &c.–

All the vessels used for medicines, drinks or nourishment, shd be cleansed the instant they are used; consequently, the same vessel or spoon shd not be used twice without its being cleaned, or used for two persons without washing.

Sister Matilda adopted most of what Dewees wrote on this subject; however, she must not have agreed with Dewees' exception that a vessel or spoon could be used twice in cases when it had been used for a substance that was not of a "nature to become offensive to any sense."[216] She did not include this.

[Advices] The Patients face & hands shd be often washed, especially when very warm, by wiping them with a towel wetted with cold water, or vinegar & water, unless there be chilliness when cold is applied – With the same view to comfort, the patient shd have his mouth frequently cleansed; by himself, if his strength will permit; and by the nurse, when this fails. This is particularly necessary in fevers wherein the tongue becomes dry and the teeth become encrusted or cased in a reddish glue.

Dewees actually wrote that "this attention is particularly grateful in the decline of such fevers as assume what is called the typhus type; that is, where the tongue becomes dry and the teeth encrusted."[217] Sister Matilda not only simplified the language for her nurse readers; she also added an additional symptom, the reddish glue, demonstrating her knowledge and most likely experience with fevers of the typhus type.

[Advices] For this purpose, yeast & water is very effectual; or a wash made of a tea spoonful of the sweet spirit of nitre, and a <u>table</u> spoonful of water. This is very acceptable to the mouth in the beginning of active fevers; where the tongue becomes loaded with a white, dense fur, [*Pg* 53] or is coated with a sticky[218] slime. The patient when able, finds comfort & amusement while performing this office for himself, by means of a tooth brush –

The following paragraph was added by Sister Matilda:

[Advices] but, where the mouth has been neglected, and the foul glue collected around the teeth, a soft mop must be gently passed along the gums, after being dipped in a proper wash, such as the yeast & water, or laudanum in water – At other times the rinsing of the mouth will do, but the mop shd be used once or twice a day. to prevent the mop from giving pain, let the soft linen be longer than the little stick you tie it on, wrapping it loosely for awhile, & then tying the thread tightly to prevent it coming off in the mouth. The mop may be an inch longer than the end of the stick and not too large, but just sufficient to carry enough of the wash on it. This precaution lessens the contagious or unhealthy tendency of the air around him –

Of Quiet in the Sick Room

[Advices] [*Pg* 54] There is scarcely any thing so distressing in the sick room, as noise. This must have the watchful attention of the nurse.

It is not enough to be quiet herself, but she must require all to observe this regulation.

> A talkative nurse is a great evil, and loquacity
> is for some the greatest annoyance.

Sister Matilda excluded Dewees' content here on equating the "superstitious" nurse with the talkative nurse and his concerns about gossip.[219] This content was covered in the Daughters' *Common Rules*.

[Advices]   In certain conditions of the nervous system, cheerful
conversation is highly beneficial, and in such cases,
an agreeable pleasantry, on a well chosen topic with
his kind nurse, will have a happy effect, but this
conversation must not be frequent or of long duration,
as excitement is almost always produced by them.

Sister Matilda's choice of language suggests a difference in intention from Dewees'. He wrote, "and in such cases, an agreeable, chatty, and well-instructed nurse, is of immense value. But even in such cases, the topics of conversation should be judiciously chosen, and their duration properly regulated."[220] While Dewees dictated specific behavior, Sister Matilda offered an explanation of the health principle of excitement underlying the behavior she advised that the nurse apply.

[Advices]   Another great misery & annoyance to the sick is when he
falls into the hands of a "bustling nurse" who is, forever
"putting things to rights" without, however, effecting the
object; and all the time makes so much noise that the patient
gets no sleep, however strong the desire – It were better, that
the hearth remained unswept, or the fire unrenewed for a
time, than the patient be deprived of his sleep, or roused
from it, as this sleep may hold an important item in his
recovery.

   Indeed a good nurse sees how to take advantage of the
times that will be least annoying to her patient – There
shd be no fixed time for, "Cleaning up the Room" As the
moment that will be of least annoyance to the sick shd be
the only one Selected.

Another great disturbance to the sick is the [*Pg 55*] creaking shoe. soft socks shd be drawn over such.

Often, near the sick, are the "Mess rooms", hear the rattling of spoons, knives, forks &c. are one continued jarring – Now the nurse shd get the habit of doing every thing quietly and without noise – And She must require the same care from all who assist her in the department – The <u>Comfort</u> of the sick, must be the <u>One</u> object and Motto of all in attendance on them <u>directly</u> or <u>indirectly</u>.

Sister Matilda created an edited version of Dewees' comments on quiet in the sickroom. The previous paragraph is one major difference in Sister Matilda's version, however; she used the term "mess rooms." This was not used by Dewees and therefore may be assumed to have been a nursing term. She also gave instructions to the nurses to include their patient attendants in learning the "one object," the comfort of the sick. She continued with her excerpts of Dewees' instruction:

[*Advices*] The door shd not be constantly on the go, if it must not remain open, then let as few come in as possible, otherwise the sick get no rest – have the door in good repair, that is, the hinges well oiled, and the door easy to open.

If your patient is sleeping, do not <u>allow</u> the door to be opened – This may be observed by pushing the feathered end of a quill thro' the key hole – This has become a speaking practice in some Hospitals – Exclude all such visitors as might endanger the safety of your patient or you may cause permanent mischief.

Of Ventilating the Sick Room

[*Advices*] [*Pg 56*] We mean by this, the removal of the foul or impure air, for that which is pure – This may be done by opening the doors and windows for a time – The frequency for doing this must be regulated by the season of the year; by the state of the weather; and the nature of the disease – In cold weather the air does not so soon become unhealthy as in warm weather, and the circulation of the air is also assisted by fire, & consequently more frequently changed.

If the weather be wet, either in warm or cold, too much air shd not, must not, be admitted immediately into the sick room – No damp air must be admitted, but, inner doors may perhaps produce the necessary ventilation – The good Sense of the Attendants must regulate this.

Fever and other acute diseases will require a more frequent ventilation than chronic affections, except when the latter is attended by profuse & offensive discharges –

The previous content on ventilation in Dewees' words was edited significantly by Sister Matilda.

[Advices] Some use burning, what they call sweet herbs, rosin, sugar, tar, frankincense &c, or decomposing vinegar on a hot shovel, for the purpose of purifying the room or air, but <u>All</u> these or others similar to them, destroy a part of the vital air, and supply its place by what is worse – These methods shd therefore be strictly prohibited.

Sister Matilda added her own content to some of the instruction that Dewees gave on purifying the air in the sickroom. She agreed with Dewees (i.e., included the content) that the substances listed destroyed a part of the vital air when burned for the purpose of purifying the air. Sister Matilda added "decomposing vinegar" to Dewees' list. Vinegar had been used as an antiseptic by the Daughters of Charity since the time of Louise de Marillac, who included the use of it in the Nurses' Daily Schedule (*See Appendix C*).

Regulating the Warmth of the Patient

Sister Matilda excluded all the comments by Dewees on regulating patient warmth. This is not surprising, given the critical tone of his statements, such as: "There is not one point in nursing, that has, so little system, or that is directed with so little judgment as the warmth of the patient. Nurses upon this point have no principles to direct them" and "she refuses to comply with the earnest prayer of the almost burnt up patient to, 'remove some of his coverings.'"[221] She wrote instead:

[*Advices*] [Pg 57] If he complains of feeling cold or chilly more covering shd be put upon him until a more comfortable sensation is restored, but after a reaction has taken place, and the patient complains of being too warm, the bed clothes must now be made lighter, or that they be gradually removed so as to gain back the pleasurable or usual state again.

Therefore the quantity of covering should always be made to suit the patient.

Examination & Preservation of the Excretions

[*Advices*] [Pg 58] This duty is too often neglected, important as it is ___ _____ A nurse should ask the physician if he desires the evacuations to be kept for his inspection, and if he does, they may be set aside, but not in the sick room – And she herself should also examine them, as well for her greater information as to be able to tell the Dr of them, in case some thing prevented his seeing them – The same case as regards the urine –

The only sentence that Sister Matilda used from Dewees' section on examination of excretions is the first sentence about the importance of the duty and that it was often neglected. After that, Dewees wrote that a nurse, "not being capable herself of drawing conclusions from the varied appearances of the evacuations, the nurse very often does not even inspect them, much more preserve them for the physician."[222] Sister Matilda taught her nurses to inspect evacuations and ask the physician if they wanted to see them. Dewees made a footnote in his book that he "almost constantly" required that evacuations be kept. Keeping evacuations was not exactly practical for the nurses and housekeepers of a hospital. Sister Matilda's suggestion that nurses ask physicians about their desires regarding preservation of evacuations would have helped to maintain better hygiene of the individual sickroom, as well as the hospital environment as a whole. She then suggested that the sisters learn from physicians and experienced nurses how to diagnosis disease and patient condition from evacuations. There is no mention in Dewees' book or in Sister Matilda's *Advices* about documenting or "charting" their assessments.

[Advices] It is well for a nurse to say simply to the Dr while he examines them; Dr, what term do you give this appearance? or if a more experienced nurse can give you this information, gain it of her ___ _____ A Diarrhoea, produces only free discharges without pain, seeming to empty the bowels entirely, when it is produced by bad food, or <u>too</u> much food – These discharges are often the cure also – But when the diarrhoea is from cold, or sudden check of perspiration &c; we see, mucus, or slime mixed with the excretion.

In Bilious Diarrhoea, the stools are loose, copious, & of a bright yellow, or green – The urine is then also deeply tinged with bile __

We see, therefore, that it is highly important to know what the discharges are, as they bespeak the character of the disease ___

Of the Patient's Sitting Up

Sister Matilda challenged Dewees' criticisms of nurses again in his section on sitting up. She excluded such remarks as his introductory statement that "an overweening anxiety on the part of the nurse to have the patient sit up, is often productive of serious consequences."[223] Whereas Dewees' book had two pages of detailed prescriptions for the activity, Sister Matilda chose to write about this task in her own words.

[Advices] [Pg 59] do not be too hasty for having the patient sit up. This action is an exercise which requires strength to suit

264

it – Exercise being a remedy, the patient's condition must make it proper, and only so much, & no more must be taken at a time – It calls for a <u>dose</u> of exercise according to the measure of strength the patient has at the time – Sitting up, is a stimulant & increases the pulse to twenty strokes more in the minute, than in a lying position, & such as often shews its unfriendly effects in fever – And when the patient is too weak for it, the heart performs its functions so rapidly, that the exhaustion that follows causes fainting in a few minutes – Therefore much care is required, in getting the patient out of bed. It is better that he rise oftener than to sit one minute longer than his strength bears comfortably; while the patient is up, some warm covering shd be put around him, & prevent a current of air from being on him, or damp air from him.

Making the Bed of the Sick

Dewees began this section on the same critical note. He wrote, "This necessary arrangement is almost always badly conducted."[224] Sister Matilda's comments agreed with the sentiment of the potential seriousness of moving a patient when he or she should not be moved; however, she did not use Dewees' bed-making content in her text.

[Advices] [*Pg 60*] The same care is necessary for this, as when he is judged able to sit up awhile – I have known persons, absolutely recovering, thrown back and die from having been taken out of bed even while the bed was being made – He may be moved about on his mattress, that is, from a warm spot to a cooler, or even the linen, but well dried, may be changed while he is on the bed – and, if he is able, a bed might be put [a]longside his own, and then be gently lifted on it, but, I repeat, when he is this weak, the change is better made on his bed.

If the strength of the patient allows it, spread the bed up twice a day for fever cases _____

265

> When the patient's condition admits of it, and
> he has been a long time in one room, or corner of
> a room, you may, with great benefit, move him to
> another, it is for him a change of air, & perhaps, views,
> but, if he gets home sick for his old place, indulge
> him, for, discontent prevents improvement __

Sister Matilda demonstrated how nurses could be creative when managing the sick room.

[Advices] A weak patient often loses ſtrength, or is kept from gaining
it by the trouble & pain they are put to for making their
evacuations, therefore, every Room, or, bed should have a
bed pan & urinal – A patient will insiſt on rising as long
as possible, but the nurse should not allow this when
they are too weak for it, and, even when they seem able,
great assiſtance may be given by the nurse – Before the
pan is offered to the sick, a pillow shd be placed under
the back, to prevent the hollow that wd otherwise diſtress
them. This neglect, is the cause of the sick objecting to
the pan __ *[Pg 61]* Every exertion muſt be ſpared the
patient, for, when every leaſt attention, requires exertion,
little by little, ſtrength is drained or used up in these
frequent, tho' seemingly small efforts – – A tumbler,
bowl, cup &c. are usually used for drinking out of, in
sick rooms, but, <u>neither</u> of these shd be found in a well-
regulated sick room, but, the <u>sick-cup</u> as it is called, shd
<u>alone</u> convey drinks while they are confined to bed __

The "sick-cup" was a Dewees recommendation for sparing the patient's energy. Sister Matilda also added that a phial could be used. A phial is a small bottle typically used for liquid medicines.

[Advices] A phial also is convenient, and this, corked, can lie
on his bed, when he wants a mouth-ful only, but,
frequently __ this, the sick can get themselves, and

they prefer it on this account, when able to get it __

Throughout the text on sickroom management, Sister Matilda (and Dewees) recommended that patients take care of themselves as soon as they were able. The nurses in a hospital were responsible for monitoring the patient's ability for self-care as well as his or her need for dependent care. This was another way that the value of self-care and becoming one's own doctor was expressed in American mid-nineteenth-century culture. The responsibility for promoting self-care continues today in the ongoing theoretical and clinical research and practice of scholars, such as those who work with Dorothea Orem's "Self Care Deficit Nursing Theory."[225]

Of Dressing Blisters

[Advices]   **[Pg 62] This is an important duty, as the efficacy and success, as well as the great comfort of the sick are all concerned in it –**

Sister Matilda described dressing of blisters as an "important" duty. Dewees referred to it as "the most useful and important part of a nurse's duty."[226] Although she included a section on blistering earlier in *Advices*, Sister Matilda added this second section, suggesting that it was a skill the sisters needed to have at the time of the writing of the text. Somewhat lengthier than other sections, Sister Matilda's section on blistering is actually an edited excerpt of Dr. Dewees'.

[Advices]   **When the circulation is languid, the spot for the application shd be first rubbed with some stimulating liquid to give the skin heat and action – The Blister shd be spread thickly so as to produce the speediest effect – Some think that if a blister rise at all, it is enough – this is a mistake – A blister spread too thin, soon dries, and only raises the cuticle, & even for this, must remain on a long time – whereas, a well made plaster, goes as deep as necessary, and in a much shorter time – To prepare the skin for the blister, it <u>must</u> be first <u>rubbed</u> with Spts [*Spirits*] of hartshorn,[227] or, turpentine,**

cayenne pepper & brandy, or same such – But where the circulation is active, & great heat is already in the spot, these must <u>not</u> be used – Again, care must be used for the blister not slipping from the proper place, for then no good is done, and as they are generally very painful, they are always necessary when ordered, and should therefore receive due attention – Blisters are better held in their place by adhesive plaster than by bandages only, for bandages must be pretty tight to keep them from slipping when the patient moves about, but the aid of adhesive plaster[228] & then, bandages <u>comfortably</u> tight, will do – When they are applied to the legs, they are kept in the right place by drawing a stocking over it – The common time for a blister to draw is, about 12 hours, but, circumstances may require a departure from [Pg 63] from [*sic*] this Rule[229] – 8 hours wd be enough for <u>children</u>, or even in less, and it shd be examined at 6 hours, & dressed if enough drawn – Again there are in some grown persons a peculiar sensibility, that calls for less than what is ordinary – Children suffer less from blisters than adults, and might not give the timely notice of its having drawn sufficiently – On the nurse, then depends the good or ill use of this important remedy – If the bandaging is too tight, the humors to be acted on cannot act, and, if too loose, they produce no action, except as they have slipped about to some wrong spot, perhaps on some bone that presses the bed, and then much unnecessary and often injurious torment is given the sick.

It is not well to spread gauze over the blister plaster _____ Sometimes, no more is <u>wanting</u> from a blister, than to excite inflammation. In this case, the blister must be often looked at, and removed as soon as it is well reddened –

Some blisters produce so much irritation or inflammation, before the time for removal, that the plaster may be removed, & thus a basilicon salve dressing, or even a soft milk & bread poultice may finish its course to the relief of the patient – blisters ordered for the legs, are meant for

the inner part or calves of the leg, and for the legs or arms,
shd be longer than wide – for the arms, the inner part also
are intended, and not so near the hand as to prevent feeling
the pulse _____ when ordered for the chest, the
seat of pain is the spot for it, but if the chest is all involved,
let it go as near the throat as possibly, [*sic*] and running
downwards, or according to the length of disease, or its
force – When for the neck, [*Pg 64*] put it on the back of the
neck, one inch below the hair, & let it run down the spine
to <u>nearly</u> the bottom part of the shoulder blades – when
for the ears, is meant, that part, behind the ear that has no
hair, or in some cases, the hair is ordered to be shaved some,
so as to give larger surface, this is done when the disease
is of long standing – When ordered for the regions of the
stomach; all the space below the breast bone, and inclining
to the left side, <u>towards</u> the middle of the abdomen, or belly,
is meant. When ordered for the Abdomen, nearly the whole
surface of the belly, is meant, or, if only one spot seems
to be affected, this then only, may be blistered _____

　　All of the following suggested measurements are taken from Dewees'
book:

[*Advices*]　The size of the blister, must vary with the size of the patient,
and their age – small, for young children, and increased
according to age. Their shape & form may vary according
to the part for their action – A large blister gives not much
more pain, while drawing than a small one, it is only more
painful as to the dressing & the position in bed - ___ for a
common sized person, the blister for the legs, shd be, from
7 to 8 inches long, & between 3 & 4 inches wide – for the
back, 7 or 8 inches long, & about 4 wide. for the chest, 7 or
8 inches long, & 6 or 7 wide – Or, for the whole chest, or
thorax, 8 or 9 inches long, & 7 or 8 broad – for the stomach,
from 8 to 9 inches long, & from 6 to 7 broad, – the greatest
size for the stomach, is, from side to side __ If the whole of

the abdomen is to be covered, from 10 to 11 inches long,
& from 8 to 10 broad – for the temples, they are rounded
& may be from an inch, to an inch & a half, in size – All
these must vary according to the size of the patient __

[Advices]   [Pg 65] Before <u>dressing</u> the blister, let every thing necessary
be in complete readiness – the plasters spread, & by the
bed – All the rags at hand; and a pair of well-cutting,
sharp pointed scissors – Snip every blister of any Size,
so to let the water run out, having a cloth under the
part to prevent the clothes or bed from being soiled –

The last part of the sentence about having a cloth under the body
part with the blister to prevent soiling of the bed or patient's clothes was
Sister Matilda's advice. Nurses typically have certain ways of performing
procedures that are protective of patient comfort and the hygiene of the
sickroom; but they also are pragmatic and try not to make additional
work for themselves. This is one example of a professional tip made by an
experienced expert to a novice.

[Advices]   the very small blisters, or portions of water, will have filled
better by the next dressing, & will not give so much pain
then – The skin shd <u>never</u> be removed from the blistered
part, however desirable the irritation may be, for the pain
caused to the patient can hardly be compensated – It wd be
better to reapply the blister immediately after its healing,
than to strip the skin off.
A blister shd scarcely ever be washed, tho' this is a
common fault.– It never does good, & often injury, by
exposing it too long to the air, produces chilliness, & is
fatiguing to the sick – ~~remove the particles of fly as stick~~
~~to the raw surface, but those on the dead skin will do no~~
~~harm, and will come off, by after dressings.~~ It is better to
leave the particles of fly on, than give the patient any pain,
or keep them longer uncovered – If a continued discharge
is desired, the basilicon ointment[230] is to be used – if this is

not necessary, simple cerate[231] is to be used – Either of these
is to be spread on, thin, old linen rags, or soft rags, at least,
& repeated twice in 24 hours, or only once if the discharge
is small – When the blister, or sore part is of big size, have
the salve dressings cut in several slips or pieces, as they can
be withdrawn without much pain – The plaster shd only
cover the sore surface, as the sound skin becomes unhealthy,
if it is covered over with the salve. [*Pg 66*] Sometimes the
sore becomes extremely painful & inflamed – this pain is
best subdued by a soft milk & bread poultice, in which is
melted a small portion of <u>fresh</u> hog's lard, or newly churned
butter, before salt has been put to it – If the poultice fail to
ease it, linseed oil & lime water, equal parts & shaken so
as to form a cream-like thickness may be often applied –
When the itching stage of a blister is very annoying – use,
an infusion of slippery elm,[232] or flax seed or very fresh
lard into which some laudanum has [*been*] mixed –

Of Relapse

[*Advices*] [*Pg 67*] The return of disease should be wisely & carefully
guarded against – Some of the following, usually give rise to
a return –
　　Stimulating food or drinks too soon indulged in – for,
if the stomach is unable to digest, it must be vomited,
or causes diarrhoea – both injure the patient, and, after
having put him to severe suffering for several hours –
<u>If</u> the <u>stomach</u> is able for it, too much nourishment is
formed, and will be too suddenly sent into the weakened
& irritable blood vessels, which usually rekindles fever.

　Sister Matilda took pages of commentary by Dewees and whittled it
into one paragraph (above), followed by Dewees' rules for the convalescent
patient, which she also summarized below:

[*Advices*] No animal substance, in any shape or form should be given

271

during fever, nor very soon after its cessation, ~~least it~~ lest
it return by the over-stimulating quality of nourishment
– When a change from the lightest diet may be made, this
change must be of the lightest kind of animal substance, as:
weak chicken water; weak beef, or veal tea; or the diluted
juice of oysters should be first resorted to – these should be
given in small quantities, and repeated at stated intervals,
day & night, if the patient is very feeble, provided, it will
not interrupt important sleep.– Three days using these
kind of nourishments, might prepare the system for a little
stronger food, and, the next advance should observe the
same moderation: the soft end of five or six oysters; a soft
boiled egg, or cold custard in its mildest form – After such
diet for three or four days, the patient may be indulged in
a small piece of boiled mutton; the breast of a partridge or
pheasant; turkey, or chicken – And after as many more he
may have a small piece of rare done beef or venison steak;
or mutton chop. At his noon meal of this kind, he may have
a tumbler of Ale, or porter & water, if this drink does not
cause headache [*Pg 68*] flatulency or sour stomach ___

During the whole stage of convalescence, the <u>bowels</u>
should be strictly attended to – one evacuation daily is
absolutely necessary; but purging must be avoided most
carefully –

As to exercise, he must accustom himself to what he is
able for in moving around his sick room, or parlor, before
he tries the open air. And a close[*d*] carriage should be first
used for this, and when he is ready for walking, and, the
<u>weather</u> <u>suitable</u>, he can be benefited by this exercise – As
soon as he is done with phials, pill-boxes, bed-pans, &c. take
them from the room so as to leave nothing in his sight that
would too much remind him of his illness __

Great care must be used to keep him from currents
of cold or damp air – and avoiding equally damp places
– He should not take a <u>full</u> drink of cold water, tho' so
desirable to a convalescent. Avoid calve's-feet, beef or

chicken jellies, and all other gelatinous substances – tho' these are so often offered to sick, they form actually the most <u>indigestible</u> portion of all animal substances, for glue it is literally, and to these are added wine, spices, sugar & acid – What <u>weak</u> stomach is ready for this? – These jellies should be banished from the sick room __

Fever ⌒

The following paragraph is in Dewees' book verbatim:

[*Advices*] [*Pg 69*] The term fever implies heat; but a mere in increase of heat does not constitute fever, since we may have considerable increase of heat, without the system laboring under this affection; and on the other hand, we may have fever with a cool, even a partially cold skin, as sometimes happens in yellow fever – <u>Generally</u>, in fever there is a sensation of chilliness, followed by an increase of heat; the pulse gives a greater number of strokes in a given time; while several functions of the body are more or less impaired, and the strength of the limbs particularly, is diminished –

The next paragraph is by Sister Matilda:

[*Advices*] Sometimes only a part of the body suffers from increase of heat in fever; as: the extremities may be cold, while the head, chest & abdomen may be unnaturally [*sic*] warm.

The next paragraph is Sister Matilda's summary of Dewees' text:

[*Advices*] The same uncertainty may happen with the pulse; its frequency by no means establishes fever; we may have a very frequent pulse without fever, or an unusually slow one, when it is really present; and this may or not may not be accompanied by increase of heat. The pulse may, therefore, be slow or frequent; strong or weak; hard or

soft, with or without fever – Fever then is occasioned
by derangement of the nervous & sensorial functions,
derangement in the circulating functions. derangement
in the secreting & excreting functions – the knowledge
of these derangemens form the true characters of fever –
Altho' there are a variety of fevers, they all have a general,
as well as a particular plan of treatment. All have to be
treated more or less upon the same general principles;
tho' certain of them may exact a specific management _ ~ ~ ~

The next paragraphs are a close adaptation of Dewees':

[Advices]   [*Pg 70*] As there is in almost all cases of fever, a strong
determination to the head, or head-ache, the patient should
be kept as quiet as possible; & should delirium attend,
company must be prohibited, also any circumstance that
might tend to augment it, & all objects removed that seemed
to attract his attention – he shd see as few faces as possibly
[*sic*], or only those employed in nursing him. the room shd
be kept pretty dark. No unnecessary conversations, and
whispering absolutely forbidden, for the patient always
believes himself to be the object of their remarks &c – –
carpet around the bed saves much annoying noise, and the
attendants shd wear socks over their shoes – In Wards of
fever, the floor might be mopped over once or twice of [*sic*]
a fine day, but not flooded over as for Scrubbing – It is also
good to sprinkle the floor occasionally with Vinegar[233] – the
bedclothing shd be regulated by the feelings of the patient –
When he is chilly, put more on him – when he complains of
too much, remove some, tho' if he be sweating, care must be
used, lest it be checked –

Cool drinks are proper for fevers – but when perspiring,
or about to do so, they shd not be <u>cold</u>. It often happens
in the higher grades of fever, the thirst calls for more
drink than the stomach can well support, then vomiting
follows – To prevent this, small pieces of Ice may be kept

near the patient & that a piece may from time to time be
taken – or if ice cannot be had, a spoonful of cold water
may be given often – the drinks of fevered patients shd be
palatable, but free from all stimulus, except in such cases
as call for stimulus - they may be some of the following:
toast-water, baum [*sic*]-tea, lemonade - current jelly in
water, molasses & water with a little vinegar, the [*Pg 71*]
water off of dried cherries, very weak milk & water, barley-
water – flax-seed tea, either with or without lemon juice.

Sister Matilda listed all of the same drinks that Dewees suggested on
page 71 of his book, with the exception of sorrel water. Sorrel (*Rumex
acetosa*) is an herb that Lydia Maria Child, who also quoted Dr. Dewees
in her book, recommended be steeped in milk. This beverage, which she
called "sorrel whey," was drunk for allaying fever, but the sorrel water was
not noted as being used in fever.[234] Sorrel is a pot herb that can be used like
spinach and has a high oxalic acid content like spinach. The acidity may
be the reason that Sister Matilda rejected Dewees' recommendation for
sorrel in fever; she suggested the cooling apple tea instead. Sister Matilda
continued her adaptation of Dewees' instructions on fever:

[*Advices*] Apple-tea, that is: warm or hot water poured on Sliced
apples, and drank when cold. We have named many, so as to
admit of choice, but simple cold water may almost always be
allowed, & is also most palatable in great heat.

In the commencement of any acute disease, little or no
food is required — Nature often, kindly assists the patient by
taking away all appetite – When nourishment is proper in
fever, it shd be given by three or four spoons ful [*sic*], large
or small, as the patient may be large or small – It shd consist
of weak milk & water: thin tapioca: sage or arrow root: gruel
of indian or oat meal; ripe fruits in moderate quantities:
when in season, such as oranges, grapes, or roasted apple
may also be given – A cup of weak tea or coffee is often
grateful to the sick, & may almost always be allowed. But in
the commencement of any acute disease little or no food is

required __

If circumstances, and the condition of the patient will
allow of it, it will be well to Change his linnen [sic] and
sheets daily, especially in those fevers that pass off by sweats,
at the same time, great care is wanting as to the perfectly
dry state of these, and the proper time and manner of doing
it. – The times for giving the remedies must be carefully
attended to, for a neglect, or mistaken condescencion [sic]
or tenderness, may allow the proper time to pass, which
another time could not supply for – the <u>time</u>, therefore,
is often as necessary to be observed, as the medicine, or
remedy itself, since, the condition of the system governs its
necessity or applications ___

In fevers, during hot weather, the fresh air will be
serviceable to the patient, and with little bed- [Pg 72]
clothing – if he be very hot, and fresh air cannot be admitted
in to the room, a sponged squeezed out of cool water may
be wiped over his forehead, & arms & body of the patient –
but, remember this, or even the fresh air is never to be used
when there is a moist skin, or tendency to sweat, and his
clothes must not be made damp by the sponging – If cough,
or other affections of the chest exist, sponging cannot be
thought of – Cool, or even cold drinks are most useful and
acceptable in fever, & may be at times changed for small
pieces of ice put in them – but given in small quantities,
tho' frequently – but, when the body is moist, these must
be avoided, and warmer drinks used – a cough only,
without sweat or moisture, does not forbid cold drinks –

The following paragraph on treatment of sick stomach follows Dewees
very closely:

[Advices] Fevers of all kinds frequently are attended by sick stomach,
or even vomiting, and the nurse too often gives an emetic as
the cure, which nearly always does great harm to the sick –
But in such cases cathartic medicines of a moderately active

kind should be given first and if these fail, external remedies may be used – The internal remedy for this feature of the disease, Nausea, may be: Calomel 8 grains, white sugar the same, divided into 8 powders, giving one every hour in a little syrup, or scraped apple until the bowels are moved – If this does not act two or three tea-spoonful [*sic*] of calcined magnesia, in a little sweetened milk may be given, or an enema may be profitable. for this, take about a pint of hot water, to a table spoonful of common salt – when the salt is dissolved, & the water about warm enough, let it be given, and repeated in half an hour, or an hour if necessary –

If these fail, take this set of remedies: rich gum arabic water. (cold) [*Note: Parenthesis and enclosed words in original document*] milk & water, about a table spoonful every fifteen or twenty minutes – Or, you may [*Pg 73*] use with more certainty of success the following julep:

> Take super saturated soda   1 ½ drachm
> powdered gum arabic   2 drachms
> oil of. mint, –   4 drops
> white sugar,   2 drachms
> water,   4 ounces–

Of this a table-spoonful may be taken every hour or half hour – Should none of these answer, take a few ounces of blood from the stomach by leeches, this may be preceded or followed by a plaster of mustard flour & vinegar until the skin smart a little, or it may be useful to apply a blister, if the vomiting be obstinate – <u>these, in case a physician cannot be had</u> ____

The underlined content above was added by Sister Matilda to the Dewees content. She then continued with her summary of Dewees on bleeding and sweating.

[*Advices*]   Altho' Bleeding is considered almost a universal remedy for

fever, in its hot stage, yet, being a remedy of great power,
it must be used with great judgement [*sic*] as to time &
quantity – Blood must not be taken when the fever has, or is
about to subside, or in a Sweating Stage – and there are very
rare exceptions to this –

There is a remedy so popular for the cure of fever, as
sweating; and none, perhaps, has been more abused, as,
there is a heat of the body which rises above sweating
point, and in this state no perspiration can be gained, and
a gentle sweating is preferable to a profuse sweat – when
a profuse sweat comes on, we should reduce it gradually
by removing little by little, the bed-clothes, or the heat
of the room, tho' this last is attended with danger – he
may cease also the drinks that had been given to effect
sweating – and when his body is perfectly dry again, then
all the clothes wet by sweating, should be replaced by dry
ones – the determination of [*Pg 74*] fever usually is to the
brain, the liver, the spleen or the lungs; & few remedies
are so proper in restoring this, as well chosen aperients,
or gentle purgatives – Besides, such matter in these cases,
are constantly forming and are necessary to be removed –
Some times there will be too much bile, again too little, &
both these extremes are to be helped by mild, but properly
selected cathartics – purgatives well chosen not only
evacuate the bowels, but the general system also, thus some
cathartics are much more useful than others – If possible, do
not not avoid having sweating and purging at the same time,
and even when not sweating, let the sick have his stockings
& warm slippers on when rising for the stool, or if he uses
the bed-pan, have a warm blanket around him & keep the
fresh air from him.

The use of blisters too, in fever must have their right
time for beneficial applications, and can only be used with
advantage when the pulse is soft, or, as some day: below
par – fever, in pleurisy, or inflammation of the liver, point
out the spot for placing the blister, but, where the disease

does not shew local injury the ancles [sic] & wrists are to
be the parts blistered – if the ancles [sic] & wrists are so
slow in circulation or cold & languid, the insides of the
thigh, & above the elbows must be the places for them – A
blister may be left on for 12 or 14 hours, if not ready to
be removed sooner, but, in many cases, they are irritable
enough to remove sooner, & may be dressed with basilicon
ointment & the blisters, hardly formed, but perhaps too
painful to endure longer, will be fully formed by the
salve – Some suffer much from strangury in blistering,
but by removing & dressing as soon as they become very
painful [Pg 75] this terrible suffering is spared them __

The next section followed Dewees' content on intermittent fever:[235]

[*Advices*] Intermittent fever is that which leaves intervals perfectly
free from fever, and they may be called according to their
recurrence: daily, or quotidian – tertian, or every other
day: again when it occurs every fourth day it is called
quartan – When it occurs in the Spring it is called, vernal;
when in the fall: Autumnal, which is usually of a severer
form – the paroxysms of intermittent fever are three: the
cold stage, the hot, & the sweating – in some the cold felt
is most intense with violent shaking – in others, some
trifling trembling only is felt. After the cold follows the
heat with dry skin, great thirst, head-ache, restlessness, the
tongue furred, the pulse frequent, & mostly hard & full –
Sometimes also, Stupor, delirium, convulsions & – After
the hot stage has had its course, a moisture is felt on the
forehead, presently it becomes general, and after sometime
no uncomfortable symptoms remain but weakness – Agues
are rarely fatal except by inducing diseases on the spleen,
liver or producing dropsical affection of the abdomen.
Warm drinks & warm applications to the stomach, feet &
legs are good for shortening the cold stage. Some Drs find
30 drops of laudanum given as soon as the patient felt the

coldness coming on, to have favorable influence, or repeated in 15 minutes if no feeling of warmth was produced – this, however, could not be used where there [*sic*] tendency of blood to the head or ſtupor – nor could laudanum be employed unless blood-letting or purging had been previously employed – After recovery from intermittent fever, great care [*Pg 76*] should be [*taken*] to prevent relapse or return of the disease. Imprudence or exposure may cause the attacks to come on about the seventh, ninth or thirteenth day, the laſt, perhaps, the moſt common. The bowels should be kept moved once a day, but by no means purged – great fatigue & dampness should be avoided for some time _____.

Bliſters are powerful helps in intermittent fever, but the[*y*] should not be used too early. [*End*]

⌒ *Nurses' Scope of Practice* ⌒

Sister Matilda not only produced a nursing text comprising her own thoughts on the nursing care of patients and on the treatment of disease, but she also constructed, albeit politely, a rebuttal for and professional commentary on the definition of a professional nurse set forth by a leading physician of the mid-nineteenth century. She had the experience and expertise to write her own text on nurses' scope of practice that not only encompassed the realm of nursing care but also in some cases reached deeply into the emerging physician domain. Sister Matilda had the level of medical as well as nursing knowledge that she needed to accomplish her ministry, especially the care of the insane. She was comfortable with her knowledge and was able to read, translate, and excerpt one of the most revered medical texts of her time for her students. Did that ease come with study or clinical experience? Most likely it was experience that helped her to critique Dr. Dewees' recommendations for patient care, especially as it related to nursing and sickroom management. As far as her critical analysis of Dewees' medical recommendations, such as who should prescribe drinks for patients, Sister Matilda may have also drawn upon her experiences from her family of origin.

Sister Matilda had two brothers who studied medicine at the University of Maryland. William graduated in 1827, just before Sister Matilda entered the Sisters of Charity at Emmitsburg; he died in 1830. Her younger brother Felix (1815–1873), whom she loved very much,[236] graduated in 1836 after writing his thesis on "Fever." The thesis was eleven pages in length, handwritten, and approximately double spaced.[237] His argument for his proposed treatment of fever was based upon Dr. John Eberle's writings. Her brothers' writings may have inspired her to write her own book, but even without her commentary on Dewees in the final sections of *Advices*, Sister Matilda's text was significantly more comprehensive than her brother Felix's thesis, which earned him a degree to practice medicine.

The Daughters recorded that Sister Matilda was considered an "oracle" even among physicians of the Baltimore healthcare community.[238] *Advices* certainly suggests the reasons that may have been so. Sister Matilda's work also may have inspired her nephew, Felix's son Oscar (1843–1889), also a physician; Oscar wrote papers on the "curable forms of insanity," on which he gave a lecture on April 1, 1873, to the Medical and Chirurgical Faculty of Maryland. Although there were no degrees for nurses in the mid-nineteenth century, let alone doctoral degrees, Sister Matilda's vast knowledge of nursing care, particularly of the insane, as recorded in *Advices*, was exemplary for her time.

CHAPTER 6

~ ♏ ~

Revising the Legend
and Repealing the Myth

Sister Matilda wrote *Advices Concerning the Sick* not only to document the procedures she employed in the care of the sick and insane but also to record her spiritual intention, the way in which she approached her care. In their remembrances of her, Sister Matilda's students confirmed that her nursing instruction had conveyed a humanity and spirituality that infused every simple assignment she taught them about patient care. Preparing toast-water became more than a daily chore for the young sisters. Sister Matilda transformed the task into a caring, enlightened ritual by instructing her nurses to seek a different level of awareness regarding the work. One student Sister-Nurse wrote of her teacher, Sister Matilda:

> She seemed always by her exterior recollection to live in the divine presence and we could not but be reminded of the All-seeing Eye, when we beheld her. . . . She would frequently come when I was preparing drinks for the sick to see how I did it. On one occasion I was preparing toast-water for them when she entered, looking at it, she said smiling: "take pains with that, and remember for who you do it. Everything we do is calculated to raise our heart to God. Even the giving of a piece of bread can recall to our minds, His love in coming to us in the holy Communion."[1]

Preparing toast-water for patients was not the most challenging of duties nor would it have been the most inspiring for young DC Nurses, who may have wished for more opportunity to exercise greater nursing skill or share their religion with others. Sister Matilda gave her students reasons for transforming the simplest of duties that might have been sheer drudgery into opportunities for conscious attention to a practice of meaningful preparation of remedies for the sick. For this enlightened exchange of instruction, Sister Matilda's students loved and respected her. The teachings for this young sister did not end with the toast-water, however. The sister wrote that when she left Mount Hope, Sister Matilda, knowing that she was esteemed by her student and "fearing that she might speak her praise," said, "Whatever you may think or feel for me, learn to keep it to your self and only speak of it to God. Live for God and love to be hidden in Him."[2] The sister did not speak of Sister Matilda publicly until after her death. It was in that teachable moment that a young sister learned how to be a Daughter of Charity who fully embraced the virtues of humility, simplicity, and charity, as well as how to be a nurse.

In the final years of her life, Sister Matilda turned her compassionate eye toward the needs of her community's leaders and her sister companions. Although she did continue to work extensively with the poor in the Emmitsburg area, Sister Matilda's gifts for nursing, religious and spiritual instruction, and helping people through difficult transitions such as illness and death also were needed within her own Community.

⁓ *Later Years of Compassionate Care, 1855–1870* ⁓

The Daughters in the 1867 *Provincial Annals* described "old Sister Matilda" in this way:

> Everyone reverences Sister Matilda and looks upon her reverently as the little figure passes. Her lips are often moving in prayer as she goes along. Yet hearts do not cluster around Sister Matilda. There is an austerity of virtue about her which excites more respect than love. But the Poor! They love her. Their wants are her peculiar

charge, her deeply religious nature spiritualizes every service she renders, and they do not fear one whose acts prove how truly she considers herself their servant.[3]

Upon returning to Saint Joseph's Central House in Emmitsburg in 1855, Sister Matilda began to give basic instructions to pupils at the charity school and to employees of the laundry service. Rev. Hippolyte Gandolfo, one of the Vincentian clergy who was a chaplain, relied on Sister Matilda for the religious instruction of the men, both white and black, employed on the farm at St. Joseph's. Just as Sister Matilda was able to translate medical jargon into simpler English for her DC Nurse students, her religious spirit was known to overflow in ways that enabled her to speak to the hired men of eternal truths and the ways of God in a way that they could receive.[4] Sister Matilda kept a shrewd and maternal eye on their conduct and assembled them for prayer in the evenings, when she also gave brief instructions on such things as their duties on the farm and the festivals of the Church.

Her spiritual instruction was also extended to the new sisters in the Community. By 1855 Sister Matilda had been nursing the sick poor and insane for twenty-five years. The "interior trials" she was said to have experienced in her early years now served as the foundation for stories she told to young sisters still in an early stage of religious formation who were sent to her for spiritual instruction. Her closest companions described her ability to share the trials of her soul that she experienced as a young sister as a "humility" that was "truly admirable."[5] The Daughters described the qualities of Sister Matilda's expertise in the nursing care of the insane which she imparted to her students: She relied on gentleness, sweetness, benevolence, and a "rare modesty" that had an "astonishing influence" over others. They wrote that she had an "irresistible charm which gained the affection and commanded the esteem of all"[6] who interacted with her. Sister Matilda was "singularly gifted in comforting the afflicted. Her kind and compassionate heart would find a balm to soothe, if not to heal, the crushed and wounded spirit. Her charity would invent a thousand ways to divert them from their troubles."[7] One sister said of Sister Matilda:

> She was an eye to the blind, a staff to the lame, a precious
> balm to the wounded heart. She wept with those who
> wept and rejoiced with those who rejoiced.[8]

From these descriptions we see that Sister Matilda exhibited many of the qualities of a talented psychiatric nurse, whose faith gave her strength of identity that enabled her to be herself fully with others. She did not flaunt her strengths nor hide her weaknesses. Sister Matilda was masterful in a full range of human emotions, which she demonstrated as needed for the good of those whom she served. She was able to discern the needs of each patient, at times providing emotional support and encouragement and other times chastisement. She celebrated and cried with her patients, demonstrating her humanity, a quality that some might not have suspected was important to the DC Nurses, whom many described as "angels" at the bedside.

In February 1857 the DC Council named several sisters to a Committee on Hospitals. Members included Sister Matilda, Sister Othelia Marshall (1816–1888), and Sister Hieronymo O'Brien (1819–1898). Two years later the council decided that Sister Matilda, age 60, would substitute during the absences of Sister Ann Simeon Norris (1816–1866), who had filled the office of treasurer of the Community for twelve years and was away periodically on business. After the union with France, Sister Ann Simeon became Mother, or "Visitatrix," of the United States Province for the Daughters of Charity based at Emmitsburg. Sister Matilda was assigned to Saint Joseph's Central House until her death, although she traveled on Community business. She also was sent to various locations in Virginia, Pennsylvania, and Maryland to serve as a nurse during the Civil War years.

Civil War, Nursing Both Sides ⌒

The American DC actively participated in the relief effort during the Civil War.[9] Of approximately 800 DC, 270 sisters provided nursing care and spiritual assistance during the War at more than sixty sites in fifteen states.[10] Regiments of both armies utilized the sisters' property in Emmitsburg before the battle at Gettysburg. At one point the sisters fed as many of the approximately 80,000 half-starved Union troops occupying Emmitsburg as they could.[11] They provided battlefield care to wounded soldiers and the dying from both the Union and the Confederate armies without discrimination.

Sister Matilda and other sisters were missioned by Mother Ann Simeon to the war in response to requests for DC Nurses. Rev. James Francis Burlando, CM (1814–1873), the provincial director of the DC Province of the United States at the time, responded to requests from medical directors and officers from both the Confederacy and the United States government for DC Nurses. Rev. Burlando stipulated to both governments the conditions under which the sisters would serve. Later in his circular of October 30, 1866, he asked the sisters to write about their war experiences and send them to him. As a result Sister Matilda wrote first-person accounts of several sites. There are also documents attributed to her that she may have recorded from the memoirs of other sisters or summarized into composite accounts of the sisters' services on the transports embarking from White House Landing, Virginia (1862), the aftermath of the battle of Antietam, Maryland (1862), and services to war prisoners in Alton, Illinois (1864).[12]

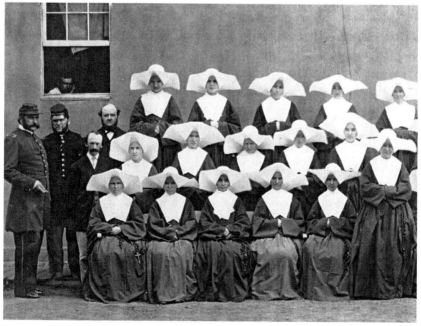

Fig. 6-1   *Daughters of Charity with officers at Satterlee Hospital 1862 – 1865*

In 1861 Sister Matilda had personal experience in nursing the sick and injured of both armies at Frederick, Maryland; Bolivar Heights at Harpers Ferry, West Virginia; and Winchester, Virginia. At Frederick she was the Sister Servant of the DC during their ministry to war victims at several locations in that city beginning in 1862. At age sixty-three she led DC Nurses into hospitals, where they took charge of the entire facility and saved the lives of hundreds of soldiers. The Daughters still endured religious prejudice from patients, especially when they first arrived at a hospital. But it did not take long for the soldiers to realize the expertise of the sisters' compassionate care. Sister Matilda distinguished herself by her untiring charity, her zeal in assisting the wounded both in body and soul. Her demeanor helped win the support of some of the individuals most prejudiced against Roman Catholics.

Sister Matilda also had assistance from medical directors, who were very supportive of the DC Nurses. When the medical director in Frederick took Sister Matilda and her companions through the hospital for the first time, he introduced the nurses to the sick by saying that "they would get their nourishment & remedies in time & proper manner now as the Srs. wd [would] do all these things for them."[13] As a result of the sisters' efforts, officers, private soldiers, and civilians of all classes of society became favorably impressed by their care of the sick and wounded of both the Union and Confederate armies. Soldiers often had to be convinced by clergy that the sisters were actually Catholic because they had "heard such terrible things" about Catholics.[14] Many of the soldiers became interested in the Catholic religion after learning that their caregivers were in fact Catholic. It was not unusual for the soldier patients to request religious instruction, pamphlets, and books on the Catholic faith; some even converted and were baptized.

Many Americans were turned around in their beliefs about Catholics as a result of the nursing care provided by the DC Nurses. A French chaplain wrote in his letters during the war that the mere presence of the sisters, the long hours they spent attending the sick was a "constant sermon" that, if it did not "enlighten the understanding of men, touched at any rate and won their hearts."[15] Just as the cholera epidemic had served to boost the reputation of the Daughters in 1832, the battlefield hospitals of the Civil War provided the sisters an opening for the promotion of a positive and pious image of Catholic life on behalf of their Church. The public had ample opportunity to compare the Daughters of Charity's works with other nurses, in particular men and Protestant women, who often had little or no preparation for battlefield nursing in the early days of the war. This helped to overcome the blind prejudices of many Americans and proved beneficial to the DC's nursing ministry.

Despite the resistance from Dorothea Dix and others who opposed the presence of nurses from religious orders during the Civil War, Jane Hoge, Mary Livermore, and others of the United States Sanitary Commission who inspected Union hospitals actually reported a prejudice against *Protestant* nurses and a strong preference for the Catholic sisters, particularly among physicians. Nurses such as Kate Cumming who were recruited to serve the Confederates during the war praised the work of the DC Nurses. She said of their work at the Cantey Hospital in Mobile, Alabama:

> The Sisters of Charity are its matrons, and we all know what they are in hospitals. And by the way, why can we not imitate them in this respect, during the war times? Here one of them is a druggist; another acts the part of steward; and in fact, they could take charge of the whole hospital, with the exception of the medical staff.[16]

The war provided more opportunities for the sisters to establish collaborative relationships with physicians. They worked side by side in hospitals and other smaller facilities such as pestilence houses (or pesthouses). The Daughters of Charity worked, for example, with Quaker physician Dr. John Terrell (1829–1922) in the Lynchburg, Virginia, Pest House performing amputations, treating patients with infectious diseases such as smallpox, and administering herbal remedies. Their work reduced the death rate significantly.[17]

The DC Nurses worked with physicians of different religions and backgrounds, keeping their focus squarely on patient care. When they were not as skilled in a particular medical task, physicians preferred to have the highly competent sisters working with them. The sisters had a reputation among physicians and surgeons for collegiality when dealing with problems in the facility. Mary Livermore had witnessed the incompetence of some of the surgeons, whom she referred to as "laggards that collided with" and "did not work harmoniously with Miss Dix"[18] or her nurses. Jane Hoge quoted one surgeon as remarking:

> Your Protestant nurses are always making a fuss, spying out some mare's-nest in a hospital and writing home that this patient is abused, that one badly treated, or the other starved; that the surgeon gets drunk, or misappropriates the sanitary stores sent to him, or some other bugaboo story, and that's why I won't have them in my hospital. He replaced them with Sisters of Charity because whatever they saw or heard, they told nothing-- the rules of their order forbade it.[19]

The sisters' rules required obedience and humility to physicians, but as is found in Sister Matilda's history, they were not reticent about questioning the orders of a physician and making their own recommendations if it would improve patient care and safety. However, the sisters' dedication to the virtues of humility and obedience would have toned down the expression of their concern and, it seems, channeled it in a way that physicians welcomed.

No Fear in Death ⌒

When Sister Matilda returned to the Central House from her temporary assignments during the war, she was assigned once again to give instructions on spiritual and practical topics to the newer members of the Community.[20] Some Sundays she gave talks to groups of sisters on an inspirational topic; she also gave instructions to the young sisters assembled in the community room at two o'clock in the afternoon. The time of day tempted some to take naps. Sister Matilda dealt with the students' inattentiveness by changing her tone suddenly and saying, "For God's sake don't sleep my Sisters! There are no sleepers in Heaven."[21] At this the sisters sat bolt upright again, backs straight, positions shifted for attentiveness until they were overcome with drowsiness again.

At one such instruction Sister Matilda spoke on the challenges, trials, and mortifications that community life brought at times and that were important for human maturation and spiritual growth. Despite having had days of personal struggle, she never lost sight of her faith. Sister Matilda again used her personal experience of spiritual desolation to illustrate her point:

> In my life I have had crosses, and thank God for them! Crosses so heavy to bear, and humiliations so deep that it has seemed at times as if both Heaven and hell were leagued against me, and as if the tabernacle before which all were kneeling was as empty to me, as any other place.[22]

One of her "crosses" may have been the challenges to the mission at Mount Hope. In 1865 the State of Maryland brought charges at the request of some patients against Dr. Stokes and Mary Blenkinsop (Sister Euphemia), the Sister Servant at the Mount Hope Retreat, for assault and false imprisonment of patients. The Daughters were represented by William Schley, R. J. Gittings, and William P. Preston. Preston was largely responsible for the outcome of the case. Sometime in June of 1865, Preston, who was not a Roman Catholic, wrote to the DC to offer his services on the defense team for the case. His daughter May was a pupil at St. Joseph's Academy at the time.

Even though she was aging and no longer missioned to Mount Hope, Sister Matilda continued to provide a nurse's support to her Community, especially those at Mount Hope. She accompanied Sister Euphemia and other sisters involved in the case to visit Preston at his home. As the first Sister Servant of Mount Hope and an elder nurse in the Community, Sister Matilda was a knowledgeable supporter of Sister Euphemia and Dr. Stokes. Although Sister Matilda did not testify in the case, Community notes state that Preston referred directly to Sister Matilda in the midst of his legal argument on February 8, 1866, when speaking to the jury about the nature of the characters of the Daughters of Charity:

> Within the sound of my voice and within this court-room, is one whom upon the bloody battlefield of Gettysburg

I saw bending over the dying and the dead—binding
up with her own hands the prostrate soldier's wounds,
or commending with her earnest prayers, his departing
spirit to the mercy of his God.[23]

Preston's defense was successful, and the Daughters and Dr. Stokes
were acquitted on February 14, 1866. The stress of the case took its toll on
the sisters and on Sister Matilda. On one occasion when she had gone with
the sisters for a long meeting with Mr. Preston the evening of February 5,
1866, Mrs. Preston noted in her diary that "Sister Matilda had traveled
from Emmitsburg to Baltimore and looked 'weak and wearied.'"[24] But it
was not only the lawsuit that had tapped Sister Matilda's strength. She
had also spent many months at the Baltimore Infirmary and the Mount
Hope Retreat nursing Mother Ann Simeon Norris during her final illness.
Although she herself never became Mother and she never was a candidate
for election after her loss of the election in 1847, Sister Matilda was a
strong supporter and nurse to those who did assume the office.

Sister Ann Simeon Norris, then treasurer, had accompanied Mother
Etienne Hall in 1851 as an American emissary to the Daughters of Charity
in Paris. The purpose of their visit was to be oriented to the customs of
the French Daughters. In her subsequent role as Community leader,
Mother Ann Simeon led the sisters through the Civil War period and
the strongest era of anti-Catholic, "know-nothing" politics. Under her
leadership, the Daughters established thirty-five new ministries in eleven
states, Washington, D.C., and Canada. Sister Matilda went with her to
Baltimore when she became ill because "it was feared Mother's extreme
amiability would not allow her to refuse any one, and the Doctor said rest
was absolutely necessary."[25] Mother Ann Simeon had a serious cancer of
the stomach, however, and rest did not help her get well. Sister Bernard
Boyle wrote of the Mother's final days, "Sister Matilda tells us, with sobs
and tears, of her angelic sweetness, her perfect resignation, her childlike
reliance in the sweet providence of God."[26] Sister Matilda wrote of Mother
Ann's reliance on her nursing counsel:

It was my happy privilege to accompany our beloved
Mother to Baltimore. O sad departure from home, and

still sadder the return. Who of us thought that six weeks only remained for us to be edified by her who had been our model, our joy and support for the six years that we were too happy to call her Mother. Of the last weeks of her life I can only say that her virtue which had left its impress on every heart, seemed to be approaching that fullness or perfection to be looked for only in Heaven. The physician soon pronounced her malady incurable: she asked me what was their opinion, I replied, my dear Mother, they fear they cannot do much towards your recovery, that to relieve you of some pain will be all they can effect.[27]

Sister Matilda witnessed Mother Ann Simeon's prayers during the preparation for the Mount Hope trial as they sat in silence together in the sickroom. She was the consummate hospice nurse, following the lead of her patient. When Mother Ann vomited black blood, Sister Matilda knew what the symptoms meant. She waited for Mother Ann to ask her what it was in the vomit and said of her reply, "I only gave her an indefinite answer, she said, 'it is cancerous blood.' On my asking if she cared if such was the case she said, 'oh no by no means.'"[28] Sister Matilda nursed Mother Ann Simeon until her death, and then she, Sister Euphemia, and six other sisters accompanied Mother Ann Simeon's body back to Emmitsburg to be buried.

Thank God

The last week in May of 1870, Sister Matilda provided nursing care to the poor near Emmitsburg. Despite her efforts, some of her patients died. The weather was damp and cold, but Sister Matilda forgot herself and spent hours in cold rooms administering aid and consoling her patients. After the last person was buried, she herself was taken ill. Sister Matilda had been sick so often and had always recovered that the sisters and her physician thought she would get well as she had before. Though she had been present at the peaceful deaths of so many patients and sister companions, Sister Matilda had always had a persistent fear of death, which was so great that even when slightly indisposed, she was nervous and fearful. But this time she was calm and tranquil from the onset. Sister Matilda did not express a single fear during her final illness, which lasted twelve days. For the sisters who survived Sister Matilda, this experience bore out the truth of the teaching of Saint Vincent de Paul that "those who love the poor in life will have nothing to fear in death."[29]

Sister Matilda spent forty-one years in the Community of the Daughters of Charity in a variety of duties in several locations. Her life experiences and her death were a source of inspiration to others. One account of Sister Matilda's death illustrates her approach to life:

> On the day she died, (Trinity Sunday,) one of the Sisters said to her, I think our Lord will take you to Heaven on this beautiful feast. "Why?" said Sister Matilda, *"am I dying?"* upon being answered, "Yes, our Lord will soon take you," she said, *"thank God -"* she kept her eyes closed and her heart united to our Lord - about a half hour before her death, she said to Mother [Euphemia Blenkinsop]: *"Oh, I am so much afraid I am not dying!"* Mother replied: "Yes, my dear, you will soon be with our Lord." She then seemed satisfied . . . A short time before her happy soul winged its flight to Heaven she asked for the little bell, blessed for the hour of death, rung it herself and said like a little child coaxing her mother for a favor: *"Come, my Mother [Virgin Mary], come and take your poor child to Heaven!"* A few minutes after, she sweetly slept in our Lord.[30]

Sister Matilda had such an influence on the young sisters that the homilist at her funeral prayed that God would send "many Daughters of Charity like Sister Matilda Coskery, loving their Vocation with that deep devoted attachment which neither humiliation nor trial can change; which consumes itself without display in the fervent accomplishment of duty, and thus God will be glorified."[31]

The last work of charity Sister Matilda undertook was the propagation of the Apostleship of Prayer among the people of Emmitsburg and the vicinity. Sister Matilda probably had access to a publication by Rev. Henri Ramière, SJ, *The Apostleship of Prayer: A Holy League of Christian Hearts United with the Heart of Jesus*,[32] which popularized a movement of apostolic prayer and evangelization during Sister Matilda's time. At its core was a program of intercessory prayer and offering of one's whole life as an apostle engaged in service. Prayer was a significant part of Sister Matilda's service later in life as she became less able to engage in nursing care and administrative duties that were more physically demanding. In this work she would have suggested prayer intentions and specific daily actions to her listeners so that they could live more fervently by gospel values in word and deed. Sister Matilda would have had increased contact with lay men and women of all ages who had a variety of presenting needs, enabling her to provide pastoral counseling, religious instruction, health education, mentoring, advice, and supportive relationships.

The Apostleship ministry work seemed to have energized her with new life. One day, after reading about the great spiritual benefits of solidarity in prayer among souls through the union that occurs in prayer among believers who are focused on particular intentions of the pope and the universal Church, Sister Matilda discovered a new field of action for spiritual service. She acknowledged, *"Oh, I could cry all the time, to think how much I might have done for my good God, had I known of this."*[33] Sister

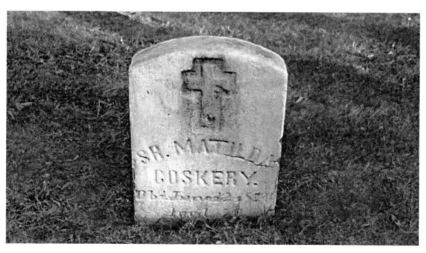

Fig. 6-2   *Grave of Sister Matilda Coskery*

Courtesy, Daughters of Charity Archives, Emmitsburg, Maryland

Matilda's reference is somewhat obscure, but she may have been referring to Ramière's text, with its focus on the solidarity of many persons united in prayer with the same intention. Her tone seems to suggest regret for untapped possibilities, perhaps as a result of new insights about ways to conduct her ministry. Her love of God had been apparent for many years. She left a legacy of a life of caring and kindness for her patients and her *Advices* book for her Nurse companions and perhaps for nurses of all faiths who would follow her on the charitable path of nursing service.

End of an Era

In the twentieth century few learned of the pioneering work of the early DC Nurses, let alone Sister Matilda's contribution to nursing and the advancement of American healthcare, particularly the care of the mentally ill. But her vision, preserved in the Mount Hope Retreat, was kept alive for a century after her death. So many social, economic, religious, and political issues challenged the survival of Mount Hope. Sister Matilda carried a vision for her dream institution through the peak years of anti-Catholic hostilities and the Civil War, during which she wrote in 1862:

> In consequence of this miserable war wh. has now devastated our country for two years, our wealthy patients from the South, (formerly our best pay & the main support of the Institute;) now utterly unable to procure a single dollar — (And yet they cannot be turned out,) the very great number of Charity-patients . . . every thing combines to cripple very much the resources of the Institution; and causes the writer of this often to say within herself: "From whence do the means come to support this family?"[34]

Building and maintaining hospitals to carry the Vincentian-Louisian-Setonian mission forward was never easy for the Community. The DC Nurses faced many challenges that were directed to them personally, professionally, and as a Community of religious women. They followed

296

their hearts' callings and made changes in the direction of their missions as needed. Their entrepreneurial spirit, grounded in their faith, guided the Community's business decisions over the years. Because of the leadership role they played in American nursing throughout most of the nineteenth century, the choices that the Daughters of Charity made had a significant impact on the evolution of the profession as well as on their Community and their Church.

Mount Hope was an example not only of what DC Nurses could do to ease the suffering of the insane but what level of contribution all American nurses could potentially make to health reforms, particularly in the realm of institutionalized care. The founding of the Catholic Health Association[35] in 1915 provided the DC as well as nurses and hospitals of other Catholic orders a forum for addressing the issues of the ongoing hospital reform movement.[36] Beginning in the late nineteenth century, the secularization of education, nursing programs, and hospital nursing staff had become equated with modernization. Secularization in nursing was a complex social concern that paralleled the difficulties Americans had been having for decades on a national level regarding the separation of church and state.

All nursing care at Mount Hope until 1925 was rendered exclusively by the sisters and their attendants.[37] By that time nurse-training programs had begun to place more emphasis on psychiatric nursing, for which they needed additional clinical sites. Education was the impetus that drew the DC into the movement toward secularization. Mount Hope opened its doors to lay nursing students. While some were concerned early on that the patients would not like the addition of lay nurses, the reality proved quite the contrary. The lay nurses actually worked well under the guidance of the sisters, and they "received invaluable experience in developing an understanding of the patient as a person, made in the image and likeness of God."[38] In 1945 Mount Hope was restructured, and it ultimately hired lay nurses. It emerged from the restructuring with a new name, The Seton Institute, by which it was known until its doors closed in 1973.

Sister Maureen Delahunt and Sister Annina Sharper were two of the Daughters of Charity missioned as nurses to The Seton Institute. Sister Annina was the Sister Servant at the time of its closing and Sister Maureen a psychiatric staff nurse. Both held Master's degrees: Sister Maureen in psychiatric mental health nursing and Sister Annina in nursing administration. In an interview in 2007,[39] they observed that while The Seton Institute had originally been a hospital for 500 patients, it had declined in the 1970s to a much smaller patient population primarily made up of religious men and women of the Catholic Church. They remember caring mostly for adult patients with depression, bipolar disorder, and catatonia and also some teens with behavior disorders. They did not, however, treat alcoholic patients, as Sister Matilda had in the mid-nineteenth century.

Care of the patients at The Seton Institute was quite different from that described by Sister Matilda. The nurses and psychiatrists no longer practiced moral therapy. And long gone was the cupping, blistering, and hops tea, although patient-nurse interaction remained. In the 1970s the nurses still did a lot of counseling with patients, but physical and occupational therapists, instead of the nursing staff, organized patient activities. The Seton Institute DC Nurses took walks on the grounds with the patients, but they did not eat with the patients. Some of the patients were treated with shock and insulin therapy, and many were given new psychotropic medications, such as Thorazine. The nurses continued the healing tradition of applying hydrotherapy treatments, such as hot baths and cold wet sheets. They also used restraint straps and isolation rooms as necessary. When asked if they used the sleeve that Sister Matilda and the early sisters had created in the nineteenth century, the sisters said that they did not.

Like Sister Matilda, Sisters Annina and Maureen identified the most important spiritual foundation for their nursing care as "respect and kindness" toward patients. They took the patients, including those who suffered from psychosis, to Mass every day. Sister Maureen said, "Those patients got better because you respected them." Both of the sisters cited the writings of Louise de Marillac as most inspirational to their work as nurses in the twentieth century. The teachings of Louise de Marillac endured, but The Seton Institute facility, built before the Civil War, had to be torn down. While the Daughters continue to be involved in healthcare today, the closing of The Seton Institute was the end of an era. Sister Matilda and the DC Nurses who followed her—and continued the dream of Mount Hope for one hundred years—lived the nursing tradition begun by Vincent de Paul and Louise de Marillac and later adopted by Elizabeth Ann Seton:

> That, then, is what obliges you to serve them [the sick poor]
> with respect as your masters, and with devotion because
> they represent for you the person of Our Lord who said,
> "What you do to the least of mine I will consider as done
> to myself." So, Sisters, Our Lord is, in fact, with that patient
> who is the recipient of the service you render Him.[40]

Sister Matilda's writings from the asylum and the battlefield, her *Advices Concerning the Sick,* and the descriptions of her life recounted by those who lived closely with her in Community, affirm the challenges and victories of a life consecrated to God for charitable service. Sister Matilda Coskery's ministry and contribution to nursing was practical, humble, and very profound in its expression of human kindness. Yet it was also anchored in simplicity. No task was too menial for the Daughter of Charity called to nurse the sick poor or insane after the examples of Vincent de Paul, Louise de Marillac, and Elizabeth Ann Seton. While not unique to the Catholic religion, these virtues, so highly valued by the Daughters of Charity since 1633, were carefully cultivated in the American sisters, who were following a centuries-old tradition. The moral character typifying the Daughters' caregiving practices and identified in the nineteenth century as "enlightened charity" are spiritual qualities understood by peoples of many faiths and cultures. Daughters of Charity Nurses like Sister Matilda, who followed the Vincentian-Louisian-Setonian tradition and nursed patients without prejudice, made a distinction between their religious doctrine and dogma and a nursing ministry of spirituality in action that appealed to many persons in need of healing. Though in outer appearances they remained connected to religious attire and the cornette, to vows, and thus to a religious hierarchy, the DC Nurses were free in spirit to exercise their faith and their humanity as they continued, year after year, to create caring conditions for the patients whom they loved as Christ himself. It was the spiritual qualities and character of all nurses, lay as well as religious, that became the central issue of the secularization movement in American nursing during the later part of the century.

⌒ *Secularization of Nursing* ⌒

Gradually, as the national wounds of the Civil War began to heal and industrialization boomed at the end of the nineteenth century, American nurses, including those of the Catholic sisterhoods, moved toward secularization of nursing education and practice. In the broadest sense of the word, secularization in nursing meant that the Daughters of Charity Nurses and nurses in other religious orders relinquished authority and control of most hospitals to lay bodies and sometimes to public authority.[41] In the late 1870s the DC left the Baltimore Infirmary after fifty years of partnership with the medical college. The State of Maryland by that time owned the college, the University of Maryland School of Medicine, which boasts to this day that it is the fifth-oldest medical school in the nation and the first to institute a residency training program, which was made possible by the partnership with the Sisters and then Daughters of Charity begun in 1823.

In the current sociopolitical climate, the Daughters no longer reside or work en masse in state-supported healthcare institutions and colleges, as they did in the nineteenth century. As state facilities moved toward secularization, the Daughters continued to create their own hospitals and educational institutions. Secularization did not preclude them from working as nurses for state institutions, however. Just as Sister Matilda and the DC had received funds for state-supported psychiatric patients, they were able to collect monies to support the care they provided to the poor and orphans who were wards of the state.

During the transition period, contractual agreements between the Daughters and hospital administrators often stipulated that they would be the *only* nurses for the institution. For example, in 1849 the *Catholic Almanac* announced that the Sisters of Charity took over the care of patients at the new Catholic hospital, St. John's Infirmary in Milwaukee:

> As the Sisters of Charity are to be the only nurses and attendants in the house, none need fear the absence of sympathy and eager vigilance. . . . Patients may call in any duly authorized medical man they please; but all food and medicine must be administered by the Sisters.[42]

As the call for secular training programs began to crescendo in the 1870s, the Daughters of Charity and nurses of other Catholic orders were challenged more and more to step aside for new lay nurses, who were in fact Protestant women educated in hospital-based training programs.[43]

There had been a call for the creation of training programs for Protestant women nurses for decades. As mentioned previously, the American Medical Association (AMA) recognized the need for Protestant women to do better in caring for the sick. Nurse Kate Cumming, the Confederate nurse who had many interactions with the DC Nurses, made a plea for better nurses and care by Protestant women. She challenged her own culture's stigma placed upon women who cared for the sick. She could not understand why a Catholic woman could "go with credit where it is a disgrace for a Protestant to go."[44] She continued, "I shall say now what perhaps I have said before, that a woman's respectability is at a low ebb when caring for the suffering will endanger it."[45]

Many Protestant women, like Kate Cumming, admired the nursing work of the Daughters of Charity. Some Protestant women converted to Catholicism just to become good nurses, but other Protestant women became jealous of the successes of the Daughters of Charity. Sisters at the St. Louis Military Hospital stated that the Ladies of the Union Aid Society who visited the hospital twice a week

> became jealous of the good that the sisters were doing. The women feared, the sisters said, that everyone would become a Catholic. The ladies even tried to make the patients call them sisters telling the soldiers they were charitable ladies who went about doing good . . . the women could not succeed because "the poor patients knew how to distinguish between real merit and big talk." In spite of the fact that the ladies could not see or understand how the sisters could have so much influence over the patients, they showed the sisters the greatest respect.[46]

The Daughters' professional and cultural authority was being challenged by Protestant women who felt the pressure to become better nurses and to occupy nursing positions in hospitals held by Catholic sisters.[47] The sisters were also faced with the growing medical dominance of which they had been aware for decades; some physicians, such as Amariah Brigham, saw it as their duty to question and resist nurses' professional authority.

While Brigham questioned the right of women nurses to administer hospitals, others called into question nurses' authority in some of the daily tasks that defined the sickroom management that had been carried out by the professional nurse for centuries. For example, stating public safety as their intent, some physicians in midcentury asserted that sick diet was their domain rather than the nurses'. Later on others began to lay claims to expertise in other duties traditionally performed and taught by nurses. For instance, one physician wrote that "it often becomes the duty of the doctor to instruct the nurse in regard to the poultices."[48] But hops and flaxseed poultices had been frequently applied in patient care, and this was a skill taught by nurses like Sister Matilda for decades if not centuries by the time this was written.[49]

Physician-authored advice and domestic-medicine books were often the platform for proliferating physician rhetoric that inflated generalized concerns about the safety of nursing practice in Britain and America. The safety of the public necessitated that *all* nurses be more obedient to university-trained physicians. But prior to the later nineteenth century, professional nurses such as Sister Matilda and the Daughters of Charity had practiced autonomously and were highly respected for their safe, effective, and compassionate care. Rev. Dubois defended the sisters' authority at the Baltimore Infirmary in the early years, saying at one point that "the sisters could do as much or more than the house doctors" and that the doctor's services were "by no means necessary for the sisters can dress wounds, bleed patients, and administer medicine."[50] This must have been difficult for physicians who, despite their good intentions, clearly sought social monopoly over healthcare. The Daughters forged ahead, courageously building and staffing hospitals and inaugurating new programs such as dietetics and nurse training.[51] By the early 1900s, 59 of the 393 nursing schools in the United States were established by religious women, and of those, 28 were begun by Daughters and Sisters of Charity in the Vincentian-Louisian-Setonian tradition.[52]

The Myth About Early Nurses ⌣

In the late nineteenth century, "modernization" of nursing was equated with secularization. Americans Lavinia Dock (1858–1956) and Isabel Stewart (1878–1963) wrote in their 1925 book, *A Short History of Nursing*, that religious orders used "ancient ways" in caring for the sick and "gradually altered" those ways by "attaching secular training schools to their hospitals."[53] Graduates of secular training programs were referred to as "trained nurses." There were no licensing boards or national exams for nurses in the late nineteenth century, but training programs typically provided their graduate nurses certificates of completion, which the nurse could then show as evidence of her qualifications. Whereas a Catholic nurse's reputation was associated with her community's history and experience, lay nurses who entered the profession independently had no strong history of public service and depended upon the reputation of their training institutions.

Dock and Stewart concluded from their historical assessment that when the Civil War broke out in 1861 there were "no trained nurses in the country."[54] If the authors were referring to all nurses when they made this statement, it would have been a highly critical and perhaps slanderous statement against Catholic nurses such as the Daughters of Charity, who had been considered highly educated and "enlightened" nurses by medical professionals, the public, and other nurses for decades. What Dock and Stewart were most likely referring to was the absence of secular or lay programs for "trained" nurses, a new title describing the lay (i.e., non-Catholic) nurse who received a formal education in a hospital—a specific *brand* of nurse, the "trained nurse" who was a graduate of a "training school" based upon the Florence Nightingale model of nurse training implemented in London.

Training schools were not new in the 1870s in America. Physicians in particular had been attempting to enroll their own schools at least since the 1820s. During that time, Joseph Warrington, a Pennsylvania physician, created the Nurse Society of Philadelphia for the study of nursing as an independent calling, a program for training working-class women in their own methods of childbirth. This provoked opposition by midwives, who were often respected healers in their communities. Warrington's attempt to establish a hierarchical model of obstetrical care in which the women he trained in his "scientific" services would be responsible to him rather than to the patient was not well attended.[55] But his notion of raising middle-class women to be the "scientifically" oriented nurses of the future did not die.

Class distinction among women nurses, as well as differences in personal character, was another focus of the secularization movement in the 1870s.[56] Like Warrington, a number of physicians at midcentury took an interest in educating young nurses from the middle class; physicians Ann Preston (1813–1872) and Marie Zakrzewska (1829–1902) were just two of the physicians who offered training programs for nurses beginning in the 1860s. But the programs had trouble recruiting Protestant middle-class women to training schools and hospital work.[57] Dock and Stewart's statement about the lack of trained nurses could also have been made in reference to the lack of success in enrolling middle-class women of good character in training programs. It would be another decade before a secular training program was developed that had significant momentum to register in history as the "beginning of modern nursing" in America. That program was at Bellevue Hospital in New York.

Scotoma and Professional Identity

Lavinia Dock and Isabel Stewart's statement about the lack of trained nurses prior to the Civil War was made in a book considered a "classic in the nursing world."[58] Their words have been repeated for more than eighty years by authors of numerous publications, by educators, and by nurses themselves. However, the phrase is most often taken out of context to mean that there were *no* professional nurses prior to the establishment of American nurse-training schools in the later part of the century. Because the history has been misconstrued, the contributions of the Daughters of Charity and other Catholic communities are most often excluded from references to the early history of American nursing, even though theirs were the contributions perceived by the public, physicians, and lay nurses as the professional ideal of the period.

What is perhaps most disconcerting is that nursing prior to training programs, particularly the opening of the Nightingale program at Bellevue Hospital in 1873, has been characterized as lacking in formal education and that nurses were slightly above domestic servants in social status, typically the "dregs" of human society. Nursing and historical texts and popular literature, too numerous to count, have perpetuated a myth that nurses prior to the 1870s were drunkards, thieves, and whores. This myth, a gross generalization significantly removed from historical context, not only has served to distance American nurses from a powerful part of their professional history found in the Catholic archives but is also a wound in the psyche of American nurses that affects professional identity. Each time an American nurse repeats a creation story in which the mothers of the profession were drunkards and whores, the wound is opened again. What is perhaps most disturbing about the adoption of the myth of pre-Nightingale nurses as drunks and prostitutes is that American nurses have allowed for the loss of a whole period of history of enlightened, powerful, entrepreneurial nursing.

There is a scotoma or memory hole[59] in the history of American nursing. Scientists and clinicians understand the importance of the exception, the unique case to the development of the body of scientific knowledge. Wolfgang Kohler, a pioneer in Gestalt psychology, wrote that "we are constantly putting aside, unused, a wealth of valuable material [which leads to] the blocking of scientific progress."[60] Oliver Sacks, whose groundbreaking work on L-dopa was a result of being able to see beyond the obvious, responded:

> But if anomalies promise a transition to a larger mental space, they may do so through a very painful, even terrifying, process of undermining one's existing beliefs and theories—painful because our mental lives are sustained consciously or unconsciously, by theories, sometimes invented with the force of ideology or delusion.[61]

The scotoma in American nursing is the early and mid-nineteenth-century period between the time of eighteenth-century Colonial nursing, when nursing existed as a community rather than an institutional endeavor, and the late-nineteenth/early-twentieth century, with its emphasis on Nightingale-trained nurses in reformed hospitals. The memory hole has been filled with images that not only serve to denigrate the profession but alter the core identity of American nurses. The best that American nursing history has had to offer nurses trying to find meaning in the difficult tasks of day-to-day caring for the sick are the victorious accounts of the "modern" Nightingale era after 1873. One British scholar's research suggests that "reformers who wanted to redefine modern nursing also lumped all old nurses together into a homogenous mass, distinguished only by its variety of failings."[62] Nelson and Gordon have referred to this disowning of nursing's past as "the rhetoric of rupture."[63]

In America neither Dock and Stewart's text nor Dock's earlier *History of Nursing* that she wrote with Adelaide Nutting in 1907 state specifically that there were no professional nurses prior to 1873 (i.e., no "mass of failed old nurses"). However, these histories, deliberate or not, did provide two building blocks for the construction of the defamation myth.

First, they did not present the Catholic history that was contrary to the myth. Neither of Dock's classic histories of the evolution of American nursing contains a chapter on the history of the American Daughters of Charity; for example, their hospital work with medical colleges beginning in 1823 at the Baltimore Infirmary, the history of the creation and administration of their own hospitals and asylums, their vocational education programs and nursing systems of care, and the exemplary work of Sister Matilda and the Daughters in the moral treatment of the insane. Other than references to the French Daughters of Charity and the influence of their founders Vincent de Paul and Louise de Marillac on the founding of the Protestant Sisters of Charity in England and America in the mid-nineteenth century, there was only one reference to the highly successful and respected care of the American DC Nurses. The Sisters of Charity are mentioned briefly in regard to their work in a Philadelphia almshouse during the 1832 cholera outbreak.

Certainly, the authors must have been more than familiar with the work of the sisters. An oft-quoted history of European-American nursing given as a lecture in 1855 and published by a Mrs. Anna Jameson in 1859 was titled *Sisters of Charity*.[64] It was Mrs. Jameson's history of nursing that was referenced by the American Medical Association in their report on nursing in 1869 that Dock cited in her books. Anna Brownell Jameson (1794–1860) was a British author most well known for her writings on benevolence, women, and the "communion of love and the communion of labour." She traveled extensively without her husband and had large social networks in Europe, America, and Canada, including one circle of friends that included Julia Smith, the aunt of Florence Nightingale. She spoke on the ability of women to overcome "the obstacles of custom and prejudice" for which she cited the success of Florence Nightingale. She wrote:

> I trust that England has many daughters not unworthy of being named with Florence Nightingale; as quick in sympathy, as calm in judgment, as firm in duty, as awake to charity; but the ability, the acquirements, the experience, the tact, the skill in judging and managing character, and overcoming adverse circumstances, at which ministers and officials were filled with wonder,--were these matters of chance? They were the result of years of study, of patient observation, of severe training. In what school? In none that England affords to her daughters; *this* is the wonder![65]

Mrs. Jameson's history contains accounts of both Nightingale and pre-Nightingale eras of professional nursing. She was knowledgeable of the nursing ministries in Europe and America and focused her remarks on the political and gender issues the women nurses faced as they went about charitable service. She detailed the protection the Sisters of Charity gave female patients from male patients and medical residents during their convalescence. She also explained how the male medical students and attendants did not complain about the care the women nurses gave in the infirmaries and dispensaries but only that it "took bread out of the men's mouths."[66] The Sisters of Charity, she said, brought to the most distasteful of nursing duties a cheerfulness that she observed stemmed from the "religious and feminine elements that influenced material administration."[67] The Sisters never became accustomed to their work in a way that would harden the heart. She cited numerous examples in which the Sisters through their embodiment of the "feminine nature to minister through love"[68] brought balance to the masculine intellect to rule through power that was prevalent among physicians in hospitals.

Mrs. Jameson echoed the call to Protestant women to seize the opportunity to become a nurse but not to make the decision lightly. She differentiated impulse from vocation followed by remarks on the lack of education for women who would be nurses:

> But I do believe that there are also hundreds who are fitted, or would gladly, at any sacrifice, fit themselves, for the work, if the means of doing so were allowed to them. At present an English lady has no facilities whatever for obtaining the information or experience required; no such institutions are open to her, and yet she is ridiculed for presenting herself without competent knowledge. This seems hardly just.[69]

These comments were made prior to the construction of the Nightingale training system. Mrs. Jameson acknowledged the presence of drunkenness, profligacy (decadence), and violent tempers and language in some nurses in England but also stated that there "were admirable exceptions, more particularly in the great London Hospitals."[70]

The second building block that Dock, Nutting, and Stewart's histories contributed to the American myth was equating the poor nursing care in dilapidated early American almshouses with the care provided in all hospitals and asylums. The care in the almshouses was custodial care at best. The term "nurse" is used in many early histories to refer to caregivers, but the almshouse workers were rarely professional nurses educated in nursing and medicine as were the Daughters of Charity. Many "nurses" were prisoners and paupers who learned on the job and often drank alcohol, either because they were alcoholics or they thought it would help ward off diseases. There were middle-class women who referred to themselves as "nurses" in the eighteenth and early nineteenth centuries who had no education and no formal nursing training by experienced nurses such as that given to new DC Nurses in the Emmitsburg Community. In addition, during the Civil War, Nutting and Dock wrote, many of the nurses were "self-taught and disciplined by dire necessity" but they "attained a high degree of practical skill."[71]

Nutting and Dock described the early almshouses, such as Bellevue in New York and Blockley in Philadelphia, as "overcrowded," "a disgrace," "desperate," and "demoralized."[72] It is no wonder that physicians called for help from the Catholic sisters. During the cholera epidemic of 1832, Nutting and Dock wrote that the bishop in Philadelphia sent for the Sisters of Charity from Emmitsburg for the Blockley Almshouse, which was in a shambles. The Sisters appeared within two hours of the call and, according to the nurses, "took in hand the whole desperate situation."[73] The surgeon general during the Civil War, Dr. William Hammond, employed the Daughters of Charity under "special instructions of his office" rather than have them report to Dorothea Dix.[74] The Protestant deaconess and secular nurses Dix recruited and managed had not yet achieved the level of experience or reputation that the American Daughters of Charity had after forty years of public service.

Even after the war, the AMA supported the Catholic sisterhoods in the United States and Canada, in particular the Daughters of Charity, whom they believed were "highly educated and refined ladies," "noble and self-sacrificing."[75] The ignorant and unfit nurses, according to Dr. Gross, who wrote the AMA report, were the mothers and daughters in private families who attempted to care for the sick themselves when they in his opinion were "wholly unfit for the discharge of so sacred a duty as that involving the health and life of a human being affected by disease or injury."[76] Gross also identified the attendants in "public institutions" such as almshouses as "superadded, not unfrequently, to the basest moral delinquencies, as intemperance, indifference to duty, and positive disregard of the orders of the medical attendant." Male nurses, he said, were notoriously "bad and incompetent" and often "drunken."[77] Gross stated that the Protestant Church was beginning to see the importance of nursing after being "so long idle in this great work."[78]

There were "nurses" who were "drunks and whores," but they were not considered by nineteenth-century American society to be professional nurses. The history of the state of American healthcare facilities that was true for the Bellevue Almshouse in New York prior to its restructuring in 1847 was not necessarily true for all state institutions, and it certainly was not true for private hospitals owned and/or administered by religious women such as the Daughters of Charity. Yet Florence Nightingale's pejorative words that British hospital nurses were women who were "too old, too weak, too drunken, too dirty, too stolid or too bad to do anything else,"[79] have often been republished in American texts. Where historians such as Susan Reverby have placed Nightingale's statement within the context of American nursing history,[80] the details of the evidence from this delicate transition in nursing history are often lost in textbook and journal publications. These typically include more general statements about the history of American nursing practice and education prior to Nightingale. For example, one author wrote, "Before the 1800's, nursing was not considered an intellectual endeavor but a service provided by religious orders or reserved for the immoral, drunken, and illiterate women of the day or prostitutes."[81] Variations of the myth, such as this, have been repeated so often that it has become the vernacular.

Perpetuation of the myth and Dock, Nutting, and Stewart's exclusion of foundational nursing history, the history of Catholic nurses, in particular the DC, who demonstrated the best of the profession—the intelligence, autonomy, and strength of America's early professional nurses—has had a profound effect on American nursing to date. Additionally, Dock, Nutting, and Stewart went one step further. They specifically predicted the demise of religious nurses. They suggested that the Sisters of Charity and the Protestant Deaconess nurses, who had formed their nursing model of care in midcentury based upon the Kaiserwerth work in Germany, would "gradually count for less and less in nursing proper."[82] For Dock and Nutting modernization entailed the secularized reform of nursing, which they believed had been defined by Florence Nightingale, who was "shaping a new order" rather than "reproducing the Sisters of Charity or the deaconesses."[83] Dock and Nutting were clearly captivated by what they perceived Florence Nightingale's work to be about . . . science.

Constructing an American Legend ⌒

At the end of the chapter in their history of the founding of the Daughters of Charity in Paris, Nutting and Dock made little to no reference to the American sisters. They wrote that the American sisters were formed by Elizabeth Seton and that the sisters' services had extended to a number of cities. In addition: "In America, they [the Sisters of Charity], as other Catholic nursing orders, have recognised and accommodated themselves to the demands of modern medical science by establishing schools for secular nurses in the hospitals under their management."[84] Although the DC Nurses had achieved renown by the public and physicians in the care of the sick, especially during the cholera epidemics and the Civil War, there was no mention of the role the American sisters had played in the health reforms and nursing innovations of early and mid-nineteenth century nurses such as Sister Matilda.

Nutting and Dock presented the ideological shift in nursing that was occurring during the late nineteenth and early years of the twentieth centuries. They not only connected modern nursing with secularization; they connected *medical science* with modernization and therefore secularization in nursing. They wrote of Nightingale's new "ideal":

> Gone forever, from the time when she applied her intellect to the problems of the Crimea was the conception of nursing as a charity, exceedingly meritorious and desiring of the heavenly reward for its self-sacrificing character. The self-sacrifice remained but under her sway nursing shone forth as part of the invincible and glorious advance of science, sanitary science, the science of health first, and of disease only secondarily. Not pity alone, but prevention foremost, not only amelioration but the reduction of suffering, was typified in the personality of this woman not only as a possibility, but a positive policy for future generations.[85]

Dock and Nutting seem to script a new history as well as predict a future for American nursing based upon their analysis of Nightingale's work, which they interpreted as an ideology founded in science rather than spirituality.

Nursing care and sickroom-management techniques remained part of the Nightingale educational model. Nightingale stressed that the training of women as nurses would not in any way compromise the roles of physicians because the nurse was not a medical man or woman. She was "there, and solely there, to carry out the orders of the medical and surgical staff, including, of course, the whole practice of cleanliness, fresh air, diet, etc. . . . Their whole training is to enable them to understand how best to carry out medical and surgical orders, including as above, the whole art of cleanliness, ventilation, food, etc., etc., and the *reason why* this is to be done *this* way and not *that* way."[86]

Nightingale also laid out her hierarchical structure of nursing with her matron/superintendent women as head nurses and educators. The "rule" she constructed for trained nurses that was, according to Dock, an "innovation" for hospital administrators, placed all nurses under the supervision of a woman rather than the physicians or hospital administrators.[87] The Bellevue board had difficulty finding a nurse to fulfill this role for the opening of the training program in America. In 1873 Sister Helen Bowden (1827–1896), a religious sister from England offered herself for the job. She was an Anglican (Protestant) sister with the All Saints Sisters of the Poor who dressed in full religious garb, including a white cornette that, though a bit floppy, bore a striking resemblance to that of the Daughters of Charity.[88] Sister Helen returned to London in 1876, after the first class had graduated, enrollment was on the rise, and American Eliza Perkins of Connecticut was ready to assume the role of matron of the hospital and superintendent of the program.

The hierarchy and rule established by Nightingale and passed to American institutions such as Bellevue were a very modified version of the *Common Rules* of the Daughters of Charity also practiced by the American DC as their 1812 *Regulations*. While the sisters vowed to be obedient to hospital administrators and all superiors including physicians, the Sister Servant, and the Infirmarian, Nightingale adopted a different tone in her instructions when discussing obedience and carrying out the orders of physicians as the "sole" nature of nursing. Neither the Daughters in France nor the American Sisters identified their role as nurses or defined their ministry as following physician orders.

Nightingale had reviewed the *Common Rules* of the Daughters in Paris when she resided with them in the mid-nineteenth century.[89] She took notes in French from those orders and transcribed some into English.[90] She also owned a "unique collection of *Regles of Religious Orders*, chiefly the French."[91] But her understanding of the religious and spiritual instruction to DC Nurses may have been skewed by the brevity of her contact with the Community, her differences with Roman Catholic belief,[92] and her concern about the potential influence of the Church in the nursing care of religious sisters.

In contemporary nursing literature American scholars in particular have identified the deep spirituality that defined Florence Nightingale and her writings. Michael Calabria, Barbara Dossey, and Janet MacRae have even suggested that there is a mystical quality in their historical analyses of Nightingale's writings.[93] Even Nightingale's letters convey an ongoing spiritual quest,[94] throughout which she wrestled with many issues from religious doctrine and societal norms for women to the difficult relationship with her sister. But despite Nightingale's deep spirituality, she was still a Protestant-born woman in a time in which anti-Catholic sentiment ran high. Nightingale was well aware of the tension between Protestants and Catholics that was permeating nursing. In a letter to her friend Lady Charlotte Canning during her 1853 visit with the Daughters of Charity in Paris, she referred to the Daughters of Charity as "the enemy":

> I am afraid my Committee will greatly disapprove of my being at Paris in the enemy's camp, instead of being very much obliged to me for acting as a spy to despoil the enemy of their good things. With the fear that they would not be as grateful to me as they ought, I did not proclaim my intention of going to Paris.[95]

Nightingale contracted measles for a second time a few weeks after writing this letter, citing "Providence" as "being in her way having twice made her ill" when trying to learn about the nursing care of the Daughters in Paris.[96] Whether Nightingale herself believed that the Catholic sisters were in fact her "enemies" or if she was using a term voiced by her family and her committee is unclear. Nevertheless, she was a leader in the secularization movement in nursing, which some Protestants perceived as an anti-Catholic endeavor.

There is no evidence that Nightingale was specifically anti-Catholic. Alternatively, she had considered conversion to Catholicism at one point in her spiritual quest. She also acknowledged the generosity and expertise of the DC and clearly respected the Vincentian-Louisian nursing tradition. However, her work in establishing a nurse-training program was intended to create opportunities for young women to become professional nurses without having to enter a Catholic, or Deaconess, religious community.

Although Nightingale believed that education was "not her genius,"[97] she was highly successful in establishing the St. Thomas training school in London as a secular model for other nursing programs in America as well. Secularization of nursing education was also a reflection of the values and the work of those aligned with the nineteenth-century women's rights movement. American women in the eighteenth and early and mid-nineteenth centuries were viewed as essentially inclined to moral behavior and inherently nurturing because of their gender. Like many of her era, Nightingale's philosophy of nursing held that women were inherently equipped for providing nursing care. She took a stance, as did many women of her time, in opposition to the women's rights movement that emphasized the similarities between the sexes. She wrote:

> I would earnestly ask my sisters to keep clear of both the jargons now current everywhere (for they *are* equally jargons); of the jargon, namely, about the "rights" of women, which urges women to do all that men do, including the medical and other professions, merely because men do it, and without regard to whether this *is* the best that women can do; and of the jargon which urges women to do nothing that men can do, merely because they are women. . . . Surely woman should bring the best she has, *whatever* that is, to the work of God's world, without attending to either of these cries. For what are they, both of them, the one *just* as much as the other, but listening to the "what will people say," to opinion, to the voices from without?[98]

That women, not men, were the natural nurses was a prevailing belief of the nineteenth and into the twentieth century. Although there are instances of American men working as professional nurses in antebellum society, it was rare that they held the institutional and community roles that the women nurses did, particularly the religious sisters. However, the Daughters of Charity were typically paid less than the male attendants in the hospitals where they provided services because their vow of poverty precluded them from asking for more than they needed for daily life. Whether hired as attendants who helped to lift patients and perform male patients' intimate hygiene care or as night watchers, men made more money than the women nurses prior to secularization reform.[99]

And while perhaps unsuccessful at helping women achieve social equality, the women's rights reform movement did impact women's political culture. Women actually lost some of their position "above politics" and their "position as the force of moral order."[100] They entered the political and social sphere of men but not as equals. Government gradually took over the roles that had been part of women's domain. This was particularly noticeable in the realm of charitable community service. Americans' "faith in scientific method and in professionalism eventually led to a devaluation of voluntary work and to the relinquishment of social policy to experts in government bureaucracies."[101]

A trained nurse was most notably distinguished from religious nurses in that she was a paid employee, whether in the home or in the hospital. A "trained nurse" was often referred to as a "paid nurse." But Florence Nightingale objected to the use of the term "paid nurse" because, she argued, it was "only the *training* of a woman that made her a Nurse."[102] Catholic sisters provided care for people of all socioeconomic levels but primarily focused their cares to the sick poor and insane, often leaving the care of the middle class and elite to the trained nurses. This posed some problems. Middle-class patients could not afford a trained nurse. An advertisement in the 1909 *Journal of the American Medical Association* stated that the new trained nurses were only providing services to the well-to-do. The ad requested that nurses in training spend their first six months working outside the hospital so that "people of moderate means" could secure "competent" nurses[103] at nurse-in-training rates set by the schools.

Nightingale, like the communities of religious sister-nurses whom she studied, believed nursing to be altruistic, a social quality that Nightingale associated with the female gender. She successfully created an image of the "professional nurse" that was by the 1870s not only widely popular in England but also in America. The legend surrounding Nightingale was composed of two contrasting images, the domestic self-sacrificing woman and the military heroine.[104] But the nurse of the future would also be an autonomous woman, free of religious authority and spiritually "called" to provide intelligent, charitable service.

Nightingale challenged the notion that women only entered nursing when "disappointed in love." She stated that women had a calling or vocation to nurse and that the professional nurse of the modern era no longer needed the religious "vow" to convince her to study nursing. She distanced her work from the Sisters of Charity (Protestant and Catholic) when she wrote in the final pages of her *Notes on Nursing*:

> It is true *we* make "no vows." But is a "vow" necessary to convince us that the true spirit for learning any art, most especially an art of charity, aright, is not a disgust to everything or something else? Do we really place the love of our kind (and of nursing, as one branch of it) so low as this?[105]

Nightingale's training model with a trained woman as superintendent was devised to ensure women autonomy in the healthcare arena. In this her acts were in alignment with the women's rights agenda. The superintendent negotiated all disciplinary action and ward issues with physicians and administrators. She encouraged those adopting her model to use their cultural authority, as she had to convince administrators that the superintendent of the nurse-training program should be a woman.

Because of the growth of American hospitals, it was not hard for the supporters of her model to convince administrators of the need for trained women nurses and women superintendents; they were cheaper than male workers. Secular nursing in America became an acceptable profession for women because of the legendary link with the Nightingale image of the "lady" nurse trained in a hospital program run by credible women and physicians. It was only a matter of time before the reputation of religious sisters, built over many decades, was transferred to graduates of the secular programs. There were, however, significant differences between the educational programs of the Daughters of Charity and the Nightingale Model.

Secularized nurses in America, whose ideal was the Nightingale

Model, were tied to physician dominance in a way that did not exist in the Vincentian-Louisian-Setonian tradition. Although the Daughters of Charity staffed hospitals in the early days, they always had input into the negotiation of their contracts with administrators, and if they felt the institution was not living up to their agreements with the community— i.e., their decisions placed the sisters' or the patients' safety in jeopardy— the sisters left. Trained nurses in the secularized program were workers for the hospital. The early student nurses were described as "industrial slaves" who were part of the "hospital machine."[106] Students often rebelled at the long hours and the level of housekeeping work required. The focus on nursing care in "reformed" hospitals had moved from a spiritually based community model represented in the nursing ministry of religious sisters to an institutional model supporting the development of biomedical science.

The Daughters of Charity, such as Sister Matilda Coskery, had historically supported medical science; they had had a deliberate hand in its evolution. But their spiritual intention and focus was always clearly the holistic corporal and spiritual care of the patient. The medical and nursing techniques and healthcare institutions, as well as the doctrine of their faith, were only the human scaffold for the work of the divinity within to heal and comfort those in need. These historical differences are subtle but important. The adoption of the Nightingale legend and its accompanying model of nursing education was a major shift in American nursing history that still influences the professional culture and identity of nurses and nurse educators in America today.

Some nurses remember having to stand up for a physician who walked onto a hospital ward in the twentieth century. This was a product of the secularization reform movement. The early Daughters of Charity were deeply respectful of physicians and other authorities, an attitude that was a manifestation of their religious beliefs surrounding their relationship to God. But there is no record of the early nurses standing for physicians simply because they walked into a room or any kind of behavior like that. For several decades following the founding of the large national medical organizations in the 1840s, nurses' work was not defined by physicians. After nursing reform in the later nineteenth century, the relationship between physicians and nurses changed significantly, seeming to fall in line with what doctors such as Amariah Brigham had in mind. American physicians amassed greater sociocultural dominance and claimed a right to define the limits of nursing work.[107] This established nursing as outside contemporary definitions of a profession as autonomous, self-directing, and holding a monopoly. History suggests the opposite was true of the DC Nurses: they were autonomous, innovative, and highly respected by physicians as colleagues and friends. It is speculative, however, that nurses, because of the nature of caring, of their close relationships with people, and their social contract to care, ever did or ever will establish a sociocultural monopoly on caregiving.

The structure of secular nursing programs mirrored the social changes of an era of rapid industrialization in which science was fast replacing God in American culture and physicians were becoming the self-appointed heads of healthcare. The doctor-nurse game was in full force. It is still talked about in the healthcare literature and in hospitals today. According to research, some nurses and educators also prefer to remain in subservient roles to physicians,[108] and some physicians prefer not to collaborate, as it will further "erode their position of authority and power."[109] Physicians are concerned, for example, about the creation of the doctorate in nursing practice. Recently, the American Medical Association House of Delegates entertained resolutions to legally limit the use of the titles "doctor," "resident," and "residency" to physicians, dentists, and podiatrists.[110] Evidently, they do not want patients calling nurses "doctor" under any circumstances.

One area in which nurses and physicians have successfully collaborated is when patients and healthcare teams are faced with moral dilemmas. In these instances, the nurse-doctor alliance "seems to enable practitioners to provide a more humane, insightful care than either individual could if acting alone; that is, the relationship is synergistic."[111] Some doctors, nurses, and educators are working toward collaborative agreements to ensure that patients have the best access to medical and nursing care and to better work together to reform the healthcare system. The collegiality of nurse-physician partnerships is foundational to the stability and success of healthcare endeavors. Numerous studies have demonstrated that doctor-nurse communication and collaboration has an impact on patient outcomes.[112]

Physicians continue to be recognized by state statutes and the

American public as the major decision makers in healthcare; there has been movement toward greater equality, however, as was present in nineteenth-century society. The establishment of the Advanced Practice Nurse (APN) role has instigated some change. APNs are a symbol of the return of some of the autonomy and freedom nurses enjoyed when helping patients earlier in the nation's history. There has been a lot of professional rivalry between APNs and physicians, especially over prescription of medicines. But gradually, individual physicians have become more accepting of APNs,[113] and many successful practice collaborations have resulted. While nurses have become better at defining their practice as the treatment of human response to illness rather than the treatment of disease, as in physician practice, to set it apart legally from physicians', the boundaries between the two disciplines are still blurred. Perhaps this is for the best, so that each professional team can have the same freedom that Sister Matilda and Dr. Stokes had to design a system of care that is able to respond dynamically to patient need. Perhaps it was the Daughters' and Dr. Stokes's mutual respect and willingness to learn from, rather than attempt to control, one another that enabled their partnership not only to stand during adversity but to thrive.

Lost in Transition ⌒

The introduction of secular training programs, a "modern" approach to nursing education, was supported by hospitals, public institutions in particular, and their physicians, who wanted finally to have a formal role in creating new nurses. Physicians exerted their authority in institutions to offer secularized nursing leaders the facilities they needed to carry out their goals. But that offer came at a price. Students and their superintendents were employees ultimately accountable to the institution, rather than the mission of a religious or apostolic community. The new nurse-training model met the needs of Protestant Americans, young women who wanted to be nurses, physicians, and the public, who wanted them to provide better nursing services. Secular programs such as the Bellevue Training School attracted more and more women as their graduates ultimately demonstrated to the public that they could provide care and manage hospitals in a way that was comparable to the standards of the Catholic and Deaconess sisters. But it was the transition that occurred behind the scenes—the accommodations and adjustments that nurses had to make to acculturate to the change—that raises some questions about the viability of the secularization reforms spawned in the late nineteenth century under the Nightingale banner. Did secularized nursing education, the Nightingale model, really *secularize* nursing, or were the programs really Protestant programs that were unaffiliated with any religious organization?

The new program was not the first attempt at secularization in nursing; secularization was a primary ideal of the founders of the Daughters of Charity. Vincent de Paul and Louise de Marillac created a community of apostolic women, unlike the nuns of their day. The women did not identify themselves as "religious," a political distinction during their time; instead, they were a confraternity or community of *lay* women who would "come and go like seculars."[114] The DC Nurses' education and the regulations that they followed prepared them for secular service. Yet the American public still identified the DC Nurses as religious women.

The sisters were affiliated with the Catholic Church and supervised by ecclesiastical superiors who handled much of the business and negotiated their contracts. It is easy to understand how the American public would associate Daughters of Charity Nurses with a religious, faith-based tradition, because they were affiliated with the Catholic religion. While from their perspective, the sisters did not proselytize and may have exercised restraint related to imparting Catholic beliefs and practices in patient care, they were certainly not completely secular by nineteenth-century definition. Although the boundaries between spiritual care and religious instruction were taught to DC Nurses by Sister Matilda, Mother Mary Xavier, and others who modeled Community *Regulations* on the subject, many recognized a need for further separation of nursing from any organized religion.

The Daughters of Charity must have accomplished some level of success in differentiating spirituality and religiosity in nursing practice. They faced anti-Catholic sentiment all the time in the early years, and yet story after story confirms why the nurses were able to thrive in the fast-growing healthcare arena.[115] Were the nurse graduates and educators of the "training" programs of the later part of the century any more secular than the Daughters of Charity? In one sense the programs' nonaffiliation with any religion made them more secular than the Catholic Sisters. It also made them more secular than those trained under the Deaconess model.

But Nightingale, whose model was the expressed ideal of secularization leaders, had trained, albeit briefly, at Kaiserwerth in Germany and in Paris with the Daughters of Charity. Her work was greatly influenced by both nonsecular experiences, especially the character development, rituals, and rule-based lifestyle followed by the sister-nurses. The women who entered the Nightingale-based training programs were to be Christians of good character. Therefore it seems that the first late-nineteenth-century nurse-training programs had only achieved a preliminary level of secularization, creating distance between nursing and organized religion and religious communities. The programs were still affiliated with Christian culture, Protestant belief in particular, and therefore remained faith based and clearly dedicated to gospel values rather than fully secular.

The Daughters of Charity were not the only community to begin to integrate the concept of secularization prior to the Nightingale educational model. Irish nurse Catherine McAuley founded the Dublin Institute of Our Lady of Mercy in 1828, a home and hospital visiting-nurse service. She and the women who joined her were Catholics and Protestants. Although they were faithful to their religious heritages and they wore religious garb, they defined their nursing organization as "secular," in that they were "concerned with the world and its affairs."[116] According to historian Therese Meehan, the women, under intense social and political pressure, were directed to form a religious order or disband.[117] The Catholic nurses became the Religious Sisters of Mercy in 1831, and Mother McAuley continued to develop her detailed system of careful nursing, which was known by many, including Florence Nightingale. Mother McAuley's system of nursing included the spiritual dimension of the patient, as did other nursing communities. Many of Mother McAuley's concepts, such as creating a restorative environment and the nurse's prudent judgment, were echoed across the Atlantic in Sister Matilda's writings.

Whether due to social, religious, or professional pressures, secularization has not been an easy goal for nursing. This raises the question whether it is really possible for nurses who care for the spiritual as well as corporal needs of the sick, poor, and insane to achieve a fully secular practice if they hold any spiritual beliefs or adhere to any religious doctrine and dogma. Trying to separate the two may be creating an unnatural schism between belief and practice in a discipline that, in the twentieth century, has been defined as a "human" and "sacred" science by nurse scholars, including Rosemarie Parse and Jean Watson.[118] The Daughters of Charity, from the earliest days of the founding of the French Community to establishment of the American, believed that they were able to set aside their religious beliefs by avoiding initiation of the discussion of Catholic instruction when ministering to patients; however, they did not stop practicing their faith, even wearing religious attire such as the cornette. They did not abandon their spirituality that they knew was valued by humanity, qualities such as kindness and enlightened charity.

Twenty-first-century nurse educators distinguish spirituality from religiosity.[119] Spirituality is the greater focus of curriculum development in secular institutions, but it is acknowledged that it is disease management rather than spirituality that has received more attention in American nursing programs in recent decades.[120] Faith-based nursing programs do attend to spiritual issues that nurses face in patient care, but they may or may not distinguish between religiosity and spirituality in nurses' approaches to those issues in practice. The American Holistic Nurses Association and nurse-authors who publish on holistic nursing often address the broader focus of spirituality as a separate context for care that reaches beyond religious belief and practice. In defining spirituality in healing and nursing, nurses draw from examples found in literature on ethics and religious studies, such as the writings of the 14th Dalai Lama, winner of the 1989 Nobel Peace Prize and numerous other international humanitarian distinctions:

> Religion I take to be concerned with belief in the claims of one faith tradition or another—an aspect of which is acceptance of some form of metaphysical or supernatural reality, including perhaps an idea of heaven or nirvana. Connected with this are religious teachings or dogma, ritual prayer and so on. Spirituality I take to be concerned with those qualities of the human spirit—such

as love and compassion, patience, tolerance, forgiveness, contentment, a sense of responsibility, a sense of harmony, which bring happiness to both self and others. While ritual and prayer, along with the questions of nirvana and salvation, are directly connected to religious faith, these inner qualities need not be, however.[121]

In a 2000 interview, M. Patricia Donahue, a distinguished American nurse historian, said about American nurses' religious history that there were three primary influences on the development of nursing that give nurses "trouble in contemporary society": religion, the military, and technology.[122] Donahue has contributed much to nursing on the topic of spirituality, tracing American nurses' roots in *spirituality* (not religion) to the Christian era.

As Dr. Donahue stated, religion in nursing has posed and continues to pose ethical and clinical challenges in nursing. Secularization seems to have been more difficult yet. Religion provides a firm structure and a set of guidelines for practice that one adopts when one works within a faith-based community, school, or organization. Economic, social, and political situations can conflict with the boundaries of religious doctrine and dogma in the realm of the healing arts . . . in nursing. Because society expects the "timeless values" of nursing—compassion, quality of care, and commitment—to be exemplified by its associated institutions and nurses, setting up rules or policies that exclude peoples of different faiths is nonproductive and potentially a threat to peace and global health. The founders of the Daughters of Charity knew the importance of community, not only of their own Community of sisters for the sake of the mission but also the relationship of their confraternity with the larger society that included peoples of all races, nationalities, gender, socioeconomic levels, and religions. The Daughters of Charity showed that nursing had the potential to evolve as an expression of the broader culture of human beings living together in global community. They may not have fully realized that potential because American Protestants were stirred to move in a new direction.

Intimate day-to-day care for the vulnerable, sick, poor, insane, and dying has propelled nurses to seek balance and boundaries between personal and professional values and beliefs. Despite numerous external pressures, early nurses wrestled with the challenges of establishing and maintaining a professional position in society in which they determined the direction of their work and ministries, evaluated the outcomes of those endeavors and held strong to patient-centered spiritual values of compassion, humility, simplicity, and charity. They did this while advocating in a male-dominated public arena for the rights of those who did not have the physical, mental, emotional, or spiritual stamina to do so for themselves. It would seem that the biggest challenge to the nursing *profession* in America and the ability of nurses to advocate for patients has been the creation of secularized training programs in which leadership could demand the loyalty of nurses to the institution and the "orders" of its affiliated physicians because the nurses were employed individually rather than collectively as a community of sister-nurses. It is not difficult to understand why some hospital nurses in the twentieth and twenty-first centuries have turned to labor unions when they have felt that their needs for proper working conditions were not being met. In the nineteenth century it was the clergy Directors and the Sister Servants instead of union leaders who were the negotiators for the sisters who worked in hospitals that were not owned by the Community. Ultimately, the Daughters of Charity realized that they would better retain their autonomy by creating their own hospitals and asylums.

Trading Autonomy for Alignment

The inauguration ceremony for the first nurse training school at Johns Hopkins Hospital occurred in October 1889. The hospital was erected on the site of the Maryland Hospital, where Sister Matilda and William Stokes first concocted the dream that would be the Mount Hope Retreat. On that day, when Isabel Hampton,[123] who was selected to lead the new training program, spoke of her vision for nursing, the Sister Servant of the Mount Hope Retreat, Sister Catharine Mullan (1833–1909) was in attendance.[124] In her speech Hampton aligned the training program, which represented the "best in nursing," with the new Johns Hopkins University School of Medicine, where the intent was to raise the standards of medicine. Johns Hopkins, founded by Quakers, was redefining the practice of medicine as an "intellectual matter" rather than a trade, and women were to take part in the endeavor. Hospital trustees chose Dr. John Shaw Billings of the United States Army Medical Corps as medical adviser. Billings rejected the Nightingale model; he was not used to working with women nurses, let alone having women in positions of authority. Although he understood the concerns surrounding the potential for young people to stray sexually, he insisted on experimenting with training some male nurses along with the women students.

The nurse in training, according to Dr. Henry Hurd, hospital superintendent, was to be given opportunity not only for work on a variety of wards but also to receive "carefully devised courses of study and systematic mental training."[125] Hurd had worked as asylum superintendent for the insane and therefore promoted the importance of kindness in nursing the sick. He, Isabel Hampton, and her assistant Lavinia Dock,[126] determined to make nursing work a career for women and to elevate its social status to that of "learned profession"[127] of women of high moral character. Physicians who supervised the nurses at Johns Hopkins, such as Dr. Howard Kelly, reminded graduating trained nurses of the "inestimable privilege" of which they were the recipients. They had been "elevated" from a class of "self-taught, selfish hired attendants" to a "new and beautiful ministry."[128]

The establishment of training programs closely aligned with Johns Hopkins and Bellevue Hospitals, and perhaps others, changed American nursing. Professionalism in nursing was no longer defined by communities of religious women with physicians as respected colleagues and consultants. Physicians' roles in supervising and training nurses had been greatly extended as they enjoyed greater economic and social authority in the quasi-secularized, Protestant institutions in which their own science-based medical training programs flourished.

Nursing was not a profession because physicians said it was so. In fact, physicians, as discussed in earlier chapters, had been vying for cultural dominance in healthcare throughout the nineteenth century, and some resisted having nurses as professional colleagues. Nurses were to be workers, the labor force. To assume greater social authority for patients, physicians needed nurses by their sides just as they had when the first medical schools decided to offer their students clinical practice as part of training. The trained nurses and their educators offered physician leaders what they had sought for some time: lay nurses who were hungry for a career. By aligning with physicians and training programs professing to graduate only women of high moral character, American women who did not want to enter Catholic sisterhoods finally had the place and means for career development. But the decision to align with medicine and its social prestige rather than religion had consequences. As the hospital world of science and technology expanded in the twentieth century, competition for funds intensified, leaving training schools and nurses "a poor second to physicians."[129]

Through the period of the Civil War, Sister Matilda and the Daughters of Charity had secured a reputation for American nurses that defined them as autonomous and enlightened. Catholic hospitals were growing, and the commitment of the Church to nursing missions was unwavering. Although the DC Nurses were responsible to their religious community and ultimately to Church authority for their ministerial actions, much of what they did was self-directed. However, at times bishops overstepped their bounds by trying to influence matters within the Community domain, including prevention of mission changes of the Sister Servant. The Daughters of Charity focused on their mission and upheld their core values and rights despite external pressures. Their relationships with physicians were collegial. Although they responded to physician "orders" and vowed humble obedience to all superiors, including physicians and hospital administrators, that obedience was always measured in terms of their spiritual commitment to God first and their advocacy of patients second. The sisters left the Maryland Hospital in 1840 because their passion for their mission "generated a desire for a level of scientific accuracy and a set of caring ethics that superseded all instruction of and obedience to physicians."[130] Before late-nineteenth-century training schools, nurses in many communities, not just the Daughters of Charity, enjoyed a much greater level of autonomy in practice. That autonomy was never achieved or perceived of as existing in isolation. The earlier nurses relied on the suggestions, advice, support, and orders of physicians, bone setters, herbalists, midwives, and an entire network of community healers.[131] Autonomy in the nineteenth century was and continues to be today a measure of professionalism.

Sociologist Elliot Freidson defines a profession as an occupation that has the "power to determine who is qualified to perform a defined set of tasks, to prevent all others from performing that work, and to control the criteria by which to evaluate performance."[132] Though they are responsible to society, professionals engage in self-directed work and are free of control by those who employ them. There is significant evidence of "professional" behavior in the history of the Daughters of Charity prior to the establishment of secular training programs. The sisters exercised a considerable amount of judgment and discernment as well as skill, which Freidson states is a barometer of professionalism. He writes that "whatever practitioners may do at work may require extensive exercise of discretionary judgment rather than choice and routine application of a limited number of mechanical techniques."[133] The educators of early training schools had good intentions of raising the standards of nursing care by Protestant women. In good faith they adopted Nightingale's model of education and her image to inspire women of moral character to enter a career without religious ties.

That severing of religious ties was also extended to history. Somehow, historical accounts of the secularized training programs for nurses of the later nineteenth and early twentieth century and the Nightingale model have become inextricably linked in the minds of many with the "beginning" of professional nursing in America. Professionalization is an ongoing process for nursing just as it has been for medicine. Exclusion and inclusion criteria for the definition are sociocultural constructions. American nursing as a culture has made certain choices about how it has defined itself and how it continues to do so.

As the secular training schools expanded their reach and grew in success after the 1873 inception at Bellevue, nurses and even physicians observed the cultural and historical shift that was occurring. At the ceremony celebrating the first graduating class of nursing students in Detroit at the Daughters of Charity's St. Mary's Hospital Training School in 1895, Dr. T. A. McGraw, who spoke about the history of nursing, suggested that, while praise was due Florence Nightingale for her work, "it should never be forgotten that the work done for the English people by her had been begun and followed up in a quieter way by the Sisters of Charity in France and Italy for 200 years before."[134] Some showed concern that the history of the important contribution of the sisters might be lost in the flurry of modernization. As the alignment of American nursing shifted from organized religion to universities and hospitals, and the ideological orientation for its reform moved from spirituality toward science, it seemed that those concerns might be legitimate.

Enlightened Reform
and Esprit de Corps

The history of Sister Matilda Coskery and the early Sisters and Daughters of Charity is in many respects a lost part of American nurses' history and *professional* identity. The sisters' contributions to "the blessed art" that is nursing are relevant, inspiring, and essential. They are relevant because the sisters in the 1800s dealt with some of the very same issues nurses face today, from staffing a hospital ward to doctor-nurse relationships to social justice. The history of their nursing ministry is inspiring because it is filled with stories of the sisters' endurance, despite great challenges to their caring missions. They started hospitals in rundown log cabins and ran their own asylum with physicians as consultants, despite public accusations of impropriety. Their reputation soared despite the political crusade of "know-nothings" because they had the courage to care for those with illnesses the public feared. Knowledge of the Daughters' early history is essential because it is a part of American nursing tradition that has been absent for more than a century.

The presence of a nursing text such as *Advices Concerning the Sick* poses the question of why American nurses chose to inscribe their "modern" history as beginning in 1873 with the establishment of a secularized program and the introduction of the educational model created by a British nurse. Perhaps American nurses' history, not unlike that of other scientists, has been influenced by religious differences. The outcome, however, has been that generations of American nurses have been deprived of a significant part of their history, of which the Daughters of Charity is only one small piece in the puzzle that is early American professional nursing. Nevertheless it is a piece that is important to the overall understanding of professional choices and policies that were established in the later nineteenth century with the advent of secular training schools and maturation of the profession's role in public life.

With maturation comes wisdom, a way of knowing that is born from experience and expertise. The Daughters of Charity Nurses possessed that wisdom. They knew that there was a curative point during convalescence; they also knew how to observe and care for the patient on the brink of healing. They practiced intelligently, with an aware spirit that required obedience to superiors and a respect for all persons that was regulated by their own discernment, a specific quality passed down from the Community founders to Mothers to Novice Mistresses and to new nurses.

The sisters' values of humility, simplicity, and charity inspired their nursing. Attention to simplicity in particular was critical to the lives of patients. Sister Matilda reminded nurses of the importance of the simplest nursing interventions, such as preparing herbal teas for patients. The preparation of teas was just one of many healing traditions, enduring time and travel between cultures, that can be traced through more than three hundred years of the sisters' compassionate care, linking American nursing with the French. The core values of Vincentian-Louisian nursing—respect for every patient and kindness as the remedy of remedies—stood the test of cultural translation across the Atlantic.

The Daughters of Charity in the nineteenth century were said to have practiced an *enlightened charity*. Their ability to demonstrate "judicious and intelligent" nursing was not the only attribute that won them this distinction, however. They were also highly devoted to their patients and exhibited a spirit of intention to care that others were said not to have possessed. The sisters were students of the devotion that St. Francis de Sales defined as "simply a spiritual activity and liveliness by means of which Divine Love works in us, and causes us to work briskly and lovingly; and just as charity leads us to a general practice of all God's Commandments, so devotion leads us to practice them readily and diligently."[1] Charity was the sisters' doctrine and devotion their intention. Enlightened charity was the product of the integration of the intelligence, respect, and thoughtfulness from the head and the devotion flowing from the heart. Heart, head, and hand, the sister-nurses made a difference in the lives of many. The spirituality that infused their nursing service is palpable in the stories of patient care by DC Nurses like Sisters Matilda Coskery, Joanna Smith, Ambrosia Magner, and Rosaline Brown.

Spirituality drew the women together into community in the first place. The early history of the Daughters of Charity Nurses demonstrates how important community was: It was manifested in mutual support for the sake of the nursing mission and the safety of women who knew that they were called to serve humanity publicly in the hospital arena that was mostly defined as a man's domain. Preservation of the spirit of community, the *esprit de corps*, was critical to each sister's spiritual path and the community as a whole. Louise de Marillac's letters are a study in community building from a seventeenth-century perspective. Community served the purpose of channeling the energies of the human ego that was humbly sacrificed for the good of the mission of the community.

The sisters had many ways of reinforcing the "unity" in community. Language was important; in the hospital setting, a head nurse was the Sister *Servant* and those assigned to her leadership were *nurse companions*. Community elders and leaders in nursing mentored the novices not only in the skills they needed to care for patients but in the spiritual practice that would buoy them when their ministry was difficult. New sister-nurses were never in want of an elder's advice because they were always assigned the company of another more experienced sister. The entire Community, often referred to as a "Company," (secular) rather than a "Congregation" (religious), was designed over the course of many years by Louise de Marillac and Vincent de Paul to be a primary place of belonging, like a home. The sisters carried the spirit of their home Community wherever they were missioned. And when controversies were not resolved, the Community adjusted, sometimes with the sisters creating new sites and branches of nursing ministry.

Recent studies confirm some of what the sisters knew intuitively about the power of community. Studies have shown that living in community reduces the risk of death due to coronary heart disease and stroke.[2] Results of a study of aging nuns, known as the "Nun Study," show that living in community, especially one in which members share a deep spirituality, provides an "ever present network of support and love," as well as security throughout life.[3] Psychologist M. Scott Peck has also written that the seeds of community are in humanity and that the establishment of community has the potential to lead to conflict resolution and global peace.[4]

The American Sisters and then Daughters of Charity sought solutions to social problems only after they had established their Community. While all religious sister-nurses had communities as their base of support, the secular, trained nurses did not. They relied upon an organization in which they were employed to provide some of the benefits the sisters enjoyed, but they did not have the spiritual community for support when controversies arose. The sister-nurses' accounts of their caring ministry showed that their foundation for decision making and for solving tough problems lay with their Community spirit. The strong esprit de corps, or support within community, enabled Sister Servants to negotiate with hospital administrators and Church governance over such issues as unsafe staffing and extending more charity to the poor. Within the security of community, sisters could more freely create solutions to their problems. They formed mutually fulfilling relationships with physicians, never guessing perhaps that an act of collegiality would challenge the status quo to the extent that it did. They left the Maryland Hospital for their own Mount St. Vincent's, followed by their patients, after trying for years to negotiate with administrators. They decided to nurse both the Union and Confederate soldiers and determined to further secularize their hospitals and educational programs when it was time to change.

History is a record of patterns of cause and effect, action and reaction to personal, community, environmental, and global change. Those patterns, the data over time, are evidence of humanity in motion on the sea of events. Sometimes the waters navigated during life changes are choppy and seem unsafe. Historical evidence provides a rudder, both clues and cautions, for present and future decisions in chaotic times. Chaos is often assigned a negative connotation. It is thought of as disturbing disorder that one experiences as a sense of being out of control. One example of this in healthcare might be the outbreak of a deadly disease such as cholera or ebola for which there is no known way to eradicate the disease before it causes death. Not knowing how to stop a disease can be experienced as chaos, especially when the disease kills hundreds or thousands of people in a short period of time. But chaos or "formlessness" in its scientific meaning is not necessarily negative or positive; it is potential or empty space waiting for fulfillment.

Chaos, more specifically the "edge" of chaos, has been the phrase used to define *this* time of millennial transition in nursing history. Nursing is at a crossroads, where many call for its reorientation, reconceptualization,[5] and reform. Nursing history is a barometer for reform and a springboard for innovation. Without awareness of nursing history, a claim for successful reform, modernization, and adapting to the "signs of the times" cannot really be made in good conscience.

Chaos seems to invoke reform. American healthcare may be in a perpetual state of chaos because healthcare reform is a subject that seems to have possessed the minds of Americans since the early nineteenth century, if not before. It was one of the most crucial social issues of Sister Matilda's time; she devoted much of her life to creating a calm, healing environment for her insane patients. Reform, it seems, was instilled as part of the existence of the sisters' Community. The sisters strived together in community through nursing and education services in a way that reformed public opinion about Catholics and in so doing indirectly affected the changing roles of women in American society. The sisters endured many hardships because they held a vision for the changes they sought. Their visions for reform were not easily deterred by exterior circumstances. Their spirituality, their inner devotion, was the quality of heart that sustained them individually and collectively. Even so, reform was still not an easy process. Bishop Bruté wrote on the subject of succession and reform to Rose White, who became Mother of the American Sisters of Charity following the death of the foundress, Mother Seton:

> Every one that succeeds others is apt to claim an exclusive talent, and to condemn her predecessors. . . . I know not, but I am pretty sure that there are abuses and imperfections everywhere. . . . For my part, here I never get any new prefect without hearing him say, he will reform, and often-times the reformer does worse than the reformed.[6]

The best ideas and intentions of health reformers are not always actualized. Sister Matilda and Dr. Stokes's decision to have women begin to nurse male patients was carried into the twentieth century, but the enthusiasm for moral therapy lost momentum within just a few decades. It was ultimately replaced with psychotropic medications as the treatment of choice. Then again, a century later, many psychiatric and long-term facilities and nurses such as reformer Esther Lucille Brown began to explore use of the physical environment for therapeutic purposes and to "restore the amenities of the era of Moral Treatment."[7] She also discussed the importance of food and eating together as a social "therapy," a practice Sister Matilda had strongly emphasized as healing to patients with mental illness and helpful to the nurses and staff working with them. Another study that spanned the course of three decades confirmed what Sister Matilda and the sisters knew about the importance of community life in the long-term treatment of psychotic patients.[8] These therapies are not really introducing a "new dimension" to patient care per se but are more of a combination of the old and new ways of caring for patients.

Reform is a creative process, which, like the concepts of secularization and professionalism, is complex and perhaps best explained within a context. Secularization is defined by the presence or absence of religion; professionalism, by the presence or absence of special skill. Reform is defined in terms of history. Whether or not healthcare is "reformed" actually depends upon a comparison between what healthcare was like before and after a specific change was introduced. "Reform" is not the change that is made to healthcare, its systems, or its people. It is a process in which the outcome is evaluated within the context of history. Sister Matilda and Dr. Stokes claimed that their approach to care of the insane, the implementation of moral therapy with kindness as the "remedy of remedies," was reforming American asylum care; but only time would tell. "Trained" nurses, it was suggested, were the products of a reformed system of American nursing. But it is clear that while major reform to state institutions and among Protestant nurses did occur, that reform did not necessarily extend to the spiritual roots of those of the Vincentian-Louisian-Setonian tradition. The Daughters of Charity did adapt to the reforms that occurred in the later nineteenth and early twentieth centuries. They began to integrate lay nurses into their hospitals and schools of nursing, but the history of that transition is outside the scope of this book. The history of secularization as it was written in the early twentieth century has affected nursing education, practice, and policy for decades. For those who plan to set future policies and practice agendas, new histories of early and mid-nineteenth-century nursing provide vital access to the experiences and expertise of the Americans who birthed professional nursing.

Ralph Waldo Emerson once wrote that "nothing great was ever accomplished without enthusiasm."[9] The Daughters of Charity nursed with devotion, enthusiasm, and a zeal that Vincent de Paul defined as the "rays of the sun" and "most pure in the love of God."[10] Their care was considered noticeably different from that of others. A passion for patient care was cultivated in each Daughter of Charity Nurse. It was self-inspired, mission driven, and generated within the Community. The sisters regularly told each other stories of healings and conversions that they witnessed in the care of patients. They quoted inspirational passages from their religious teachings to each other and then put their words into action by their work. It is in this spirit that Sister Matilda wrote *Advices*, and it is in this spirit that we have written this history.

History is revelation. We are enthusiastic about the implications of this history to nurses, novice and experienced. We are hopeful that this history will clarify the intentions and practices of some early religious nurses and their role in the development of professional nursing in America. We are grateful for the opportunity to spend so many years inside the world of American nurses who were pioneers in every sense of the word. And we pray that there have been parts of this history that have informed if not inspired new visions; for what one nurse has done in her time, any can do in theirs.

Appendix A:
Rules and Regulations for the Maryland Hospital, 1833

Courtesy, Daughters of Charity Archives, Emmitsburg, Maryland

Patients:

1. None other than lunatic patients are to be admitted into this institution unless by the express direction of the Board of Visitors.
2. Lunatic patients can only be admitted upon the order of a Court of Competent Jurisdiction - or upon the certificate of two regular physicians.
3. Cases of Delirium Tremens and Drunkeness may be admitted on an emergency without the required Certificate, provided however they are furnished as speedily as possible after the individual has been admitted.
4. In all Cases security for the board and other expenses of the patients must be given, and no patient can be permitted to remain unless regular payment for the board and other expenses is made.
5. Pauper lunatics sent by authority of the cities or counties under the provisions of the Acts of Assembly, are to be received at the rates established by said act; but provision must be made by the Sheriff or his agent for the regular payment of such rates, and for proper and sufficient clothing.
6. In default of payment by any City, County or guardian the patient must be sent to his proper place of residence.

7. Patients are to be received at the Hospital by the Sister Superior, and lodged in such rooms as may be chosen by the friends or may be proper to their care.
8. The personal effects of the patients are to be placed under the care of the Sister Superior, and in no instance can a patient be allowed to retain clothes, trunks, etc. in his room without the permission of the Standing Committee.
9. All patients must conform to the rules and usages of the Hospital and submit to the management of the Sisters of Charity, and by the Sister Superior in such things as she may direct; and it is expressly enjoined on them to behave respectfully to the sisters and all attendants -- all disrespect to be reported to the Board of Visitors.
10. Patients are to rise at _____ OCLK A.M., dine at _____ OCLK P.M., sup at _____ OCLK P.M., and retire to their rooms at _____ OCLK P.M., except such patients as may be designated by the Medical Attendant for particular reasons.
11. No patients shall be allowed fire, lights or Segars - Tobacco and Snuff may be allowed under the directions of the Medical Attendant for particular reasons.
12. No patients shall go without the enclosure of the Hospital without the consent of the Medical Attendant, and at the same time he must inform the Sister Superior or her substitute that he has such permission to leave the Hospital and for what length of time.

Medical Attendant:

1. It shall be his duty to reside in the Hospital and devote all his talents and benevolence to the benefit of his patients, attending them at all times, day and night when necessary.
2. It shall be the duty of the Medical Attendant to see each patient as soon as admitted and obtain all possible information about the nature of the disease.
3. Should he think it for the benefit of the patient that his room should be changed, he must request the Sister Superior to cause such change to be made as he may think necessary.

4. The Medical Attendant must endeavor to give satisfaction to the friends of the patients whenever called on by them for information.
5. Should the president object, the Medical Attendant shall not permit another Medical gentleman to see a patient even though the Medical Attendant should be willing thereto.
6. The Medical Attendant must consult with the President in all important cases--reporting to him all wants in his department.
7. It shall be the duty of the Medical Attendant to conduct the plan of Medical & moral treatment agreed upon between himself and the President particularly as regards air, exercise, diet, confinement, occupation, amusement, reading, conversation, etc.
8. No patient can be confined or punished without the consent of the Medical Attendant, unless necessity should require for obvious reasons that the Sister Superior should do so; and even in this he must be the judge whether the confinement or punishment must be continued.
9. The Medical Attendant must keep a prescription or diet book and state in it the progress of each case. By this book the Sisters are to be governed in attending the patient.
10. The Medical Attendant must also keep a register of the patients, according to the Custom of all Hospitals, and report once a year to the Board of Visitors in Writing, the result of his treatment, giving as full a statement as he can.
11. The Medical Attendant may in his discretion take the patients to walk, to ride, to fish, or to Church, observing proper care that his indulgence does not go too far.
12. It is the duty of the Medical attendant to classify the patients as regards their association with each other at table and in the parlors and lodging.
13. The Medical Attendant is especially enjoined to maintain the authority and respectability of the Sisters of Charity; the end and principle of the whole system being to advance the cause of humanity. It is evident that this cannot be done without a good understanding between the Medical Attendant and the immediate attendants upon the patients.

14. Should differences of opinion occur between the Medical Attendant and the Sisters, the President is to be umpire unless an appeal to the Standing Committee or the board be desired by either party.

Sister Superior:

1. To the Sister Superior is confided the entire domestic management of the institution.
2. The Sister Superior will received all patients on their arrival at the Hospital and arrange with their friends what room they are to occupy and at what price.
3. The Sister Superior will call upon the Medical Attendant to see the patient as soon as practicable after his or her arrival.
4. Should the Medical Attendant advise the removal of the patient to a room different from that occupied by the patient at the time, the Sister Superior will cause the removal to be made accordingly.
5. All monies paid on account of patients will be received by the Sister Superior.
6. The Sister Superior must require before the patient is admitted the usual certificate of insanity except in the cases herein before excepted.
7. The Sister Superior will demand and receive the security for the payment of the expenses of the patient.
8. She must keep a book in which the names, ages, residences, time of admission and discharge, price of board and security are all to be entered.
9. The Sister Superior must be governed in the charges made by her by the direction of the Standing Committee.
10. The Sister Superior will, under the direction of the President, make all purchases and keep regular accounts to be open at all times to the inspection of the President and Board of Visitors.
11. Collection which the Sister Superior cannot make, she will request the President to make, furnishing him the accounts therefore.

12. The Sister Superior will appoint the Sisters to their several duties according to her knowledge of their disposition and capacities.

13. The Sister Superior shall have the power to select her servant to be employed in the Hospital but shall retain none that the President shall not approve of.

14. The general domestic economy of the Institution being thus in charge of the Sister Superior, she is required to keep the President, as the executive officer of the Board of Visitors, advised of all matters having bearing upon its interests that may come to her knowledge.

15. The Sister Superior must from time to time inspect the rooms of the patients to see that they have proper attention. She must inculcate in the Sisters the necessity of mildness and forbearance to the patients, indeed those having more immediate care of them, to talk to & amuse them, and to endeavor by every effort of moral management, to interest and soothe the patient's mind, sitting in their rooms with them when opportunity admits-- and in short, doing what they can by kindness and charity to soften the hard lot of insanity.

16. The Sister Superior must consider the President as the official organ of the Board, and consider herself as acting for the Board under his advisement.

The Sisters of Charity:

1. It shall be their duty to attend to the sick and insane under the direction of the medical attendant, in the execution of his prescriptions and in doing all in their power to aid him in relieving the patients.

2. They shall attend to all such duties in the economy of the house which the Sister Superior shall direct.

3. The Sisters will always have the privilege of keeping the Chapel and of having Mass whenever they think proper, as well as of seeing their acquaintances and friends.

The President:

1. This officer represents the Board in the intervals between its meetings, and is the executive officer of the institution.
2. It is the duty of the President to lay down the plans of medical and moral treatment for the patients.
3. He is responsible for the attendance of the Medical Attendant and must consult with him in all cases of difficulty.
4. He must see that the patients are well attended, fed and accommodated, that proper attention is paid to them, and they are gently and humanely treated.
5. He must see that order & cleanliness prevail in the institution and that proper economy is observed in its expenses.
6. He must see that proper attention is paid to the collection of all dues to the institution--that the books and accounts--medical and financial--are correctly kept, and must endeavor to keep the institution out of debt, by a proper regulation of the charges.
7. It is the duty of the president to attend to the improvement of the grounds and preservation of the buildings.
8. The president shall give such advice as he may think proper to the medical attendant and Sister Superior in their several departments, & should any difference of opinion arise between them, he is to be the umpire, unless an appeal is made to the Standing Committee or to the Board.
9. The president must call the Board when required & must consult the Standing Committee on all important points, and act by their authority and the rules of the Board.

Standing Committee:

The Standing Committee shall consist of the president and two members of the Board to be appointed annually by the Board. They shall report to the Board at every meeting of that body. They shall advise with the President on all matters of importance and aid him as far as practicable in the performance of his duties in the care and superintendence of the institution.

General Regulations:

1. No male person shall visit any female patient unless accompanied by a Sister.

2. Should any patient be on the point of running off or showing violence to the Sisters or attendants, the Sister Superior, or any Sister, if she deems it necessary, may confine such patient and then inform the medical attendant of the fact, whose province it is to determine whether the patients can with propriety be kept confined.

3. No coercive means will be permitted in the institution other than solitary confinement, low diet, shower bath, the muffs--and deprivation of some accustomed gratification--and only under medical advisement.

4. No servant will be permitted under any circumstances to use violence with a patient--dismissal must follow a violation of this rule.

5. The persons employed must be polite and cheerful in their intercourse with the patients, but must never behave towards them as companions.

6. Servants are forbidden to carry letters or newspapers from or to the patients--all such must go through the hands of the Sister Superior and the Medical Attendant.

7. The male patients must be confined to such parts of the house as the President may direct. They must never go upstairs. They are required to show politeness to each other and to the Sisters and all other attendants.

8. The use of segars and pipes is prohibited to all persons connected with the institution.

Appendix B:
Advices Concerning The Sick
by Sister Matilda Coskery

Courtesy, Daughters of Charity Archives, Emmitsburg, Maryland

[*Pg 1*] When a patient is brought to the house, place him according to sickness. If his condition would be disagreeable to others, put him by himself, or as far off in the ward as possible, without however letting him know why.

If he is very sick or weak do not stop to question him about his sickness, as the one at the door shd know his disease, & he may be questioned as to the treatment after he has rested.– Then learn from him what has been done for him as to medicine, blistering, bleeding, dieting, etc.–

Often the weakness of the sick Poor, is from hardship as to food clothing or labor & exposure, so a little light broth shd be given to them soon after they come in.

If he is faint-like, give him a little wine, or toddy. Always keep a bed or two ready, so that the poor sick may not be kept waiting. If he is able & needs a foot wash, put a handful of common salt, or two tablespoons of mustard, or a pint of wood-ashes, into a bucket of warm water, & only wash, not bathe, the feet before getting into bed, let them be dried well. If he has no clean linen, & needs one, loan him one, that his condition may be comfortable. If he is too weak to have the foot wash, let him rest, & when he is more refreshed, let his face, neck, hands, arms, feet & legs be wiped with whiskey, weak spirits of camphor or bay rum. Whatever be his condition, do not let him wait long for a drink if he is thirsty, but give him that that suits his sickness.

If he has fever & ague, he may have almost anything, unless his bowels are too free, in this case, give him barley-water, rice-water, toast-water,

344

gum-water, or water alone, and if he is not too feverish, he may have port

[*Pg 2*] wine with a small piece of ice in it, but never much drink at a time, or the bowels become more free. If the bowels are in good state, he may have jelly-water, lemonade, cream of tartar-water, apple-water, or plain water.– Apple-water, or apple-tea, as it is called, is made by slicing a few ripe apples thinly, pouring a pint of boiling water on them, and when cool, mix as much cold water with it as just leaves the pleasant taste.– If he seems in a sinking state, give him wine or brandy toddy, rub his temples with camphor - put mustard plasters on his ancles [*sic*] not the bones & wrists, & if there be pain of chest or bowels, put a plaster there also. If a patient has had bowel complaint for a long time, great care must be had to his food & drink. If allowed dry toast & tea, the tea shd be fresh & made palatable. – When he may have toast & tea, any of the following things are allowed too, & serve as a change for him, since all these watery things become distasteful to them when they are confined to them. They are as follows: thick rice, or barley water, seasoned with loaf sugar & milk – or arrow-root, sago, tapioca – well cooked & seasoned as the others – Also thin pap, which is made by boiling milk & water thickened with wheat flour, and, very well boiled, & with the sugar, & milk you may also add a few grains of salt for seasoning. When the diet is of this kind, do not make too much at once, for it is unpalatable if old; & the stomach sickens on it, which may cause him to sink, as he is not allowed other food. If he is very low & prostrated, he may have a tablespoonful about every 15 or 20 minutes, but if not so low a teacup ful every 2 or 3 hours; or as best suits the stomach. . . . Tea shd be made every few hours, or stand in an earthen vessel & kept covered – given hot not warm. –

[*Pg 3*] Toast sh [*should*] be <u>browned</u> slowly, <u>not</u> <u>burned</u>, but prepared in a way to be palatable. If they may have it, let it be what they <u>can</u> take, or, as you wd [would] like it brought to yourself, to a sick Parent, and, especially as you shd prepare it for Jesus Christ, who says: "What ye do to these ye do to me" – and: "<u>I</u> was sick, hungry, thirsty, sad &c, and you consoled & ministered to <u>me</u>." When such kind of food is continued for some time, you may give them a greater relish for it, by taking a chicken bone, strip the meat off it, and lay it on a <u>clean</u>, ~~gr~~ <u>hot</u> gridiron, till it schorches [*scorches*] or cooks, or if it had been cooked til it gets hot – sprinkle a few grains of fine salt on it, & let him have it hot – At first he will be almost angry that you wd bring him a bare bone, but after he has tasted it, he will prefer the bare bone to all the other things he gets – and the salty taste of the juice gives him a better appetite for the sloppy, watery things he is allowed – Once or twice a day he may have a bone if he wishes.– Sometimes a very small thing that saves or destroys life.–

In fever, the face, hands, arms & feet shd be often wiped with whiskey, bay- rum or weak spirits of camphor. If he is in his senses & strong enough to use a mouth-wash, let it be by his bed, to rinse his mouth often with, and his tongue may be scraped with a thin whale-bone to prevent it from becoming coated. But if this is already so, & the dark glue is around his teeth, it must be gently removed by a soft mop, & the same for the tongue, as whalebone cd [*could*] not be used on the sore tender tongue – neither cd the brush then be used for the teeth in that condition. But, they must be cleaned little at a time, not at once. By keeping the mout[h] clean, there is less danger of the

[*Pg 4*] disease spreading to others. In all contagious sickness, care shd be taken against receiving their breath into the lungs or stomach – This can easily be avoided, nor need the poor sick know it.– When there is tendency to contagion, let spirits of camphor be often sprinkled on his bed, dampen a towel with it also & leave it about his bed.

If he is allowed cold water, give it fresh & in a <u>clean</u> glass or cup. Not too full or in too large a cup, or he spills it. If he is allowed but little at a time, give him the right quantity only. If he is very weak & has constant thirst, it is handy for him to have his drink in a phial on his bed, as he prefers this to being served, especially as he can take it without fatiguing himself. When they cannot take much drink & the mouth is hot & dry, he may hold water in his mouth & then spit it in the basin.–

If ice, or cold cloths are ordered to the head, place a dry sheet about his neck, shoulders & pillow to prevent them from getting wet; or he may have lung disease by the time his fever is cured. Ice shd be in a bladder or silk-oil cloth bag, which holds the water from running over him as it melts. If cold cloths are used, have two towels, fold them the size you want, & wring one out of the cold water dry enough to keep from dripping

– spread it, or lay it in its folds over the forehead– and in 10 minutes or so - turn it over, laying the upper side next the head, presently changing it for the one that is in the basin, wringing it as the first one, but do not put the warm one in the basin in the fold, or it will soon make the water as warm as the head–but open it & fan it a little when it will be as cool as the water, & it need not be put in the water often, for this fanning makes it cold – keep changing the towels in turn till it is enough. If he shudders from chilliness, stop the cold cloths immediately &

[*Pg 5*] take the wet sheet from him, covering him up for the time, as this shivering is sometimes from some great change in his condition.– If it shd continue long, give a little warm toddy, wine or something to warm him, wipe the forehead dry as soon as he shivers and rub camphor on the temples.– If the ~~the~~ chilliness is only a few minutes & the head shd become hot again, you may apply the cold again — The fanning of the wet towels, often prevents the nurse from taking cold that the dabbling so much in the ice water wd expose her to.–

The shivering, chilliness is apt to occur in Mania a Potu cases, and must have prompt attention, and as often as it comes on the same means of checking it must be used - and when the heat returns, repeat the cloths. in some these changes occur in 10 or 20 minutes of each other, give them a teaspoon of brandy, or if they do not ~~even~~ occur so often a table spoonful – however it may be, care must be had, not to give too much brandy – you must judge of that. —

Never let them sit up to have their sheets or linens changed when they are very low or in a sweat – But wait for more strength or till the Dr says it may be done safely – Health & life is more than cleanliness – At such times avoid washing around his bed also.– A small thing near the <u>crisis</u> of the patient, is very often the cause of death, for being at its height, & on the point of changing for better or worse, one little right matter neglected or one little wrong thing done, takes from him his last chance for recovery. This is what Drs call the curative point, and mostly rests in the hands of the nurse & attendants. —

Avoid plaguing them with unnecessary attentions, these are hateful to God & man, but doubly so now, as life hangs on what is

[*Pg 6*] what is right & proper; more, or less than this is injurious at this critical point.– The sick are weaker than we in body, but strong enough in mind, to see when we work for God, & when for Man. —

Others again who serve the sick, are so very neat, that the poor patient dare not turn in his bed, for fear of rumpling the bed clothes. —

Do not raise a window or open a door too near them when sweating or in diseases that are increased by fresh air - & when smoothing the quilt do not fan or flirt it about their head, if sweating it checks it & if low takes the breath. – If visitors see them in wet weather, do not permit them to loll, or rest their wet arms on his bed. — If the illness has been long, it helps them to move to another room once or twice, staying a week or two in each, but, shd they become house-sick for the room they had left, let them return to it, this indulgence will help them more then, than the stay there. Every reasonable gratification is an important means of recovery, because it excites to content of mind, for the absence of which nothing supplies; and makes you more able to benefit soul & body.– Do not let them wait for their remedies, nourishment, drink or other comforts, for by this delay, besides the harm you may do the body, you irritate & discourage them — Where a disgusting dose is to be given, & the stomach is weak, you may put a small mustard plaster on the pit of the stomach 5 or 10 minutes before giving it, which will prevent their throwing it up again. Have something to give immediately after it, such as a bit of orange or its dried peel - apple - clove, allspice &c— if salts is given, cold water, apple or lemonade is good – and salts may be mixed or dissolved in lemonade; and worked off with it or cold water - but all the other purgatives require warm drinks to make them active enough – but if there be Tendency to loose bowels, much drink shd not be given; and these ought to be one movement from the bowels before drink is taken, unless there be great thirst, then a

[*Pg 7*] mouthful or two may occasionally be taken. or if the nature of the medicine does not prevent it, he may hold water in the mouth & then spit it out. When the convalescent take something for an action of the bowels only, he need not keep from drink or food unless he prefers it.– When medicine is too active it may be checked by a little port wine - or black coffe[e] without cream or sugar, & if it continues, give a few drops, 5 or 6 drops of laudanum occasionally – Or a mustard plaster over the bowels – if the sick is too weak for this, warm some whiskey, rum or brandy & dip a flannel several times folded & put it on as hot as he can bear it – have a second flannel to put on when the first cools.

When they are weak from frequent sweatings, they may be sponged 2 or 3 times a day with warm spirits of camphor, but whilst sponging, keep the air from them by having them well covered at this time.–

When pills are given have them of one size, or the smaller one will dissolve so long before the larger that no effect will be produced, and not allowing for this, stronger will be given which may do him harm; or be too much for him.

Emetics

When an emetic is given have two large basins, a bench or chair to put one on by the bed-side - place a chair, with the back against the bench for the sick to rest his hands or head on whilst vomiting. If he has no handkf [*handkerchief*], hand him a clean towel to wipe his mouth & face with. As soon as he has had one little vomiting or Severe gagging, give him a big drink of <u>warm</u> water, say about a pint & swallowed in big mouth-fuls, as this makes him vomit more easily & may prevent cramps. After each vomiting spell give <u>warm</u> water – if they do not seem easy to vomit you may make the water saltish with table-salt or put a little mustard in it. After he has puked 4 or 5 times freely, give no more water, let him rest if he can, but if the gagging continues put a small mustard plaster over

[*Pg 8*] the pit of the stomach and give a few mouth fuls of strong black coffee, that is coffee without cream.– Two or three hours after, he may take a little light nourishment if he wishes.– As thirst usually follows vomiting, he shd not take right cold drinks even the same day unless the Dr allows it – he may have toast-water that has the cold air off a little at a time.

Blistering

When a fly plaster is ordered, put it <u>on the place</u>, & <u>at the time</u> ordered for it. Have all things ready by the bed-side before his clothes are opened.

If the Blister plaster is large & the weather very cold, warm it some before applying it. fix it comfortably tight to prevent its slipping about. If the plaster is for the abdomen, side or back, sprinkle a little powdered opium over it, or dampen it with laudanum to prevent strangury. If this occurs, give him a tea-spoonful of sweet spirits of nitre in a cup of warm flax seed tea, or water once in 2 or 3 hours if continues so long.– When it has drawn enough, have all the dressings ready before openin[g] his blister. with sharp pointed scissors cut off the blistered skin – do not tear it off - warm the salve rag or the coldness of it on so hot a sore may cause congestion. twice a day will do for salve dressing. If it is to be kept running, let the morning dressing be of the drawing kind & the milder for the evening. or if it must have sharp salve every time, let the last or evening dressing be early enough to have the smarting gone before sleeping time. — When they take a distressing tormenting burning, they may be soothed by mopping them with a mixture of lime water & mild oil of equal parts–shaken well together to form a kind of cream. Never let the dregs or lumps of lime be

[*Pg 9*] in the water. After this has quited it, the dressings may be put on again.– When cabbage leaves are the dressings, take the tender, small green ones. pare the coarse stems out of them, scald or crimp them on red hot coals & then squeeze them in a towel in yr. [*your*] hand, keeping them warm until the place is ready for them. they shd be laid on about 4 or 6 thick, or they will dry too soon, be very painful & do no good; & 3 times this dressing shd be made daily.—

Mustard Plasters

Mix the mustard with <u>hot</u> <u>water</u> by the sick bed, as the hotter they are applied the quicker relief they give. For the instep, ancle [*sic*] or wrist one teaspoonful of the dry mustard flour is enough, but for the chest, abdomen or side a tablespoonful – let the paste, be thick so as not to run & wet the clothes, or have a large wet rag over the sick – have an old thin muslin or gauze rag to lay over the mustard to keep it from sticking to the skin, for when they make sores, they are hard to heal.– the time for leaving them on must be as circumstances call for. Some can only bear them a few minutes, & if relief is soon given they may be removed – 15 or 20 minutes if they are not too painful, is not too long. for a tender, delicate skin this cd be too long if they burned much– A child cd not bear it long, & for a child a little corn-meal had better be mixed with the mustard-flour.– Never put them on the bony part of the ancle, [*sic*] that is the ancle [*sic*] bone or shin bone, but on the side of the ancle, [*ankle*] on calf of the leg, or the instep.– When a mustard <u>poultice</u> is ordered, make a stiff corn meal mush, & after it is spread 2 inches thick

[*Pg 10*] on a rag, sprinkle mustard freely over it, if the pain be very great. but, if not, do not put on so much - but have the thin gauze over this. If mustard is not ordered, but only the hot mush, spread a little soft grease over the mush. A weak patient cd not bear so heavy a poultice – and as it must be thinner it must also be changed more frequently, as it cools quicker than a thick one.– Always make enough for 2 - so that one may be kept warm while one is on, & when warm poultices ar[*e*] needed, cold ones do harm – have a big dry cloth spread over the poultice to keep the clothes & bed-clothes dry & clean – When they are very important know whether they are to be kept on during the night – if not, or at any time you are to leave them off, have a large, folded flannel warmed, & lay it where the poultice had been.– When poultices might serve, but the sick are very weak & sick, it does well to warm whiskey, rum, spirits of camphor or other such spirits, & apply it on a hot flannel folded several times – keeping a warm one on all the time.–

Try to prevent bed-sores, for <u>no one is able</u> to tell the violent, excruciating pain they cause, & when once formed can hardly be cured.– When a delirious patient, after being long in bed shows more restlessness, examine the back – rather it shd be examined sooner & all means used to prevent them.—

Teas, Tonics &c.

Make them strong, & in a clean vessel, have the water boiling – keep them covered while boiling or steaming. When done, strain & cover it. In warm weather do not make too much at a time, & keep it in a cool place. Nurses are often careless in these things, thinking they are only simple matters, thus, they prepare them negligently,

[*Pg 11*] & are irregular in giving them – or give them after they are sour & mouldy, and this makes the stomach sick, or getting them irregular does no good. The Dr thinks it is the fault of the tonic & changes it for something stronger, perhaps, brandy or some other thing that does real harm– He loses confidence in that tonic, names it to his students and Medical friends, who likewise discontinue it, & in all these cases that fall into their hands, some stronger thing is given, when the thing itself was right, in right hands. How often, these, seemingly small things, are the beginnings of the death-bed & in many, many cases, Life & Death is [*in*] the hands of the nurses, more than in the Physicians.

Foot-Baths

For a common foot-bath take hot, or right warm water, put into it one table spoonful of mustard, or a handful of coarse salt, or a pint of wood-ashes. Have it ready before the sick gets out of bed. Have cold water near, in case he says it is too hot, but, in pouring it in do not splash it on his feet. Let him sit comfortably, a blanket around his shoulders & something over his lap to keep him warm. 150 [*15*] or 20 minutes is long enough – have two towels to wipe them, either wipe both at once, or have one in the water while the first is getting dried – do this as quickly as possible & do not let him step on the floor, but get immediately into bed. If he becomes sick or faint-like, take him out of the water at once. Never let him take it if he be sweating, for, sweating is what you wish to gain by the bath,

[*Pg 12*] and by rising at that time it is checked; & gives new cold, perhaps congestion.– A purgative medicine and a foot-bath ought not be given in the same night.

Injections

When only an action from the bowels is desired, warm water alone will do, or warm soap suds is better. A common injection for strong persons in slight sickness is: about a pint of warm water with one tablespoonful of table salt, the same quantity of molasses & lard. When a stronger one is necessary epsome [*Epsom*] salts may be used instead of table salt or castor oil instead of lard. let the salt be entirely melted. rinse the pipe with hot water, or its coldness will cool the mixture too much. Just before filling the pipe with the mixture, draw the handle suddenly in & out of the pipe a few times to get all the air out of the tube. Then, put the small end into the mixture, holding it under the surface so as that the air cannot get into it. let the pipe fill, or as much as you need, by drawing the handle steadily & slowly. when you take it out, keep the finger on the small end of the tube until the patient is ready to help themselves – but if they are too weak for this, they must be previously fixed for it by having the hips raised by a pillow or something. If the hips are not raised the mixture will return when the pipe is withdrawn. When the pipe is placed, inject the mixture steadily & when the bowel has received it keep the pipe perfectly still for a minute or two, or if you take it suddenly away the contents follow it. Very soon the patient wishes to rise because the bowels seem disposed to act, but this feeling is only from the mix-

[*Pg 13*] ture, and they must force themselves to wait half an hour or so, if possible, or, only the injection will pass & then it must be repeated, whereas by waiting a more natural action will be gained.– but if no good is derived, it must be repeated in about 2 hours – often the 2 one is more successful.–

When particular injections are required the Dr names the things that is to compose it, as in bad bowel complaint, starch & laudanum are used, and in some cases any injection wd be given after each movement of the bowels – You shd know from the Dr whether they shd be given cold or warm.

Opiates

Usually in about half an hour after an opiate has been given, it shd compose or dispose to sleep. But if there be loud talking or other noise around him, the opiate cannot act favorably, & on the contrary, does harm & after a certain time, will not act however quiet things may be. care shd be taken therefore, to prevent their being disturbed at this time.

Cleanliness

Keep the drinks that stand by their beds covered from dust & flies – do not have it in heavy mugs, or so full that they spill it in taking it. wipe away slops & spills off the table or other things that serve to collect flies. do not let poultice or sore rags lay about or soiled clothes – empty the spit cup or basin frequently and return it quickly & clean. The chamber vessel should

[*Pg 14*] [be] removed after each action from the bowels, unless the Dr is to examine it, in this case, have two vessels, setting one aside till the Dr sees it, & leaving the other by the bed. – When the bowels are too free, or if purgative medicine has been given, have two vessels with lids for their use.– In like manner, two basins when an emetic is given.– If mud or dirt is on the floor around the bed, do not have much of the floor wet at a time, & none at all if there be danger, or unless the Dr says it can be done without danger. Never let a love for cleanliness expose yr. [*your*] poor patient, & thus endanger also, yr. [*your*] conscience, for in some sicknesses a little damp air might cause relapse & death.– There shd be changes of clothing kept in the house for such as come in, in soiled clothes and have no change, pay great attention to all clothing sheets & bedding being perfectly dry before using them.

General Remarks

Do not use any kind of metal spoons in medicine or sour drink, but pewter or silver. if these cannot be had brittania [*sic*] is next best – neither let ~~such stand in this~~ medicine or sour drinks or eatable stand in tin or metal cups. When one is very weak, & wishes to wet his mouth often, he may be relieved by leaving the drink in a phial on his bed. this he can get without fatigue & he prefers this to being waited on—

It is always in our power to render them many little services by small attentions & little by little they help towards recovery, and the charity that accompanies

[*Pg 15*] them does much for their content of mind.

In Summer, have large pieces of coarse bobinet lace or cat-gut propped on a frame or sticks over their head & shoulders & so as that their arms & hands will also be kept from the flies – then they can use their hands inside of it – even when they are not sleepy, they cannot rest, & fatigue themselves by driving the flies off themselves. – There shd be several of these for every ward, so that one might be washed after a consumpted or fever patient, before giving it to another. If you are ready to put their room in order, but find the patient sleeping or nearly so, wait for awhile, especially if they stand in need of sleep from having had but little his rest will do him more good than a clean room or all your other care might do: this is what we would do for a sick friend or Parent, do not let the visit of friends cause him to be awakened, if he has suffered for sleep, let friends wait; when they are weak, all means for gaining strength must be afforded them, and in nervous complaints, it is so necessary that they would die from this matter being neglected.–

Let every phial or box of medicine have its name on it and the quantity to be given, or serious mistakes will be the consequence: do not let dangerous medicines stand about ~~unlockehed~~ unlocked, such as laudanum or others.

As the recovery and life itself often depends on the sustaining effects of nourishments and drinks the greatest care must be taken in these things, they must always be properly and plateably [sic] prepared or their weak stomachs not being able to keep or take them, they will sink in spite of all the Dr can do; and when you see them so prostrate, it will probably, and most likely, be too late to raise them or get back the strength and little appetite they had. What a misfortune to answer

[Pg 16] answer [sic] for!!. These things, if they had been prepared with St. Vincent's spirit, that, is for his Jesus, such as the poor sick could have taken, how much better the fruits would be for them and the negligent nurses! let true practical charity season every thing they require, otherwise we are guilty of injustice by with-holding from them their means of cure.

When spirits of camphor is used for sponging the skin, the diluted will do, that is, the gum camphor is dissolved in whiskey, some brandy, rum &c.–

When spirits of camphor is used inwardly, the gum is disolved [sic] in good Alcohol as long as it will disolve in it, and when the gum remains undissolved, it is strong enough. When a sudden distress finds you unprepared for the occasion, let this event & its anxiety teach you to be prepared for all things as much as possible; for instance, to be without adhesive plasters, bandages, lint, cups, injecting pipes, mustard, the medicines in common use, &c. &c. makes too much delay in urgent cases that would call for these.

Experience teaches in time, but too many are sacrificed by this method of teaching. A low tone of voice, with cheerful, kind manners must be strictly observed & practised [sic] by those who wait on the sick.

Mania a Potu or Delirium Tremens

Delirium Tremens, which is the lighter stage of this malady is produced by intoxication. The trembling stage should be attended to in time for fear of the worst condition. As soon as such a patient is brought in take him to his room, having learned from

[Pg 17] from [sic] his friends as to the violence or otherwise state of his mind, & if necessary have all things, that he would be disposed to break or throw at you removed from the room such as bowls, pitchers, looking-glasses, tables, &c. have a trusty person to undress them, handing each piece as he takes them off: the patient usually objects to stay or undress &c., but the attendant says, it is necessary that he gets some sleep and therefore she entreats and insists very politely & helping off with coat, vest, &c. and leaving the hired man to finish the remains out-side the door to take the clothes from him, for fear the patient hides something he should not keep; it is better to put the clothes on a chair until all is there, and then hand the chair out-side saying, they will be put away, or they will get dusty &c. as they sometimes hide things in a belt under the shirt, have a night shirt ready for him, that he may be more comfortable; thus you may be satisfied whether you have left any thing about him. When they object strongly to taking off their cravat, boots &c. you may fear they have a special reason: in some cases you must not insist then, but stay in the room as though through politeness &c. until you may ask him again that he takes them off, and saying always that you know that they cannot be [e] asy with them on: sometimes they only have money that they are trying to keep from their friends, but you should try by all means to satisfy yourself that they have no intention to hurt themselves, yet this fear you have must not enter into their thoughts, or you would do them more harm by this than you could ever repair.

All insane or delirious persons should [have] the same examination upon coming in; and even if friends assure you that they have nothing of dangerous matters about them, do not fail going through this precaution: experience teaches the necessity; after this provision for destroying themselves comes into their mind as soon as they find the

[Pg 18] the [sic] friends are determined to take them from home and though they give no reason for the friends thinking of it, they prepare themselves now, and will try to secret razors or pen=knives [sic] &c. under pretence [sic] of pairing their nails &c.=, pocket=comb with nail=pail=[sic] in it, thumb=lance, opium=phials, powders, small=ropes &c. &c, Sometimes a favorite pocket=hkf [handkerchief] will be kept unknown to the friends on purpose for hanging himself, or his suspenders may do. With the insane the thing they first thought of using for this is the one thing they try to secure and this should be a great point of information to gain, for this one thing may be kept from them, they may in time lose the intention: but in the minia [sic] a potu, if the thought or desire to destroy himself exists, he will do it by any manner, even to beat his brains out against the wall if left alone.–

If the mania=a=potu patient wishes he were dead you may be on the watch, for the next thing to effect it: the greatest prudence is necessary; if you saw that they had kept something, but do not know what, you must judge of the propriety of insisting on seeing it, for this would let him know what you feared and would make him more determined, fearing let he would be watched &c, and so lose the chance, or if he had no thought of killing himself before he is now put in the mind of it by your suspicion and thinks he ought to do it since you thought of it: so the better way is to stop a while longer and not leave him alone until you are certain about it; but by providing the night shirt you have the best way of knowing whether he hides any thing or not. Never reproach those suffering from intoxication, for their own thoughts are often more than they can bear, even when you may feel nothing: in most cases it is better to

[Pg 19] to [sic] console them saying that others have reformed from this vice or habit and became the joy & credit of their family and that they must now make strong resolutions and imitate them in their last state since they had fallen into their first state &c. &c.

As they get more out of their senses they think they see enemies going to kill their parents, wives, children &c, or that some one is aiming a gun or blow at them, this makes him dodge about & try to hide and often he tries to kill himself, rather than let one who was once his friend, kill him &c. these excessive fears excites and heats the already injured brain until it can bear no more, and his fright makes him sweat so much that if he is confined in a strict way, or held down, he will surely die. At times they think hell-flames are all around them, then they reproach themselves & deplore the shame, disgrace they bring their friends to, and the loss of their soul. Reason comes & goes almost in the same moment, their terror, horror & torment are not to be expressed.– Now in this misery and despair, it is plain to be seen that the kindest, mildest, persuasion is the only course to pursue. You cannot have greater objects for your charity. Let every attendant see in this poor creature a beloved Father or Brother, and act accordingly.

They should not be left alone even when they are calm, for often self-reproach is keenest then, & remorse like a fiend is more fiercely at work, – remembering past joys, respect, honor, dear friends &c., and now the horrid future he is about to enter, all all [sic] rack his mind so that he seems to see only one thing to do which is to destroy himself!

For God's sake do not laugh at them or suffer others to treat them with contempt,

[Pg 20] though this shd be the hundredth time he has been brought to yr. [your] care, you may save the soul the last time, and this done, all is right. Perhaps, crushed by frowns at home, he hopes to find pity from the Daughters of Charity as channels of mercy from Jesus & pity from Mary, & cheered & sustained by you, he may, like Magdelaine rise to fall no more, instead of leaving this life Judas, saying: only hell remains for me.– Tell them to take courage, that this will pass off, and they must now resolve to serve God and pray for grace to avoid falling again.– that they must now do as the Dr & Srs. [Sisters] tell them and all will soon be right, that they will then go home and give their dear friends great happiness by showing them how well they will do the remainder of their lives.-

These seem like simple advices, but only experience can tell their value. —

When they have not sense enough for such things, but violent in trying to get away, have two strong, but <u>kind</u> men, and a Sister present to direct them. Let them pick up the patient & put him on the bed, or he may sit in an easy chair, comfortably, but not held rudely – Some hired men kneel on the patients chest or abdomen to hold him down, or holding his hands in theirs clenched & pressed down hard on the bowels or chest of the poor patient so as to cause his death, even after the delirium has passed off. This hard usage causes the patient to say hard things to the men & then there is no limits to their cruelty.-

Our good Savior did not break the bruised reed. We shd imitate Him.

[*Pg 21*] After the Dr has named the kind, quantity & frequency of the opiates & stimulants, there is still much depending on the attendants, as in many cases these remedies increase excitement & shd therefore be <u>dis</u>continued until the Dr comes again, & telling why these were not given– Hop tea is a good substitute as opiate & tonic; & often serves better than opiates or spirits. Chicken soup is a good remedy, also, because it strengthens them.

An old, worn-out drinker will not be able to digest his fill of water, but a stronger one may drink as much cold water as he craves, unless it causes too much vomiting or pain.—

If he will be still enough, or even when he is jumping & dodgeing [*sic*] about, you may begin to ask him the most familiar questions, speaking in a mild, moderate tone, but with earnestness, as though you wished very much to know, & do not smile, or allow others present to do so, or you will do no good. Let yr. [*your*] questions be short & such as wd give his understanding no trouble to answer. Such as: What is yr. [*your*] christian name? What was yr [*your*] Father's? Are you married? What is yr. [*your*] wife's name? how many brothers have you? how many Sisters? What is yr [*your*] oldest brother named? then the next & so on with the Sisters. Then have you children? how many? What the oldest's name? And so with the others. Then, what street is yr [*your*] house in? Is it brick? What no? how many stories high &c. &c. &c.

[*Pg 22*] At first he will give no attention to you, but, the questions being so short & easy to answer, he answers at last in hopes you, will then let him be. But as soon as he has answered the first one, then, with the same calm but earnest manner, ask him another, keeping to <u>that</u> one until he speaks in reply. If you were to speak loud or hurriedly, he would confound yr [*your*] voice with those he imagines he hears, and therefore you wd not gain his understanding. —

But if often asking him, he seems too busy to hear you, having to dodge to avoid that gun, axe &c, say quietly: All is right, dont fear &c – Then begin the questions again.–

Immediately after he has answered one question, you will see some improvement, and if he is not a worn-out drinker, or in danger of congestion, he will be cured by these questions, for soon, your voice has more influence over his senses than his fancied terrors; & he, who to all appearance had but an hour to live, is, if he is carefully spoken to, entirely out of danger in an hour after he begins to answer the questions. –

If he shd show sleepiness, of course you wd stop speaking & give him every chance for sleep.– Do not grow weary of this simple method, for the demon is not weary in trying to put some new folly on the poor brain, in order to prevent your success, so the good Samaritan must not give up first; for while life is in the body the soul & body may both be saved.

~ --------

If he is a Catholic, the presence of a Priest may help to bring him to his senses, as often happens, even though he may have been

[*Pg 23*] negligent in christian duties when sober, for the horror he has now of hell, makes a hope Spring up in his mind on seeing a Priest, and often the[*y*] are able to make a confession– In many, intemperance is their only fault or vice, and God, seeing their hearts and human weakness, does not reprobate them as readily as men do who see neither.

Some patients will remain all the night kneeling by a hat or coat on a chair, thinking he is making confession to a Priest.–

A Priest shd be sent for, for them although some Priests, not knowing much about the state of delirium, say they can do nothing for them, and almost wonder at being sent for, but, having sent, begin then to question yr [*your*] poor patient so as to have him calmer by the time he arrives, but conjure the Priest to stay with him awhile, even if he is yet very wild and excited. Your questions in this occasion may be of confession, as: When was you at Confession? do you not wish to go now? Who did you go to? But, quiet him in any manner, so that composure be gained. Do all you can, and if you fail as regards yr.[*your*] patient, you will have at least did all you cd for his soul & so avoided sin by neglect.–

Do not put restraints on them unless obliged to do so to prevent their killing themselves or others – but if you must do so, and they get angry at it, say to them kindly: My dear friend you oblige us to do so, for, you need composure & you will not take it, but as soon as your fever is off, we will set you free &c. Say too: If you were my Father or Brother, I wd do the same – we do this for your benefit, not to irritate or trouble you. &c

[*Pg 24*] Let us indeed bear in mind how we wd do our very best for a dear Father or Brother, and wd not suffer them to be badly treated or laughed at.– Our Vocation is Charity, we must, as St. Paul says: put on the bowels of Jesus Christ wherewith to serve His suffering members; our fallen Brethren.– Always speak to yr [*your*] patients in a kind, sympathising [*sympathizing*] manner, you thus excite their courage & confidence and lessen their wretchedness. What a blessed duty!

If such patients are determined to kill themselves, they will pretend to sleep, thinking the attendants will then leave him, & thus leave them to their opportunity. In one instance a man did so for ~~th~~ two or three days & nights, after which the man attendant went to his breakfast, without being replaced by another, and the Patient rose immediately, but his hands being confined some, he commenced beating his head against the door case; a Sr. [*Sisters*] passing heard the blood falling on the floor & went in. The Dr was called to sew up & dress the cut, but, the Patient did all he cd to prevent the Dr from doing him a Service.– But time & care restored him & every such case as was brought to the Hospital while he staid there, he wd stand by their bed to give himself a new fear of ever falling again, and as far as we were informed several years after, he never did.–

The word suicide or <u>self</u>-destruction must never be used in their [*presence*], or any other weak-minded patient.– When opiates excites when given internally, sleep may be gained by rubbing laudanum in the hair & eyebrows, laying also a little lint or rag wet with [*it*] near enough for him to smell it.–

[*Pg 25*] If you have not a Physician's prescription to treat him, you may, with great advantage, perhaps, give the following, as it has often produced speedy cure.–

Take, Castor oil –	2 ounces
" Spirits of Turpentine	½ ounce
" Elm emulsion	4 ounces
" Laudanum	1½ ounces

Mix and give him one tea-spoonful very two hours until he sleeps.

When cups are to be applied on the head, temples or any other place near the bone, the lancets must be set very shallow, or the gristle that covers the bone will be injured. It is better for the Dr to apply them when done on the temples. If it cannot be set shallow, beare very little on the scarificator whilst cutting.

Have near the bed, a table with a lighted candle, two basins, one holding hot water, the other empty for the blood. the cups in the hot water – about 20 or 30 pieces of soft paper, tissue or news paper in size of a silver dollar, a sponge in the water – a soft towel on the table to pass the cups quickly over when

[*Pg 26*] taking it from the water. When the place to be cupped is ready, dampen the parts with a hot sponge squeezed out of the hot water – then take a cup in one hand, one of the little papers lit & blazing in the other, throw it in the cup & place it quickly on the spot – then another in the same manner until all are on, or as many as you intend to use. Have the scarificator ready while these are drawing, and when the cups have drawn the flesh pretty well into them, begin taking them off, taking off the one you put on first. You may take all of[*f*] before you begin to cut them, or you can cut one at a time, putting on the cup again before you take another off.–

As soon as you cut the place, light a paper as in the first instance & put it over the bleeding spot. If you take all the cups off before you cut any, cut all before you put on any; or the raised flesh will flatten down too much & thus too the bone wd be in danger.–

When the cup is filled, or even half full, or that you see the blood is not coming any more, squeeze your sponge again & remove the cups carefully, holding the sponge near so as to catch the blood if it shd run – And, wetting the spot again, with the hot sponge, put the cup on again, unless you have as much as was required. – If you do not know well how to cup, do not be ashamed to ask one who does know, for you may not get as much blood as wd benefit the patient. If you did not take the quantity ordered, let the Dr know it that he may know what else to do. Always have a large, dry cloth to prevent the clothes of the sick or the beg [*bed*] from getting wet or bloody.

[*Pg 27*] Dry the scarificater [*sic*] & strike it into a <u>mutton</u> tallow to prevent rust. Dry the moisture from the skin of the patient with a soft towel & then lay a soft rag over it if necessary.–

When cupping is ordered for the back, <u>avoid</u> the <u>spine</u> (back-bone), but cup each side of it. <u>Avoid</u> also the shoulder blade. <u>Do</u> <u>not</u> cup on the side of the neck or the front, (the throat) and even for the temples, it is better to have the Dr, as some times it is hard to stop the Blood, there being so many veins and so little flesh there.–

When <u>Dry</u> cupping is ordered, the cups are used as in the other, but the scarificator (the lancets) are not used consequently no blood is to be taken, as a better circulation is all that is wanting in this case, & often gives great relief.–

[*Pg 28*] *A Few Remarks on Insanity.*

When an Insane or Melancholy Patient is proposed for admission into the Hospital, gain all the information you can concerning previous health, disposition, temper, whether quick & angry- minded or the contrary, natural character, habits, business, &c. – Request also the friends to make you acquainted with any thing that the[*y*] noticed as being different from what the patient used to be – telling them that a very small matter as they think, may help very much to restore him provided the Dr or Sisters were to know it. – Ask them especially, what he did or said that first made them think that his mind was getting wrong. – This information is so necessary that, Some Institutions have printed forms to be used by those who receive them. The following are some of them in addition to those above named:

What is his age? How long since you first saw a change in him?

What was it that made you fear that something was wrong with him? What did he do or say that made you think so? Was he ever this way before this time? How long ago & how long did it last? how old was he then? What did you think caused it then? had he had trouble of any kind, or sickness, & what sickness & of how long standing. Is he married? is his wife living or how long dead? did other deaths occur that distressed him greatly? had he difference with members of his own family or neighbours? how did he behave during this disagreement? Is he kind in his family? had he loss of property or injustices done him, or spiteful enemies that talked hard of him?

[Pg 29] how did he bear these things? Was he disappointed in his affections? What was his general health before this strangeness came on? Are any of his Relations in this way? Was he much with them, & how did it affect him? What was his appetite before this, & how is it now? how much did he use to sleep, & how much now? Was he often from home? Was he a drinking man, & how long & what was his usual condition? how long since he quit it? has he smoked, chewed or snuffed Tobacco greatly? & how long since he quit it, or is he a great snuffer yet? did, or does he chew opium, or has he used laudanum or Paregoric often? has he quit these & how long ago? and is there a change in him Since? Was he free & pleasant among his friends, or Sad & gloomy before this? Does he desire to be alone now? what seems to be his greatest desire? desire to wander from home? Seem to fear friends? Does he hate or love some one particularly? who is that one? how long has he had a Drs care & what was done for him? Was he bled, cupped, blistered, leeched &c? how often or has he lost much blood in any way? has he been dieted, how long & what was the kind of food & how much was he allowed & how much did he take, or did or does he still desire more food than the Dr allowed him? Was he freely purged? What used to be the State of the bowels & what are they now? did the Dr order opiates, such as Morphine, Laudanum, or what kind of opiates, how much & how did they seem to affect him & how long did he use them, and how long since he quit them? how was he different in taking, or not taking them? Does he

[*Pg 30*] or has he at any time since he is so, wished he were dead? has he tried to hurt others? or himself? and how? for usually, the way they first tried to kill themselves, will be the one they will think of most, & perhaps if the thing or kind of thing were kept out of their way, they might forget their intention entirely. this has been told after their recovery. But in some this desire to kill themselves is so fixed that it seems to be itself the derangement – these will use any means in their power & no Sane person cd think of their inventions.–

A gentleman so disposed was brought to the Hospital. His friends told us that he had expressed the wish to kill himself, because he thought he was a disgrace to the family &c., but that they had no fears of it, since a very emminent [*sic*] Dr them that such as intended to do so, never told their wish or intention – As friends seemed easy, we hoped for the best, at the same time kept it in mind to use what care we cd prudently, for if the Patient suspects that you fear it, he is sure to do it, thinking then that he must since you have thought of it. – the means this unfortunate man had intended was to hang himself with a Silk pockt [*sic*] hdf. [*handkerchief*] he had about him & which he never sent to the wash with his soiled linen. this we were ignorant of, but, with this, seeing it daily & pondering over it he succeeded – had this been told us by friends, we knowing the importance of taking it from him, wd have managed some way of getting it, without exciting his suspicion, and we have cause to believe he wd have

[*Pg 31*] given up the idea, as he seemed to be improving in mind

——— — —

When the Patient is a Female their age and condition of general health must be particularly enquired into.

The best writers on Insanity; say: that kindness is the main remedy, because this method treats them as if they were Sane: this excites to self-respect, for the poor patient feels there is something wrong with him, but seeing he is treated like others – his remarks and wishes attended to, he begins to think he is not out of his mind, or that if he has been so, he must be better now, since he is considered & respected like others. This bright hope makes him try to deport himself in the best manner, he suppresses rising emotions. Even Idiots love kindness, and may be improved by it.–

Kindness in paroxisms [*sic*] of great excitement is of the best results, and in their rage and fury, no harsh word or treatment should be used with them. but whatever may be the force or restraint you may be obliged to use with them, let it be done as to a loved parent or Brother – Saying to them kindly! My dear Friend, do not be angry with us for this, you are so out of humour, that we are obliged to do this. When you are better, all will be right again. You have fever, makes you do as you do, and when it passes off, you will be comfortable again – Why, the thing you wish to do, would not be for your good, or we would be too glad to gratify you – We like to see you happy. If you were my own dear Brother, I could not grant it – It is because we love and respect you, that we

[*Pg 32*] refuse you now, &c.&c — Such mild remarks as these, calm their feelings, though they may rave on – And when these paroxisms occur they do not injure them, if they are treated kindly during them, for, it is harshness in their treatment that does them harm. They forever remember what bitter things were said to them and by whom – An excitement you can always explain to them, by calling it fever, and this raises their broken spirits, but they know they must have been very bad to have brought such things as they remember was said or done to them.–

This debases them so in their own mind, that they say: I know I am crazy, as they treated me as such, I can destroy myself at any rate – Even though it may not go so far, they are always depressed at remembering the contempt or hard things said to them – O break not, the bruised reed! But if you are kind, gentle, patient under all their violence and abuse, they love and respect you as Angels of consolation, and each paroxism will be lighter, as they recollect your tender compassion for them. thus too, they lose their dread of these attacks, and improve rapidly. _____

We should bear in mind that God leaves us our reason, whilst He takes it from our patient, but shall we outrage this God of Charity by making a cruel use of ours over His poor Servant, who, without sense, is put under our care by Him?

Or will we by anger, add our own violence to theirs? Their attacks of excitement hurt their constitution, whilst your harshness, hurts their mind!

[*Pg 33*] Even those who are subject to greatest violence, have a sense of self-respect, on which you may still rebuild their tottering mind, but, your contempt by hard treatment & manners towards them destroys this, and strength of scattered reason cannot be rallied again.

Could we push back in to the deep, a struggling, drowning, fellow creature, a Brother? – Too often the attendant thinks they ~~they~~ are not capable of feeling while in this state of rage, thu[s] what is the use of rudness [*sic*], but to exercise your own vexation? You have not kept your reason calm, and they would gladly be able to give you no trouble! Ah let us not love a cruel authority! It is better by far to be without reason, than abuse it by a bad or uncharitable use of it! _____

An angry man feels & remembers all hard things said to him, because, the hard ones, or hard things, pain us. this is why these are longer on the mind than other things. On the contrary, gentle, mild, pity &c, is so sweet to the poor chained brain, that it soothes and binds the wounds they endure. His power of thinking, feels muffled, or as groping about in the dark, confusedly. Your mild tone of voice, is like a ray of light, or taking the hand of a blind man, saying: this way, my friend. Thus you loan them your reason, till their's [*sic*] returns.

like the strong friend gives his arm to his sick, or weak friend. – This is a glorious application of our faculties – His is the part of the good Samaritan.–

We should never show that their bad speeches or manners towards us had pained us – especially as they sometimes [*Pg 34*] say such horrible things that it would be a great mercy to help them forget them –

They seeing you are always the same kind friend towards them, begin to think, those hateful things were only dreams.___ But should they make an apology for improprieties of speech or manner, say pleasantly: O if I had had your fever, I might have done far worse, do not think of it. I do not care for what my dear Brother said to me last month in his ship-fever &c.

These precious words are registered in Heaven, as they are on the grateful heart of your poor patient. How then does the Heart of your Jesus view them! ___ And if in the course of time, they, or their grateful Friends may come to know & embrace the true Religion, it will be because its truths were written in honey. But a hasty, self-opinioned, or negligent & unfeeling attendant, prevents good from being done. She serves him as a Swine-herd, without respect to him, or merit to herself, and by one short word or remark, makes quick work of the Slender chance that had been carefully Studied in better hands – This chance gone, all future care, perhaps, may be useless – like the tender plant in taking root, must have time, tender care, and preserved from the boisterous winds, or it withers, never to be restored.– The diseased mind is like an Infant trying to walk – if another child leads him, he will be injured by falling and vexation, but if one capable of directing his crooked steps is with him, all will soon be right.

Happy, happy lot of the Sister of Charity, whose duty is, Service to the Insane!

[Pg 35] Conversation is a matter on which much depends for the Insane. What they say should not be abruptly contradicted, or turned into ridicule, contempt &c, as though at first thought we saw it wrong – but seem to be pleased with their remark, or considering it, even to add your own to it, and then presently, as if you took another view of it, propose that which might be better . . .

that is if this is necessary, for if the thing is trifling, let it remain as they first said, for this respect for their opinion is very useful to them – it is another stone in your building, especially as being picked from among the ruins of what once stood higher.

But if the thing is bad & would lead to ill consequences, Seem to be thinking about it. and then as though you just saw it right, propose the contrary quietly.

When first little remarks of theirs meet with our attention & respect they begin little by little to speak more freely to us of themselves or of other patients.

– thus you gain their confidence, and, becoming better acquainted with them & those of whom they speak, (for often they know each other better than we yet know them) [Note: Parenthesis and enclosed words in original document] and this information becomes very profitable to them if we make a right use of it – but we must not show much eagerness to know from one patient of another, or they will become Suspicious and guarded on these things. – They often become the confidents of each other, for the Dr and Srs are looked on as instrumental in keeping them there, &c. and so they are slow in trusting them.

once they receive always from you

[Pg 36] a kind, respectful bearing, seeing you so towards all, also (For they are quick sighted in partialities, indeed, in all our weak points) [Note: Parenthesis and enclosed words in original document] they lose their distrust and begin to view you as their best, often their only friend – In a word, we only succeed with them by taking God's way with them, that is: Justice, Charity, clemency, or in His own words: "Do to others, as you would have them do to you."

The tendrils of the plant will run wild without support, and so do the thoughts of the insane when they converse only with each other.

But should the attendant be an improper prop, they are badly off.– But by prudence we may gain a timely knowledge of the strange things they had planned among themselves, and thus prevent terrible consequences.–

It require [sic] great prudence also, for selecting right topics for conversation, as you must avoid what excites or exasperates them. One thing or subject is odius [sic] to one & indifferent to another, you must be like an able Pilot on dangerous waters – often a little misplaced word or sentence tears open a closing wound that had taken much time & care; or excites another to violence.

With the Melancholy or desponding patient, it is well to advise them never to speak of their troubles to the other patients, who believing what they say, are apt to confirm them in their sad impressions.

And if they wish to speak of them constantly to you, you would do better to say to them: "Now

[Pg 37] my dear friend, I believe you distress yourself too much by speaking always of your troubles, so I cannot let you do so, but if you cannot join in other subjects of conversation, at least try to entertain yourself on what others are talking about." Do not grow weary of giving this advice, for a little gained, is a great thing.

After they have refrained from speaking of it or from warning it a couple of days or so, do you, yourself say to them kindly: "Well how is your poor heart now? don't you think you can bear your troubles now better than when it first came to you? I think you will soon be better – I know what sadness is, and bitter as it is, it is only a sickness of the mind, as fever is of the body, and like fever too may be cured, but we must have patience – It will pass away.

Our Heavenly Father can heal us when all others fail, but He knows the best time for healing our poor wounded hearts – You have had bodily sickness, and you got well again & so you will of this – take courage – many have been like you, and are well and happy now – when you get well and go home to your people, you will be so brave, that if any of your dear friends should be in trouble, you will be their comfort & encouragement, for the mind is like other things it becomes stronger by having been seasoned by keen trials and afflictions. I can bear much more now, having had trials of the mind.–

Believe me, a sickness like this, wonderfully fortifies the mind for coming troubles, or common occurrences of life."

[Pg 38] Such things said kindly to them occasionally help them so much, that you might call them the means of their restoration.

– Consequently, when these assistances of consolation are omitted, the Melancholy becomes derangement & fixed.–

The diseased or the troubled mind is like a fractured limb, which does not often heal without help – So too much pains cannot be taken to become a proper aid to the fractured or shattered mind._____

Be careful that the gloomy or sad patient is not made the sport and derision, of the rough, jolly wit of the unthinking class of Patients, for the very being associated with such, they consider a degradation & painful to their too sensitive feelings.–

Some attendants, for want of experience, think it well to turn them into ridicule, but it is injurious, and to such as were disposed to destroy themselves, it would increase the desire to do so, and thus shew their abhorrence of such low jesting and gross annoyance as they now deem it. "Break not, the bruised reed."

It is often advantageous to permit one low-spirited patient to talk to you of her troubles in the presence, or hearing of another like her without your seeming to know she is there. The one who hears the other speak of herself as the worst off in the world, and also hears your replies, thinks just as you do in her case – She becomes for the time entirely occupied in listening to her, and is surprised that anyone can be so mistaken, since she herself is the only one so truly wretched. She continues to listen to her woes, so as most to forget her own for a moment – She

[Pg 39] thinks about it, believes her entirely mistaken, & that your advices to her were perfectly right, and in a day or two, she will begin to tell you of the reality of her own case, but the other she heard speaking, was only imaginary, &c.–

Slowly and gently, draw the comparison & gradually you will weaken the strength of her opinion on such & such points, she used to be positive on. – She, who before this would not speak to any one, now seeks the company of her fellow-sufferer, and if they are not left too long together at a time, will very much improve each other without their knowing it.

——— ——

Associations of males and females is not of advantage to either side, and should be carefully avoided.

——— ——— ———

The word: suicide or self-destruction should never [be] used in their hearing.

The word: punish for every slight fault or mischief they do, will make your government odius [sic] to them, and threats exasperate them. When shower baths are necessary, do not let them think they are given as a punishment, but only as a remedy & for their benifit [sic] or health &c.

– If they resist so far as to get in a great heat, they should not be put in, or the consequence may be death, as has happened. Or if you might fear, that other reasons, (with females) [Note: Parenthesis and enclosed words in original document] should prohibit it – Do not fear that giving up to their objections, will make them more outrageous another time, thinking, that they conquered you, &c.

no, no, if you show

[Pg 40] no impatience in mood or manner, they will think you give up, because you pity & feel for them, and this supposition will make them love you, and this may bring about the beginning of their good deportment, and again we see the fruits of kindness, for [it] is, and forever will be, the remedy of remedies, whereas, showering, or such things, are in most cases only a power of subduing the body, but often hurts the poor head by giving some new aversion for you & any who have any control over them, as also it is often too great a shock to the Brain.

Only time, daily associations and experience can teach us of how much we can help, or injure them. According as a thing is precious or valuable, so does it call for care and attention. Now what price would we take for our Reason? Then let us pray and labor, & labor and pray for light and charity, by which we may be able to help our dear fellow creatures in this blessed work of Mercy.

The great St. Francis de Sales cured the most violent, by, patience, kindness and prayer.

[Pg 41] General Remedies include 1st Arterial Stimulants; sometimes called: Incitants, which, while they raise the actions of the System above the standard of health, shew their influence chiefly upon the heart & arteries: 2nd Narcotics, which especially affect the cerebral (brain) [Note: Parenthesis and enclosed words in original document] functions, & are either stimulant or sedative according as they increase or diminish action; 3d Antispasmodics, which, with a general stimulant power, exert a peculiar influence over the nervous system, by the relaxation of spasms, the calming of nervous irritation &c., without any special & decided tendency to the Brain; 4th Tonics, which moderately and permanently exalt the energies of all parts of the frame, without necessarily producing any apparent increase of the healthy actions; 5thly Astringents, which have the property of producing contraction in the living tissues with which they may come in contact.–

Local Remedies may be divided into four sections: those affecting the function of a part; namely, 1st Emetics, which act on the stomach, producing vomiting; 2nd Cathartics, which act on the bowels, producing a purgative effect; 3rd Diuretics, which act on the kidneys, producing an increased flow of urine; 4th Antilithics, which act on the same organs, preventing the formation of calculous (gritty or stony) [Note: Parenthesis and enclosed words in original document] matter; 5th Diaphoretics, which increase the cutaneous discharge; 6th Expectorants, which augment the secretions from the pulmonary mucous membrane, or promote the discharge of the Secreted Matter.

[*Pg 42*] [*Nothing written on this page.*]

[*Pg 43*] For the sake of convenience, in the absence of proper instruments, we often make use of means of measurement, which, tho' not precise, afford results sufficiently accurate for ordinary purposes –
There are certain household implements, corresponding to a certain extent with the regular standard measures.

Custom has attached a fixed value to these implements, that is well to be familiar with.

A tea cup is about 4 fluid ounces or a gill.
A wineglass holds 2 fluid ounces.
A good sized table spoon, ½ a fluid ounce.
A tea spoon (60 drops) [*Note: Parenthesis and enclosed words in original document*] holds a fluid drachm.

One drop is called a minim, or sixtieth part of a fluid drachm – but, as some liquids form larger drops than others, the safer method is, to use the minim measure in important cases.
As the abbreviations are mostly from the Latin, we give them here in english, as also the signs of the weights.

℞	*stands for, take*	*Collyr.*	*Means, an eye water*
āā	" *of each*	*Cong.*	" *a gallon*
lb.	" *a pound*	*Decoet*	" *a decoction*
℥	" *an ounce*	*Ft.*	" *make*
ʒ	" *a drachm*	*Garg.*	" *a gargle*
℈	" *a scruple*	*Gr.*	" *a grain*
O	" *a pint*	*Gtt.*	" *a drop*
f ℥	" *fluid ounce*	*Haust*	" *a draught*
f ʒ	" *fluid [d]rachm*	*Infus.*	" *An infusion*
ℳ	" *Minim*	*M.*	" *Mix*
chart	" *a small paper*	*Mass.*	" *A Mass*
coch.	" *a spoonful*	*Mist.*	" *A Mixture*
qs.	" *sufficient*	*Pil.*	" *A pill*

[Pg 44] Pulv. means a powder

S.	"	*write*
Sf[?]	"	*a half*

374

[*Pg 45*] The office of "Nurse" is one of awful responsibility if its duties be properly considered; for on the faithful discharge of them, will the Life of a fellow being, in very many instances, almost exclusively depend.–

How much intelligence, good sense and fidelity are therefore required, that the patient may profit by her attentions; or that [s]he may not be injured by her self-willedness or neglect! Where there is a Medical Attendant, the duties of a Nurse are reduced to two simple, but highly important rules; the observance of which Should be most rigidly insisted upon. First, to do every thing that the Physician orders to be done, and this in the strict letter of the commands. Second, to do nothing herself, nor permit any one else to do, that which he has not ordered; for it is fairly to be presumed, that the Physician will direct to the best of his knowledge, whatever he may think is essential to the welfare of his patient. —

There are however, exceptions to these remarks, that the Medical faculty admit of, that is; when the nurse is <u>experienced</u> and faithful, and has also shewen herself equal to her duty, she may, and should, withhold medicines, drinks &c, which she observes acts contrary to the designs or wishes of the Phyn, but, this liberty is only to be exercised between his visits, and she should relate to him as soon as he comes of what she had done, & why.– The injury usually done in nursing is, by being in the <u>advance</u> of the Phyn when improvement appears, for then, She, of her own accord, allows him more nourishing drinks, food &c, or tests his strength too fast by having him

[Pg 46] rise too soon, often &c.– Could all the consequences of ill timed omissions or commissions, as regards nursing, be laid down, or sufficiently remembered, the remedy would be gained – It is believed that a majority of relapses in acute diseases is owing to the injudicious employment of what is considered a very innocent indulgence of something, "more palatable": as in one case, three table spoonfuls of chicken water, created so much fever, and so severe a renewal of the pain of Pleurisy, that severe bleedings were required to subdue them; tho' when it was given, even the Phyn thought the patient convalescent – Therefore, it is in the injudicious use of animal substances, either entire or in solution, that Nurses most frequently effect the mischief complained of above – In the same way they venture on seasoning their nourishment with, "a little dash of Wine or Brandy", tho' contrary to the positive orders of the Phyn — Is it then surprising that fever should have so many Victims, when the force of the disease is aided by the attendants on their recovery?

[Pg 47] Hitherto we have spoken only of the Patient, let us now pay some attention to the Sick Room. If "good nursing is half the cure", let us see in what it consists.

The Phyn acknowledges that his attentions upon the sick would be altogether unavailing, were his directions not obeyed by the Nurse, and this, in the most faithful manner, for the Phyn sometimes rests his hopes on what may seem small in the mind of the nurse, she must therefore follow his directions most implicitly; except as in circumstances before alluded to– On the nurse depends most important responsibilities; the faithful administration of the medicines, in <u>time</u> and manner; the giving drinks and nourishments; attention to comfort and cleanliness; keeping the room quiet; procuring its proper ventilation; preserving a proper temperature of the air of the room; regulating the warmth of the Patient; the examination and preservation of his excretions; her management of his sitting up; making of the bed; the proper attention to the utensils for the evacuations; the mode of giving him drinks; the application & dressing of blisters; the administration of enemata; & management of the patient during Convalescence.she should possess moral honesty, that she may completely understand her situation as regards those, whose orders from the nature of her office, she has voluntarily bound herself to obey. Her duty consists in passive obedience; and when she refuses this, she breaks a contract; and if she follow her own promptings in the management of the patient, she betrays a trust, by which, she may counteract the best devised plan of treatment. The nurse shd be cleanly in person, apparel & habits. She shd after each meal rinse her mouth, that the breath, or flavor of what she had taken disturb the weak stomach of her patient –

Her hands must be always clean –

_____ too much duty must not be given her, or she may fail at a moment, when of all others, her services may be most necessary.

[Pg 48] To prevent this, ~~her~~ her health, strength & constitution shd be consulted, that no more be put upon her than she will be able to bear – In cases of long protracted illness therefore, other assistance shd be added, so as to give her occasional rest.

This is better than to withdraw her entirely, for she having become acquainted with his strengths, habits & disposition, is, during his sickness, almost necessary for him, as also, any matter of pain or annoyance wd now cause him to feel, that it is from the change of nurses. This interfering with his quiet & content, interrupts improvement, besides the reality of very frequently being seriously important to the patient –

When the disease is acute, no or very little talking or conversation shd be allowed in his room – If some conversation may be, let it always be of a cheerful nature, in a tone of voice that the patient may hear it distinctly without straining his attention – and never relate a thing of fatal or sad termination – whispering must <u>never</u> be used in the sick room – The nurse must speak to her sick in a low, kind, gentle and respectful manner – just loud enough to be heard without the patient being obliged to ask her what she said – Therefore she shd speak plainly, simply and in proper terms – She shd never be "<u>talkative</u>"- Sickness may become supportable by a nurse of kind, willing & amiable deportment, & the obligation of gratitude is long felt by the object of her affectionate care – So important is this, that it is often necessary for recovery, & the contrary has de<u>stroy</u>ed the nervous, sensitive or debilitated sufferer ⁓⁓

[*Pg 49*] The power of medicine over disease, is owing to its proper selection. This belongs to the Phyn, but it depends too often upon the nurse, whether it be efficacious or otherwise – In many cases, life itself is at the mercy of the nurse, as she may faithfully or negligently perform her duty. How necessary is it then, that this important personage, shd feel the responsibility attatched to her situation; & be influenced by a conscientious regard, for the proper fulfilment of the duties, her position has imposed upon her.–

In insisting on the entire conformity of the Nurse to the directions of the Phyn however, we repeat, there are exceptions to this rule –

The patient as well as the Phyn are occasionally indebted to the nurse, for a judicious, or weltimed [*sic*] suspension, or perseverence [*sic*] in remedies, beyond the strict <u>letter</u> of her orders; and especially, when such departures have proceeded from a genuine exercise of judgement [*sic*];

and not from a preference for her own method, carelessness &c.–

Variety of constitutions may deceive or escape the expectation of the Phyn, no one can be certain that his remedy will act up to his desires; consequently were the medicine not suspended, or sometimes urged, beyond the common direction, much injury might follow.–

In such instances, the judicious interference of the nurse, may be highly valuable & fortunate. But she shd not presume on a frequency of these, as they are rare.

Much depends on the mode of giving the medicine – A cheerful, persuasive manner on the part of the nurse, with disposition to lessen its nauseating effect, by having some little thing

[*Pg 50*] of pleasant taste to present immediately after swallowing the disgusting dose. good sense must prevent her from insisting on his taking it at a moment when he discloses he cannot retain it, as in case he had just vomited, or been greatly disposed towards it, wait, in this case, even 10 or 15 minutes over time appointed

[*Pg 51*] *Of Giving Drinks and Nourishments.*

Greater errors are committed in the use of drinks and nourishments, than in the neglect, or mal-administration of medicine. A nurse may suppose that thirst must be allayed whenever it is great & then allow free drinks unmindful of quantity or quality –

This is sometimes of very serious moment, as it either overloads the weak stomach, or causes it to be vomited, much to the inconvenience or injury of the patient. An over quantity causes oppression; an improper quality may seriously injure him.–

The nurse, therefore, shd never depart from the quantity or quality of the drinks prescribed.

The same care is necessary in point of food or nourishment – too much of the right kind wd be as bad as to give what had been objected to – If the over quantity remains undigested, he suffers much pain, and if it digest[s], it may afford too much nutriment to the system at a time when it requires less – Nothing shd be thought small in the mind of the Nurse, where the benefit or injury of her patient is in question –

APPENDIX B

Of Cleanliness in the Sick Room

[*Pg 52*] Pure air is so necessary for the sick room, that every means must be used to preserve it.

On the nurse, this duty almost entirely depends. Every thing disgusting smell or sight must be removed as soon as possible – The evacuations removed immediately from the room; the body, & the bed clothes shd be as frequently changed as circumstances will allow. Fresh air shd be admitted as freely as the condition of the sick will allow of; no filth to remain on the floor, tables, bed, hearth &c.–

All the vessels used for medicines, drinks or nourishment, shd be cleansed the instant they are used; consequently, the same vessel or spoon shd not be used twice without its being cleaned, or used for two persons without washing.

The Patients face & hands shd be often washed, especially when very warm, by wiping them with a towel wetted with cold water, or vinegar & water, unless there be chilliness when cold is applied – With the same view to comfort, the patient shd have his mouth frequently cleansed; by himself, if his strength will permit; and by the nurse, when this fails. This is particularly necessary in fevers wherein the tongue becomes dry and the teeth become encrusted or cased in a reddish glue.

For this purpose, yeast & water is very effectual; or a wash made of a tea spoonful of the sweet spirit of nitre, and a table spoonful of water. This is very acceptable to the mouth in the beginning of active fevers; where the tongue becomes loaded with a white, dense fur,

[*Pg 53*] or is coated with a sticky slime. The patient when able, finds comfort & amusement while performing this office for himself, by means of a tooth brush –

but, where the mouth has been neglected, and the foul glue collected around the teeth, a soft mop must be gently passed along the gums, after being dipped in a proper wash, such as the yeast & water, or laudanum in water – At other times the rinsing of the mouth will do, but the mop shd be used once or twice a day. to prevent the mop from giving pain, let the soft linen be longer than the little stick you tie it on, wrapping it loosely for awhile, & then tying the thread tightly to prevent it coming off in the

379

mouth. The mop may be an inch longer than the end of the stick and not too large, but just sufficient to carry enough of the wash on it. This precaution lessens the contagious or unhealthy tendency of the air around him –

[Pg 54] *Of Quiet in the Sick Room.*

There is scarcely any thing so distressing in the sick room, as noise. This must have the watchful attention of the nurse.

It is not enough to be quiet herself, but she must require all to observe this regulation.

A talkative nurse is a great evil, and loquacity is for some the greatest annoyance.

In certain conditions of the nervous system, cheerful conversation is highly beneficial, and in such cases, an agreeable pleasantry, on a well chosen topic with his kind nurse, will have a happy effect, but this conversation must not be frequent or of long duration, as excitement is almost always produced by them.

Another great misery & annoyance to the sick is when he falls into the hands of a "bustling nurse" who is, forever "putting things to rights" without, however, effecting the object; and all the time makes so much noise that the patient gets no sleep, however strong the desire – It were better, that the hearth remained unswept, or the fire unrenewed for a time, than the patient be deprived of his sleep, or roused from it, as this sleep may hold an important item in his recovery.–

Indeed a good nurse sees how to take advantage of the times that will be least annoying to her patient – There shd be no fixed time for, "Cleaning up the Room" As the moment that will be of least annoyance to the sick shd be the only one Selected.–

Another great disturbance to the sick is the

[Pg 55] creaking shoe. soft socks shd be drawn over such.–

Often, near the sick, are the "Mess rooms", hear the rattling of spoons, knives, forks &c. are one continued jarring – Now the nurse shd get the habit of doing every thing quietly and without noise – And She must require the same care from all who assist her in the department – The

Comfort of the sick, must be the One object and Motto of all in attendance on them directly or indirectly.

The door shd not be constantly on the go, if it must not remain open, then let as few come in as possible, otherwise the sick get no rest – have the door in good repair, that is, the hinges well oiled, and the door easy to open.–

If your patient is sleeping, do not allow the door to be opened – This may be observed by pushing the feathered end of a quill thro' the key hole – This has become a speaking practice in some Hospitals – Exclude all such visitors as might endanger the safety of your patient or you may cause permanent mischief.

[Pg 56] *Of Ventilating the Sick Room.*

We mean by this, the removal of the foul or impure air, for that which is pure – This may be done by opening the doors and windows for a time – The frequency for doing this must be regulated by the season of the year; by the state of the weather; and the nature of the disease – In cold weather the air does not so soon become unhealthy as in warm weather, and the circulation of the air is also assisted by fire, & consequently more frequently changed.–

If the weather be wet, either in warm or cold, too much air shd not, must not, be admitted immediately into the sick room – No damp air must be admitted, but, inner doors may perhaps produce the necessary ventilation – The good Sense of the Attendants must regulate this.–

Fever and other acute diseases will require a more frequent ventilation than chronic affections, except when the latter is attended by profuse & offensive discharges –Some use burning, what they call sweet herbs, rosin, sugar, tar, frankincense &c, or decomposing vinegar on a hot shovel, for the purpose of purifying the room or air, but All these or others similar to them, destroy a part of the vital air, and supply its place by what is worse – These methods shd therefore be strictly prohibited.

[Pg 57] *Regulating the warmth of the Patient*

If he complains of feeling cold or chilly more covering shd be put upon him until a more comfortable sensation is restored, but after a reaction has taken place, and the patient complains of being too warm, the bed clothes must now be made lighter, or that they be gradually removed so as to gain back the pleasurable or usual state again.–

Therefore the quantity of covering should always be made to suit the patient.

[Pg 58] *Examination & preservation of the Excretions.*

This duty is too often neglected, important as it is ___ _____ A nurse should ask the physician if he desires the evacuations to be kept for his inspection, and if he does, they may be set aside, but not in the sick room – And she herself should also examine them, as well for her greater information as to be able to tell the Dr of them, in case some thing prevented his seeing them – The same case as regards the urine –

It is well for a nurse to say simply to the Dr while he examines them; Dr, what term do you give this appearance? or if a more experienced nurse can give you this information, gain it of her ___ _____ A Diarrhoea, produces only free discharges without pain, seeming to empty the bowels entirely, when it is produced by bad food, or too much food – These discharges are often the cure also – But when the diarrhoea is from cold, or sudden check of perspiration &c; we see, mucus, or slime mixed with the excretion.–

In Bilious Diarrhoea, the stools are loose, copious, & of a bright yellow, or green – The urine is then also deeply tinged with bile __

We see, therefore, that it is highly important to know what the discharges are, as they bespeak the character of the disease ___

[Pg 59] *Of the Patient's Sitting Up.*

do not be too hasty for having the patient sit up. This action is an exercise which requires strength to suit it – Exercise being a remedy, the patient's condition must make it proper, and only so much, & no more must be taken at a time – It calls for a dose of exercise according to the measure of strength the patient has at the time – Sitting up, is a stimulant & increases the pulse to twenty strokes more in the minute, than in a lying position, & such as often shews its unfriendly effects in fever – And when the patient is too weak for it, the heart performs its functions so rapidly, that the exhaustion that follows causes fainting in a few minutes – Therefore much care is required, in getting the patient out of bed. It is better that he rise oftener than to sit one minute longer than his strength bears comfortably; while the patient is up, some warm covering shd be put around him, & prevent a current of air from being on him, or damp air from him.

[Pg 60] *Making the Bed of the Sick* –

The same care is necessary for this, as when he is judged able to sit up awhile – I have known persons, absolutely recovering, thrown back and die from having been taken out of bed even while the bed was being made – He may be moved about on his mattress, that is, from a warm spot to a cooler, or even the linen, but well dried, may be changed while he is on the bed – and, if he is able, a bed might be put [a]longside his own, and then be gently lifted on it, but, I repeat, when he is this weak, the change is better made on his bed.–

If the strength of the patient allows it, spread the bed up twice a day for fever cases _____

When the patient's condition admits of it, and he has been a long time in one room, or corner of a room, you may, with great benefit, move him to another, it is for him a change of air, & perhaps, views, but, if he gets home sick for his old place, indulge him, for, discontent prevents improvement __

A weak patient often loses strength, or is kept from gaining it by the trouble & pain they are put to for making their evacuations, therefore, every Room, or, bed should have a bed pan & urinal – A patient will insist on rising as long as possible, but the nurse should not allow this when they are too weak for it, and, even when they seem able, great assistance may be given by the nurse – Before the pan is offered to the sick, a pillow shd be placed under the back, to prevent the hollow that wd otherwise distress them. This neglect, is the cause of the sick objecting to the pan __

[Pg 61] Every exertion must be spared the patient, for, when every least attention, requires exertion, little by little, strength is drained or used

383

up in these frequent, tho' seemingly small efforts – – A tumbler, bowl, cup &c. are usually used for drinking out of, in sick rooms, but, <u>neither</u> of these shd be found in a well-regulated sick room, but, the <u>sick-cup</u> as it is called, shd <u>alone</u> convey drinks while they are confined to bed __

A phial also is convenient, and this, corked, can lie on his bed, when he wants a mouth-ful only, but, frequently __ this, the sick can get themselves, and they prefer it on this account, when able to get it __

[*Pg 62*] *Of Dressing Blisters.*

This is an important duty, as the efficacy and success, as well as the great comfort of the sick are all concerned in it –

When the circulation is languid, the spot for the application shd be first rubbed with some stimulating liquid to give the skin heat and action – The Blister shd be spread thickly so as to produce the speediest effect – Some think that if a blister rise at all, it is enough – this is a mistake – A blister spread too thin, soon dries, and only raises the cuticle, & even for this, must remain on a long time – whereas, a well made plaster, goes as deep as necessary, and in a much shorter time – To prepare the skin for the blister, it <u>must</u> be first <u>rubbed</u> with Spts [*Spirits*] of hartshorn, or, turpentine, cayenne pepper & brandy, or same such – But where the circulation is active, & great heat is already in the spot, these must <u>not</u> be used – Again, care must be used for the blister not slipping from the proper place, for then no good is done, and as they are generally very painful, they are always necessary when ordered, and should therefore receive due attention – Blisters are better held in their place by adhesive plaster than by bandages only, for bandages must be pretty tight to keep them from slipping when the patient moves about, but the aid of adhesive plaster & then, bandages <u>comfortably</u> tight, will do – When they are applied to the legs, they are kept in the right place by drawing a stocking over it – The common time for a blister to draw is, about 12 hours, but, circumstances may require a departure from

[*Pg 63*] from [*sic*] this Rule – 8 hours wd be enough for <u>children</u>, or even in less, and it shd be examined at 6 hours, & dressed if enough drawn – Again there are in some grown persons a peculiar sensibility, that calls for

384

less than what is ordinary – Children suffer less from blisters than adults, and might not give the timely notice of its having drawn sufficiently – On the nurse, then depends the good or ill use of this important remedy – If the bandaging is too tight, the humors to be acted on cannot act, and, if too loose, they produce no action, except as they have slipped about to some wrong spot, perhaps on some bone that presses the bed, and then much unnecessary and often injurious torment is given the sick.–

It is not well to spread gauze over the blister plaster _____ Sometimes, no more is <u>wanting</u> from a blister, than to excite inflammation. In this case, the blister must be often looked at, and removed as soon as it is well reddened –

Some blisters produce so much irritation or inflammation, before the time for removal, that the plaster may be removed, & thus a basilicon salve dressing, or even a soft milk & bread poultice may finish its course to the relief of the patient – blisters ordered for the legs, are meant for the inner part or calves of the leg, and for the legs or arms, shd be longer than wide – for the arms, the inner part also are intended, and not so near the hand as to prevent feeling the pulse _____ when ordered for the chest, the seat of pain is the spot for it, but if the chest is all involved, let it go as near the throat as possibly, [*sic*] and running downwards, or according to the length of disease, or its force – When for the neck,

[*Pg 64*] put it on the back of the neck, one inch below the hair, & let it run down the spine to <u>nearly</u> the bottom part of the shoulder blades – when for the ears, is meant, that part, behind the ear that has no hair, or in some cases, the hair is ordered to be shaved some, so as to give larger surface, this is done when the disease is of long standing – When ordered for the regions of the stomach; all the space below the breast bone, and inclining to the left side, <u>towards</u> the middle of the abdomen, or belly, is meant. When ordered for the Abdomen, nearly the whole surface of the belly, is meant, or, if only one spot seems to be affected, this then only, may be blistered _____

The size of the blister, must vary with the size of the patient, and their age – small, for young children, and increased according to age. Their shape & form may vary according to the part for their action – A large blister gives not much more pain, while drawing than a small one, it is only more painful as to the dressing & the position in bed - ___ for a common sized person, the blister for the legs, shd be, from 7 to 8 inches long, & between 3 & 4 inches wide – for the back, 7 or 8 inches long, & about 4 wide. for the chest, 7 or 8 inches long, & 6 or 7 wide – Or, for the whole chest, or thorax, 8 or 9 inches long, & 7 or 8 broad – for the stomach, from 8 to 9 inches long, & from 6 to 7 broad, – the greatest size for the stomach, is, from side to side __ If the whole of the abdomen is to be covered, from 10 to 11 inches long, & from 8 to 10 broad – for the temples, they are rounded & may be from an inch, to an inch & a half, in size – All these must vary according to the size of the patient __

[*Pg 65*] Before <u>dressing</u> the blister, let every thing necessary be in complete readiness – the plasters spread, & by the bed – All the rags at hand; and a pair of well-cutting, sharp pointed scissors – Snip every blister of any Size, so to let the water run out, having a cloth under the part to prevent the clothes or bed from being soiled –

the very small blisters, or portions of water, will have filled better by the next dressing, & will not give so much pain then – The skin shd <u>never</u> be removed from the blistered part, however desirable the irritation may be, for the pain caused to the patient can hardly be compensated – It wd be better to reapply the blister immediately after its healing, than to strip the skin off.–

A blister shd scarcely ever be washed, tho' this is a common fault.– It never does good, & often injury, by exposing it too long to the air, produces chilliness, & is fatiguing to the sick – remove the particles of fly as stick to the raw surface, but those on the dead skin will do no harm, and will come off, by after dressings. It is better to leave the particles of fly on, than give the patient any pain, or keep them longer uncovered – If a continued discharge is desired, the basilicon ointment is to be used – if this is not necessary, simple cerate is to be used – Either of these is to be spread on, thin, old linen rags, or soft rags, at least, & repeated twice in 24 hours, or only once if the discharge is small – When the blister, or sore part is of big size, have the salve dressings cut in several slips or pieces, as they can be withdrawn without much pain – The plaster shd only cover the sore surface, as the sound skin becomes unhealthy, if it is covered over with the salve.

[*Pg 66*] Sometimes the sore becomes extremely painful & inflamed – this pain is best subdued by a soft milk & bread poultice, in which is melted a small portion of <u>fresh</u> hog's lard, or newly churned butter, before salt has been put to it – If the poultice fail to ease it, linseed oil & lime water, equal parts & shaken so as to form a cream-like thickness may be often applied – When the itching stage of a blister is very annoying – use, an infusion of slippery elm, or flax seed or very fresh lard into which some laudanum has [*been*] mixed –

[*Pg 67*] *Of Relapse* –

The return of disease should be wisely & carefully guarded against – Some of the following, usually give rise to a return –

Stimulating food or drinks too soon indulged in – for, if the stomach is unable to digest, it must be vomited, or causes diarrhoea – both injure the patient, and, after having put him to severe suffering for several hours – If the <u>stomach</u> is able for it, too much nourishment is formed, and will be too suddenly sent into the weakened & irritable blood vessels, which usually rekindles fever.

No animal substance, in any shape or form should be given during fever, nor very soon after its cessation, ~~least it~~ lest it return by the over-stimulating quality of nourishment – When a change from the lightest diet may be made, this change must be of the lightest kind of animal substance, as: weak chicken water; weak beef, or veal tea; or the diluted juice of oysters should be first resorted to – these should be given in small quantities, and repeated at stated intervals, day & night, if the patient is very feeble, provided, it will not interrupt important sleep.– Three days using these kind of nourishments, might prepare the system for a little stronger food, and, the next advance should observe the same moderation: the soft end of five or six oysters; a soft boiled egg, or cold custard in its mildest form – After such diet for three or four days, the patient may be indulged in a small piece of boiled mutton; the breast of a partridge or pheasant; turkey, or chicken – And after as many more he may have a small piece of rare done beef or venison steak; or mutton chop. At his noon meal of this kind, he may have a tumbler of Ale, or porter & water, if this drink does not cause headache [*Pg 68*] flatulency or sour stomach ___

During the whole stage of convalescence, the <u>bowels</u> should be strictly attended to – one evacuation daily is absolutely necessary; but purging must be avoided most carefully –

As to exercise, he must accustom himself to what he is able for in moving around his sick room, or parlor, before he tries the open air. And a close[d] carriage should be first used for this, and when he is ready for walking, and, the <u>weather</u> <u>suitable</u>, he can be benefited by this exercise – As soon as he is done with phials, pill-boxes, bed-pans, &c. take them from the room so as to leave nothing in his sight that would too much remind him of his illness __

Great care must be used to keep him from currents of cold or damp air – and avoiding equally damp places – He should not take a <u>full</u> drink of cold water, tho' so desirable to a convalescent. Avoid calve's-feet, beef or chicken jellies, and all other gelatinous substances – tho' these are so often offered to sick, they form actually the most <u>indigestible</u> portion of all animal substances, for glue it is literally, and to these are added wine, spices, sugar & acid – What <u>weak</u> stomach is ready for this? – These jellies should be banished from the sick room __

[Pg 69] *Fever*

The term fever implies heat; but a mere in increase of heat does not constitute fever, since we may have considerable increase of heat, without the system laboring under this affection; and on the other hand, we may have fever with a cool, even a partially cold skin, as sometimes happens in yellow fever –

<u>Generally</u>, in fever there is a sensation of chilliness, followed by an increase of heat; the pulse gives a greater number of strokes in a given time; while several functions of the body are more or less impaired, and the strength of the limbs particularly, is diminished –

Sometimes only a part of the body suffers from increase of heat in fever; as: the extremities may be cold, while the head, chest & abdomen may be unnaturally [sic] warm.

The same uncertainty may happen with the pulse; its frequency by no means establishes fever; we may have a very frequent pulse without fever, or an unusually slow one, when it is really present; and this may or not may not be accompanied by increase of heat. The pulse may, therefore, be slow or frequent; strong or weak; hard or soft, with or without fever – Fever then is occasioned by derangement of the nervous & sensorial functions, derangement in the circulating functions. derangement in the secreting & excreting functions – the knowledge of these derangemens form the true characters of fever – Altho' there are a variety of fevers, they all have a general, as well as a particular plan of treatment. All have to be treated more or less upon the same general principles; tho' certain of them may exact a specific management ˜ ˜ ˜

[*Pg 70*] As there is in almost all cases of fever, a strong determination to the head, or head-ache, the patient should be kept as quiet as possible; & should delirium attend, company must be prohibited, also any circumstance that might tend to augment it, & all objects removed that seemed to attract his attention – he shd see as few faces as possibly [*sic*], or only those employed in nursing him. the room shd be kept pretty dark. No unnecessary conversations, and whispering absolutely forbidden, for the patient always believes himself to be the object of their remarks &c – – carpet around the bed saves much annoying noise, and the attendants shd wear socks over their shoes – In Wards of fever, the floor might be mopped over once or twice of [*sic*] a fine day, but not flooded over as for Scrubbing – It is also good to sprinkle the floor occasionally with Vinegar[233] – the bedclothing shd be regulated by the feelings of the patient – When he is chilly, put more on him – when he complains of too much, remove some, tho' if he be sweating, care must be used, lest it be checked –

Cool drinks are proper for fevers – but when perspiring, or about to do so, they shd not be <u>cold</u>. It often happens in the higher grades of fever, the thirst calls for more drink than the stomach can well support, then vomiting follows – To prevent this, small pieces of Ice may be kept near the patient & that a piece may from time to time be taken – or if ice cannot be had, a spoonful of cold water may be given often – the drinks of fevered patients shd be palatable, but free from all stimulus, except in such cases as call for stimulus - they may be some of the following: toast-water, baum [*sic*]-tea, lemonade - current jelly in water, molasses & water with a little vinegar, the

[*Pg 71*] water off of dried cherries, very weak milk & water, barley-water – flax-seed tea, either with or without lemon juice.

Apple-tea, that is: warm or hot water poured on Sliced apples, and drank when cold. We have named many, so as to admit of choice, but simple cold water may almost always be allowed, & is also most palatable in great heat.–

In the commencement of any acute disease, little or no food is required — Nature often, kindly assists the patient by taking away all appetite – When nourishment is proper in fever, it shd be given by three or four spoons ful [*sic*], large or small, as the patient may be large or small – It shd consist of weak milk & water: thin tapioca: sage or arrow root: gruel of indian or oat meal; ripe fruits in moderate quantities: when in season, such as oranges, grapes, or roasted apple may also be given – A cup of weak tea or coffee is often grateful to the sick, & may almost always be allowed. But in the commencement of any acute disease little or no food is required __

If circumstances, and the condition of the patient will allow of it, it will be well to Change his linnen [*sic*] and sheets daily, especially in those fevers that pass off by sweats, at the same time, great care is wanting as to the perfectly dry state of these, and the proper time and manner of doing it. – The times for giving the remedies must be carefully attended to, for a neglect, or mistaken condescencion [*sic*] or tenderness, may allow the proper time to pass, which another time could not supply for – the time, therefore, is often as necessary to be observed, as the medicine, or remedy itself, since, the condition of the system governs its necessity or applications ___

In fevers, during hot weather, the fresh air will be serviceable to the patient, and with little bed-

[*Pg 72*] clothing – if he be very hot, and fresh air cannot be admitted in to the room, a sponge~~d~~ squeezed out of cool water may be wiped over his forehead, & arms ~~& body of the patient~~ – but, remember this, or even the fresh air is never to be used when there is a moist skin, or tendency to sweat, and his clothes must not be made damp by the sponging – If cough, or other affections of the chest exist, sponging cannot be thought of – Cool, or even cold drinks are most useful and acceptable in fever, &

may be at times changed for small pieces of ice put in them – but given in small quantities, tho' frequently – but, when the body is moist, these must be avoided, and warmer drinks used – a cough only, without sweat or moisture, does not forbid cold drinks –

Fevers of all kinds frequently are attended by sick stomach, or even vomiting, and the nurse too often gives an emetic as the cure, which nearly always does great harm to the sick – But in such cases cathartic medicines of a moderately active kind should be given first and if these fail, external remedies may be used – The internal remedy for this feature of the disease, Nausea, may be: Calomel 8 grains, white sugar the same, divided into 8 powders, giving one every hour in a little syrup, or scraped apple until the bowels are moved – If this does not act two or three tea-spoonful [*sic*] of calcined magnesia, in a little sweetened milk may be given, or an enema may be profitable. for this, take about a pint of hot water, to a table spoonful of common salt – when the salt is dissolved, & the water about warm enough, let it be given, and repeated in half an hour, or an hour if necessary –

If these fail, take this set of remedies: rich gum arabic water. (cold) [*Note: Parenthesis and enclosed words in original document*] milk & water, about a table spoonful every fifteen or twenty minutes – Or, you may

[*Pg 73*] use with more certainty of success the following julep:

Take super saturated soda	1 ½ drachm
powdered gum arabic	2 drachms
oil of. mint, –	4 drops
white sugar,	2 drachms
water,	4 ounces–

Of this a table-spoonful may be taken every hour or half hour – Should none of these answer, take a few ounces of blood from the stomach by leeches, this may be preceded or followed by a plaster of mustard flour & vinegar until the skin smart a little, or it may be useful to apply a blister, if the vomiting be obstinate – <u>these, in case a physician cannot be had</u> ____Altho' Bleeding is considered almost a universal remedy for fever, in its hot stage, yet, being a remedy of great power, it must be used with great judgement [*sic*] as to time & quantity – Blood must not be taken when the fever has, or is about to subside, or in a Sweating Stage – and there are very rare exceptions to this –

There is a remedy so popular for the cure of fever, as sweating; and none, perhaps, has been more abused, as, there is a heat of the body which rises above sweating point, and in this state no perspiration can be gained, and a gentle sweating is preferable to a profuse sweat – when a profuse sweat comes on, we should reduce it gradually by removing little by little, the bed-clothes, or the heat of the room, tho' this last is attended with danger – he may cease also the drinks that had been given to effect sweating – and when his body is perfectly dry again, then all the clothes wet by sweating, should be replaced by dry ones – the determination of

[*Pg 74*] fever usually is to the brain, the liver, the spleen or the lungs; & few remedies are so proper in restoring this, as well chosen aperients, or gentle purgatives – Besides, such matter in these cases, are constantly forming and are necessary to be removed – Some times there will be too much bile, again too little, & both these extremes are to be helped by mild, but properly selected cathartics – purgatives well chosen not only evacuate the bowels, but the general system also, thus some cathartics are much more useful than others – If possible, do not not avoid having sweating and purging at the same time, and even when not sweating, let the sick have his stockings & warm slippers on when rising for the stool, or if he uses the bed-pan, have a warm blanket around him & keep the fresh air from him.–

The use of blisters too, in fever must have their right time for beneficial applications, and can only be used with advantage when the pulse is soft, or, as some day: below par – fever, in pleurisy, or inflammation of the liver, point out the spot for placing the blister, but, where the disease does not shew local injury the ancles [*sic*] & wrists are to be the parts blistered – if the ancles [*sic*] & wrists are so slow in circulation or cold & languid, the insides of the thigh, & above the elbows must be the places for them – A blister may be left on for 12 or 14 hours, if not ready to be removed sooner, but, in many cases, they are irritable enough to remove sooner, & may be dressed with basilicon ointment & the blisters, hardly formed, but perhaps too painful to endure longer, will be fully formed by the salve – Some suffer much from strangury in blistering, but by removing & dressing as soon as they become very painful

[Pg 75] this terrible suffering is spared them __

Intermittent fever is that which leaves intervals perfectly free from fever, and they may be called according to their recurrence: daily, or quotidian – tertian, or every other day: again when it occurs every fourth day it is called quartan – When it occurs in the Spring it is called, vernal; when in the fall: Autumnal, which is usually of a severer form – the paroxysms of intermittent fever are three: the cold stage, the hot, & the sweating – in some the cold felt is most intense with violent shaking – in others, some trifling trembling only is felt. After the cold follows the heat with dry skin, great thirst, head-ache, restlessness, the tongue furred, the pulse frequent, & mostly hard & full – Sometimes also, Stupor, delirium, convulsions & – After the hot stage has had its course, a moisture is felt on the forehead, presently it becomes general, and after sometime no uncomfortable symptoms remain but weakness – Agues are rarely fatal except by inducing diseases on the spleen, liver or producing dropsical affection of the abdomen. Warm drinks & warm applications to the stomach, feet & legs are good for shortening the cold stage. Some Drs find 30 drops of laudanum given as soon as the patient felt the coldness coming on, to have favorable influence, or repeated in 15 minutes if no feeling of warmth was produced – this, however, could not be used where there [sic] tendency of blood to the head or stupor – nor could laudanum be employed unless blood-letting or purging had been previously employed – After recovery from intermittent fever, great care

[Pg 76] should be [taken] to prevent relapse or return of the disease. Imprudence or exposure may cause the attacks to come on about the seventh, ninth or thirteenth day, the last, perhaps, the most common. The bowels should be kept moved once a day, but by no means purged – great fatigue & dampness should be avoided for some time _____.–

Blisters are powerful helps in intermittent fever, but the[y] should not be used too early. [End]

Appendix C:
A.88 — Hospitals[1]

Sullivan, Louise, DC. , ed. and trans. *Louise de Marillac Spiritual Writings:*
Correspondence and Thoughts. New York: New City Press, 1991.

Courtesy, Daughters of Charity Northeast Province, Albany, New York

In the name of God, the Daughters of Charity shall rise precisely at four o'clock. They shall make their beds after having made their act of adoration and after having dressed. At a quarter to five, they shall begin meditation. They shall conclude it at five-thirty, and then they shall recite the Litany of Jesus and two decades of their rosary.

They all shall come to the hospital at six o'clock. They then shall empty the night vessels and basins and make the beds of the sick. Before going to the hospital, they shall each have taken a piece of bread and some wine except on days when they receive Holy Communion. On these days, they shall content themselves with the scent of vinegar, putting some vinegar on their hands. This shall only be necessary until they become accustomed to the air in the rooms of the sick.

At seven o'clock the sisters shall have the sickest patients take a bouillon or a fresh egg for breakfast. The less sick shall take some fresh butter or cooked apples.

The Daughters of Charity shall hear Mass every day. Beforehand, however, it is necessary to have the ordered medicines given to the sick. Also, there must be great care to give bouillons at the precise times.

The Daughters of Charity who have need of breakfast shall go immediately and then return to the sick in order to console those who

---

1. Because of a large tear in the manuscript of this passage, the lines are incomplete. However, they have been completed through reference to corresponding passages in the copy of the Rule of Angers, evidently written by Louise de Marillac (Note of Sister Geoffre).

are close to death. They shall provide for those sick in need of instruction concerning salvation, so that they can make a general confession of their entire life. This should dispose the sick to go to confession and to receive Communion every Sunday, as long as their illness persists. It should also prepare them to receive Extreme Unction at the proper time. Those sick who will recover should be moved nevermore to offend God. If they should fail in this, they should be prepared to go to confession as soon as possible.

The Daughters shall see that the sick have dinner precisely at ten o'clock. If they are in charge of the food for the sick, they shall provide at least some veal and mutton, with a bit of beef. In the evening, some roasted and boiled meat shall be provided. At least four bouillons and three fresh eggs per day shall be given to the sick who do not eat meat.

After having cleared the table of the dinner of the poor, a Daughter Shall remain at the hospital. The others shall dine precisely at eleven o'clock after having made their particular examen. During dinner, each shall take her turn reading. After Grace has been said, they shall recite a decade of their rosary. Immediately afterward, two of them shall return to the hospital. Their recreation shall be in recreating with the sick. The daughter who had remained at the hospital shall go to the second table with the reader. After having said Grace as the others did, and after having cleared the table, these two shall go to the hospital for recreation with the sick. The other two shall go to their quarters and work at whatever needs to be done, doing as much for the linens of the poor as for their little Community.

If there is no Company of Ladies which brings the afternoon collation, the Daughters shall all come to the hospital at precisely two o'clock in order to give the sick poor a few little sweets such as toast and cooked pears.

Those who have work to do shall go to their duties, or if there is nothing urgent to be done, they shall go to the bedsides of the sick and shall try to move the new arrivals to make a general confession, instructing them beforehand on the manner in which they are to confess their sins.

At four o'clock, they shall wash the sick. They shall change soiled bedsheets, empty the vessels, and put the beds of the sick back into some order without the sick getting out of bed.

At five o'clock, they shall serve supper to the sick. After supper, the same sister will remain in the hospital that did so at dinnertime. The others shall go to supper after the particular examen which should take a good quarter of an hour. This examen shall be in the form of repetition of meditation, unless they make a half hour of meditation followed by the particular examen at a later time. There shall be reading during supper.

After Grace, which shall be at about six-thirty, the sisters shall go to the hospital. The sister who had remained at the hospital shall go to supper with the reader. Those sisters who have just returned to the hospital shall make sure that the sick are all in bed at seven o'clock, and that there is water, some wine and a few little sweets for those who need them. At seven-thirty, all the Daughters shall come to the hospital to make their general examen aloud in the midst of the poor. They shall recite the Litany of the Blessed Virgin and shall give holy water to all the sick.

At eight o'clock, they shall go to prepare the necessities for the next day's service of the sick. They shall finish their rosary, make an act of adoration, and then go to bed at precisely nine o'clock. One sister shall stay on night duty and shall see to it that none of the sick die without having received the Last Sacraments. Until the sick first awaken, she shall recite her rosary and shall read the subject of her meditation.

The sister on night duty shall have a book to read, so long as it does not interfere with her service of the sick. After having made her meditation at three-thirty, she shall go to awaken the other sisters at four o'clock. If she wishes, she may have breakfast and then go to bed, rising at 9 o'clock in order to hear Mass. Another sister shall take her place in the hospital, and she shall make her meditation in the same manner as the others.

All the sisters shall take their turn staying awake at night to watch over the sick.

The Daughters shall not go out into the city and shall conduct themselves with great modesty in the Motherhouse. They shall often recall the presence of God and shall speak modestly and gently with externs. They shall act in the same way among themselves and with the sick.

I think that something should be said concerning the sisters' associating with the religious.

It is hoped that the sisters shall have at their disposal some preserves, some fruit, some sugar and some wine so that the sick are not left with something sour if they desire some nourishment outside of mealtime.

The sisters shall take proper care of the linen of the sick.

In the hospital, there should be several holy water fonts and at least two oratories in the form of small altars.

The sisters shall have four Crucifixes to leave with the sick who have received Extreme Unction. A plenary indulgence is applied to these Crucifixes through the ejaculatory prayer "Jesus, Mary."

They shall have four pieces of coarse cloth to put on the beds of the sick for extraordinary confessions of persons who are not from the Motherhouse.

At the hospital, there should be some small copper tubs in order to facilitate the emptying of basins. There should be two larger tubs, always filled with water, attached to the wall. These should empty into ditches or elsewhere and be used to wash the basins and vessels.

In the hospital, there should be two censers which may be lit when needed. In these should burn only sweet fragrances, such as juniper or bay seed. Sometimes old bread crusts may be burned in the furnaces. Red hot gridirons should be quenched with vinegar.

It is hoped that the girls destined to join our Company would have their beds in the hospital in order to accompany the sister on night duty.

The Daughters must care for the table napkins, spoons, cups and plates used in serving the sick their meals. The order that the sisters must retain some for their service is not noted here.

I am not speaking of the act of adoration which, it seems to me should be made with the poor each morning. Likewise, I am not speaking of the Benedicite and the Grace of the sick, for I do not wish to know what the men religious do. And then it seems to me that there are so many things to say in order to inspire the sisters in their actions that I should speak of these topics from time to time.

If I remember other things, I shall write them, if it pleases God.

Appendix D:
Missions of Sister Matilda Coskery and Highlights of Antebellum American History

1799   Sister Matilda (SM) born in Frederick County, Maryland

1828   SM entered Sisters of Charity of St. Joseph's
           Andrew Jackson elected president
           SM received the Holy Habit August 15

1831   SM made vows December 25 for the first time
           Jackson re-elected president

1831–33   SM #1 Mission to Mount St Mary's Infirmary, Emmitsburg, MD
           Cholera Epidemic (1832)
           Black Hawk War (1832)

1833–38   SM #2 Maryland Hospital for the Insane, Baltimore, MD
           American Anti-Slavery Society founded (1833)
           Whig Party formed (1834)
           Anti-Catholic Riot in Boston (1834)
           Southeastern Native Americans removed on "Trail of Tears"
             (1835–9)
           Van Buren elected president (1836)
           Battle of the Alamo (1836)

APPENDIX D

1838–40   SM #3 Richmond Infirmary (SS=Sister Servant), Richmond,
          Virginia
          Publication of Sarah Grimke's Letters on the Condition
             of Women (1838)

1840–47   SM #4 Mt. St. Vincent / Mt. Hope Retreat, Baltimore, MD (SS)
          Economic depression (1837–1843)
          Harrison elected president
          Dorothea Dix begins exposé of prison conditions (1841)
          Dix petitions Massachusetts legislature on behalf of insane (1843)
          Robert Hartley founds N.Y. Assn. for Improving the Condition
             of the Poor
          Philadelphia Bible Riots (Anti-Catholic Riots) (1844)
          Polk elected president (1844)

1847–49   SM #5 St. Patrick's Asylum, Rochester, New York (SS)
          Potato famine in Ireland (1845–1849)
          Mexican War (1846–1848)
          Seneca Falls Women's Rights Convention (1848)
          Taylor elected president (1848)

1849–50   SM #6 St. Mary's Asylum and School, Norfolk, Virginia (SS)
          Cholera epidemic (1849)
          Know-Nothing Party formed (1849)
          California Gold Rush (1849)

1850–52   SM #7 St. Mary's House for Invalids, Detroit, MI (SS)
          Fillmore assumes presidency after Taylor's death (1850)

1852–53   SM #8 Baltimore Infirmary, Baltimore, MD (SS)
          Pierce elected president (1852)

1853–55   SM #9 St. Peter's Asylum and School, Wilmington, DE (SS)
          Republican Party organized (1854)
          Know-Nothing party emerges (1854)

SM #10 St. Vincent's Asylum, Washington DC (SS)
SM Temporary Patient at Baltimore Infirmary
John Brown's Pottawatomie massacre (1855)

1855–70   SM #11 St. Joseph's Central House, Emmitsburg, MD.
SM Taught at Poor School
SM Treasurer during absence of Sister Ann Simeon Norris
Buchanan elected president (1856)
SM Appointed by Council to serve on Committee on the
    Hospitals (1857)
Gold Rush in Colorado (1858)
John Brown's raid on Harpers Ferry (1859)
Civil War (War Between the States) 1861–1865
SM was Civil War Nurse (1861)

1870   SM Died and buried in Emmitsburg at St. Joseph's

Appendix E:
Suggestions for Teaching
Early American Nursing History

One of the most rewarding experiences of teaching nursing is to be in the position to witness the awakening of a student to the historical impressions that professional nurses have made on society and culture. Stories from history serve as the most noble of teachers. Learning the history of one's profession is strengthening because it improves one's sense of identity and belonging. While all students who learn nursing history can become the story keepers of the profession, some go on to become the storytellers, those who research, record, and retell the past so that others may better understand the patterns of the profession in the hope that enlightened decisions will be made that will positively shape its future.

It is important that students critically explore their nursing traditions as part of the foundation for their development as nurse scientists, clinicians, and educators. The National League for Nursing (NLN) Position Statement: Innovation in Nursing Education: A Call to Reform (2003) states, "All levels of nursing education, undergraduate and graduate, are obligated to challenge their long-held traditions and design evidence-based curricula that are flexible, responsive to students' needs, collaborative, and integrate current technology."[1] Those who study early nursing history are given the tools and the opportunity to examine nursing traditions so that they are better able to fulfill what the NLN has suggested we are "obligated" to do. Students of early history, a period typically underrepresented in the nursing curricula, are given a broader historical framework from which to investigate nursing traditions.

The experience of studying nursing history can be likened to cultural immersion. To fully understand the past that one is studying, one releases all associations with present culture to allow oneself to be absorbed into the past, with its own peculiarities of being. Time and space become the portal of travel as one projects one's consciousness into another period. All facets of one's present life become assumptions. One's thoughts, observations, feelings, beliefs, and judgments must be turned consciously into questions to ensure that the entrée into a previous time is untainted by the presentist lens. This is not easy, as the ego that keeps us rooted in the present moment would have us compare the past to all that is around us and in us in this moment. It is to this preparation of the student that the teacher's first efforts are directed.

What follows is a brief sampling of some of the educational strategies and resources that I, Martha Libster, have used over the years to help students and practicing nurses connect to the profession's early healing traditions, which are very different from today's. My premise for this work is twofold: first, that those who take the opportunity to learn from the past are better able to create strongholds for creating their personal and professional future and, second, that the foundational humility and gratitude necessary for perpetuating the spirit as well as the work that is *nursing* is instilled in students and practicing nurses through the study of the elders, those who have walked the professional path before.

Preparation for Historical Study

1. Centering: identifying body, mind, and spirit with the present moment. I like to lead students through mindfulness exercises, such as eating an orange with one's senses fully engaged over a period of ten minutes. This allows the students to relax and release any defenses that would bar them from listening closely to the history they may be reading.

2. I define early American nursing history as the period before the 1870s, when the adoption of the Nightingale Model became the dominant nursing education culture and the focus of nursing practice was shifted from the community to the hospital. I begin the students' cultural and historical immersion with some reading from the period that serves as a marked contrast to contemporary life. For this, I have chosen such readings as McBride's *Women of the Dawn*.[2] The process of reading about the caregiving practices of healing women of the Abenaki Nation and other tribes, allows students of nursing to begin to broaden their present definitions of caregiving and nursing and to examine their preconceptions about the early history of American nursing.

Objectives

Examples of some of the objectives for a course on early American nursing state that the students will be able to

1. Analyze the role of the nurse of eighteenth- and nineteenth-century America in constructing a caring community within the broader sociocultural context of the history of the American healthcare system;
2. Differentiate the elements of nursing practice that were defined as "expertise" when compared with women's roles as family caregiver;
3. Evaluate the influence of eighteenth- and nineteenth-century American nursing history and traditions on contemporary nursing knowledge, practice, and American health policy;
4. Utilize the nursing metaparadigm to examine the health beliefs and practices of early American nurses.

Examples of Student Responses to Their Study of Early Nursing History

Author's Note: Thank you to my students, whose enthusiasm for learning history has been my inspiration and my delight. The following quotes are used with permission.

It is interesting to learn of things that earlier nurses did to help create the opportunities we have today. It was exciting to learn how nurses worked with so little resource, but provided quality care.

—T. M.

The historical work we learned with Dr. Libster presents a remarkably different picture of the early/mid-nineteenth-century nurse (or protonurse) from what I've encountered before. It evokes a much more dynamic world in which women actually enjoyed status and even (in the case of midwives) power as they extended their strength from the domestic sphere into the community.

—M. E. W.

When I read about the early nurses, I am impressed by their willingness to share and work together. This seems to be a difficult task in our current climate.

—C. W.

I thought nursing began with Florence Nightingale until I took a doctoral course in the history of nursing in the eighteenth and nineteenth centuries. It was then that I realized that nurse educators do not give a thorough history of nursing to students. Through the study of history, I have learned that there is an identity of nursing. History is a story worth telling, but no one will realize its worth if it is not told.

—A. P.

Studying the history of nursing has changed me not only professionally but personally as well. Learning a portion of the history of nursing has helped me to understand and refine my identity as a nurse and as a nurse researcher. As I immersed myself into the eighteenth and nineteenth centuries, it was exhilarating to experience the art of caring demonstrated by these nurses. It is empowering to envision the nurses' autonomy, commitment to their patients, and the care they provided in the absence of the knowledge and technology we hold today.

—A. M.

This history course was a transformational and awakening experience that made me more sensitive to my relationships with clients, families, communities, and health workers I work with. It revealed to me some of the solutions for the present nursing crisis.

—S. S.

I vaguely remember reading about Colonial women applying home remedies like poultices and salves before taking this course. What I did not expect was the personal growth I experienced during the quest for hidden histories of women and men who established American nursing traditions and during the times my professor challenged me to question what appeared to me to be the obvious. I now have more pride in my nursing career and not only feel that I am connected to the past nurses who have come before me but that I have more to offer the nursing students that I am instructing.

—S. B.

Course Activities and Study Modules

Module 1: Introduction

Topics:
Historical immersion and the purpose of storytelling. Exploring the questions, "What is a nurse?" and "How is a nurse identified in early history?"

Books:
Women of the Dawn[3]
Sisters of Charity and the Communion of Labour: A Lecture. History of early nursing written in 1855 by Anna Jameson.[4]

Module 2: Colonial America

Topics:
Health beliefs and nursing. Social healers and professional boundaries.

Book:
The Healer's Calling: Women and Medicine in Early New England.[5]

Module 3: Nineteenth-Century American Healthcare

Topics:
A culture of pluralism, health reform and self-care. Sickroom management as the laboratory of the nurse. Nursing expertise and creating healing environments. Cultural authority and professional autonomy.

Books:
Enlightened Charity: The Holistic Nursing Care, Education and Advices Concerning the Sick *of Sister Matilda Coskery, 1799–1870*
Herbal Diplomats: The Contribution of Early American Nurses (1830–1860) to Nineteenth-Century Health Care Reform and the Botanical Medical Movement[6]

Module 4: What Is "Medicine"?

Topics:
Gender. The power of prescription.

Book:
Sickness and Health in America[7]

Module 5: The Bridge to Contemporary Practice

Topics:
Industrialization and the integration of technology and tradition.

Book:
Devices and Desires: Gender, Technology, and American Nursing[8]

Endnotes

Preface – Endnotes

1 Martha Libster, *Herbal Diplomats: The Contribution of Early American Nurses (1830-1860) to Nineteenth-Century Healthcare Reform and the Botanical Medical Movement* (www.GoldenApplePublications.com, 2004).

2 This is the term used throughout the book to describe the nursing heritage that immigrated to America from the community founders in France, Vincent de Paul and Louise de Marillac.

3 Historically, the Daughters of Charity have been referred to as a Company of Servants of the "Sick Poor." See Louise Sullivan, DC, ed. and trans., *Louise de Marillac Spiritual Writings: Correspondence and Thoughts.* (New York: New City Press, 1991). Sister Matilda Coskery refers to the Sisters' care of the "sick poor" in her *Advices* book. While we recognize that the more appropriate phrase today might be "poor and sick persons," we have chosen to use the historical terminology that was important to the Sisters of the period represented here.

4 Edward Hallett Carr, *What Is History?* (New York: Vintage Books, 1961), 86.

Introduction – Endnotes

1 The Baltimore Infirmary became University Hospital and is now known as the University of Maryland Medical Center.

2 Letter from Dr. Pattison to the Mother at Emmitsburg in Arthur Lomas, "As It Was in the Beginning: A History of the University Hospital," *Bulletin of the School of Medicine, University of Maryland* 23, no. 4 (1939): 192. Archives of the University of Maryland Health Sciences & Human Services Library.

3 The word "insane" was a proper medical term in the nineteenth century, used when referring to those with mental illness. See chapter 3 for further information about nineteenth-century psychiatry.

4 William Stokes, *First Annual Report of the Physician of the Mount Saint Vincent's Hospital for 1843.* 1844. Archives of the Daughters of Charity, St. Joseph's Provincial House, Emmitsburg, MD, # 11-2-39.24.

5 William Stokes, *Report of the Mount Hope Institution near Baltimore. 1846–1888.* Archives of the Daughters of Charity, St. Joseph's Provincial House, Emmitsburg, MD, #11-2-39.18.

6 This institution developed over the years using different names: 1840–1844, Mount Saint Vincent's Hospital; 1844–1856, Mount Hope Institution; and 1856–1944, Mount Hope Retreat. From 1945 until its closure in 1973, it

was The Seton Institute. For ease in reading, it will generally be referred to throughout this book as "Mount Hope."

7   Stokes, *Report of the Mount Hope Institution near Baltimore*, 19.

8   Dorothea Dix, Memorial of Miss D. L. Dix to the Hon. General Assembly in Behalf of the Insane of Maryland. March 5, 1852. Archives of the State of Maryland Web site, http://www.msa.md.gov/.

9   Stokes. *Report of the Mount Hope Institution near Baltimore*, 19.

10 Ibid., Report for 1845, 25.

11 Catherine Barmby, "On Forbearance, 1839," in *Women and Radicalism in the Nineteenth Century*, ed. Mike Sanders (London: Routledge, 2001), vol.1:313.

12 Ibid.

13 Roy Porter, *The Enlightenment*, 2nd ed., (London: Palgrave, 2001), 2.

14 Ibid., 7.

15 Matthew Ramsey, *Medical Fringe & Medical Orthodoxy, 1750–1850*, ed. W. F. Bynum and Roy Porter (London: Croom Helm, 1987), 84.

16 Stokes, *Report of the Mount Hope Institution near Baltimore*. Report for 1845, 24.

17 Ibid., 25.

18 Defined by the Catholic Encyclopedia online (http://www.newadvent.org) as "a voluntary association of the faithful, established and guided by competent ecclesiastical authority for the promotion of special works of Christian charity or piety." See 124a in Pierre Coste, CM, and Vincent de Paul, *Regulations for the Sisters of the Angers Hospital*, ed. and trans. Jacqueline Kilar, DC, and Marie Poole, DC, vol. 13b, *In Correspondence, Conferences, Documents*. (New York: New City Press, 1985–2008), 13b:3. Archives of the Daughters of Charity, St. Joseph's Provincial House, Emmitsburg, MD. See also 125 in Coste and de Paul, *Regulations for the Sisters of the Angers Hospital,* 13b:5.

19 Catharine Esther Beecher and Harriet Beecher Stowe, *The American Woman's Home or, Principles of Domestic Science: Being a Guide to the Formation and Maintenance of Economical, Healthful, Beautiful, and Christian Homes* (Piscataway, New Jersey: Rutgers University Press, 2002), 254.

20 Anna Jameson, *Sisters of Charity and the Communion of Labour: A Lecture Delivered Privately February 14, 1855 and Printed by Desire* (London: Longman, Brown, Green, Longmans, and Roberts, 1859), 37. Google Books.

21 Thomas Webster, Mrs. Parkes, and D. Meredith Reese, *An Encyclopaedia of Domestic Economy: Comprising Such Subjects as Are Most Immediately Connected with Housekeeping; as, the Construction of Domestic Edifices, with the Modes of Warming, Ventilating, and Lighting Them; a Description of the Various Articles of Furniture; a General Account of the Animal and Vegetable Substances Used in Food, and the Methods of Preserving and Preparing Them by Cooking; Making Bread; Materials Employed in Dress and Toilet; Business of the Laundry; Description of the Various Wheel-Carriages; Preservation*

of Health; Domestic Medicines, &C. (New York: Harper & Brothers, 1845), 19. Old Sturbridge Village Research Library, Sturbridge, MA. "Sick nurses" refers to nurses of the sick.

22 As cited in Jameson, *Sisters of Charity and the Communion of Labour,* 47. Author's Note: The term "Sisters of Charity" is used by Jameson to refer both generally to nurses in religious life and also the actual order of Daughters/Sisters of Charity following the Vincentian-Louisian tradition. The term "Sisters of Charity" is only used in this book when referring to the Vincentian-Louisians. When quotes that mention the Sisters of Charity are utilized, all have been fact checked and are known to refer only to the Sisters of Charity (Emmitsburg before 1850), the Daughters of Charity (Paris), or the Daughters of Charity (Emmitsburg after 1850).

23 S. D. Gross, *Report of the Committee on the Training of Nurses.* 1869. American Medical Association Archives, Chicago, 165.

24 Rt. Rev. Frederick Rese, Correspondence to Mother Rose White at Emmitsburg. November 2, 1834. Daughters of Charity Archives, Mater Dei Provincialate, Evansville, IN.

25 Catholic Church of the United States, *The United States Catholic Almanac, or, Laity's Directory for the Year*: May 15, 1849, 130–131. University of Notre Dame Library, Microfilm Collection. 1817, 1822, 1833-ongoing.

26 Sister Matilda Coskery, *Cradle of Mount Hope: Historical Account of Mt. St. Vincent Hospital / Mount Hope Retreat.* n.d. Archives of the Daughters of Charity, St. Joseph's Provincial House, Emmitsburg, MD, #11-2-39.

27 Sister Matilda Coskery, *Advices Concerning the Sick* (Emmitsburg, MD: Archives of Daughters of Charity, St. Joseph's Provincial House, n.d., c. 1840).

28 As will be described later, the Sisters of the Vincentian-Louisian tradition were different from other communities of religious women in that they were not cloistered; that is, remaining within the convent. They are also formally recognized by the Catholic Church as a *society of apostolic life* dedicated to following in the footsteps of Jesus Christ.

Chapter 1 – Endnotes

1 Vincent de Paul was canonized (recognized as a saint by the Catholic Church) in 1737. Louise de Marillac was canonized in 1934.

2 Châtillon-les-Dombes is now Châtillon-sur-Chalaronne.

3 Daughters of Charity. Origins of the Company. 2004. Archives of the Daughters of Charity, St. Joseph's Provincial House, Emmitsburg, MD.

4 Louise Sullivan, DC, ed. and trans., *Louise de Marillac Spiritual Writings: Correspondence and Thoughts.* (New York: New City Press, 1991), 320.

5 Raymond Deville, "Saint Vincent and Saint Louise in Relation to the French School of Spirituality," *Vincentian Heritage* 11, no. 1 (1990): 29.

6   De Sales as cited in Wendy Wright, ""Hearts Have a Secret Language": The Spiritual Friendship of Francis de Sales and Jane de Chantal," *Vincentian Heritage* 11, no. 1 (1990): 47.

7   Ibid.: 47–48.

8   143 *Regulations for the Sisters of the Angers Hospital*, in Coste and de Paul, *Regulations for the Sisters of the Angers Hospital*, 13b:108.

9   #1407 in Pierre Coste, CM, and Vincent de Paul, *Saint Vincent De Paul: Correspondence, Conferences, Documents*, ed. Jacqueline Kilar, DC, Marie Poole, DC, et al., 14 vols. (New York: New City Press, 1985–2008), 4:259. Archives of the Daughters of Charity, St. Joseph's Provincial House, Emmitsburg, MD.

10 #1407 in ibid.

11 Susan Dinan, *Women and Poor Relief in Seventeenth-Century France: The Early History of the Daughters of Charity* (Burlington, Vermont: Ashgate, 2006), 104. See also Edward Udovic, CM, "Caritas Christi Urget Nos': The Urgent Challenges of Charity in Seventeenth Century France," *Vincentian Heritage* 12, no. 2 (1991).

12 The Daughters of Charity motto is "The Charity of Christ Impels Us." Holy Bible, 2 Cor 5:14.

13 143a "Contract with Saint-Jean Hospital in Angers," in Coste and de Paul, *Regulations for the Sisters of the Angers Hospital*, 13b:114.

14 Sisters of Charity. Origins of the Company, in ibid.., 13b:108.

15 114, "Rules for Sisters in Parishes: Care of the Sick; Virtues of Barbe Angiboust," Pierre Coste, CM, and Vincent de Paul, *Rules for Sisters in Parishes*, ed. Jacqueline Kilar, DC, and Marie Poole, DC, In *Correspondence, Conferences, Documents* (New York: New City Press, 1985–2008), 10:537. Archives of the Daughters of Charity, St. Joseph's Provincial House, Emmitsburg, MD.

16 Deville, "Saint Vincent and Saint Louise in Relation to the French School of Spirituality," 35.

17 Betty Ann McNeil, *The Vincentian Family Tree* (Chicago: Vincentian Studies Institute, 1996), xvii.

18 The term mission is also used in the DC Community as a verb. To be "missioned" is to be sent officially by a superior to accomplish a particular work of the Community in a specific location.

19 L. 160. Louise de Marillac to Sister Élisabeth Martin, October 1646. In Sullivan, ed. and trans., *Louise de Marillac Spiritual Writings: Correspondence and Thoughts*, 182.

20 Those sisters who served with the Sister Servant on a mission were referred to as "companions." Nurses who served on a mission with a Sister Servant in a hospital were also referred to as "companions."

21 Sullivan, ed. and trans., *Louise de Marillac Spiritual Writings: Correspondence and Thoughts*, 397.

22 Ibid., 427.

23 Ibid., 771.

24 "On the Spirit of the Company" #51 in Pierre Coste, CM, and Vincent de Paul, *Saint Vincent De Paul: Correspondence, Conferences, Documents*, ed. Jacqueline Kilar, DC, Marie Poole, DC, et al., 14 vols. (New York: New City Press, 1985–2008), 9:467. Archives of the Daughters of Charity, St. Joseph's Provincial House, Emmitsburg, MD.

25 Sullivan, ed. and trans., *Louise de Marillac Spiritual Writings: Correspondence and Thoughts*, 532.

26 Ibid., 406.

27 Ibid., 155.

28 Ibid., 20.

29 501.Vincent de Paul to Louise de Marillac in Coste and de Paul, *Saint Vincent de Paul: Correspondence, Conferences, Documents*, 2:164. See also 37. "Humility" in Coste and de Paul, *Saint Vincent de Paul: Correspondence, Conferences, Documents*, 11:46.

30 149a. "Common Rules of the Company of Sisters of Charity Called Servants of the Sick Poor Which They Must Keep to Perform their Duty Well by the Grace of God," in Coste and de Paul, *Regulations for the Sisters of the Angers Hospital*, 13b:148.

31 Regina Bechtle, SC, and Judith Metz, SC, eds., and Ellin Kelly, mss. ed., *Elizabeth Bayley Seton: Collected Writings*, 3 vols. (Hyde Park, NY: New City Press, 2000–2006), IIIb:501.

32 Ibid.

33 Sullivan, ed. and trans., *Louise de Marillac Spiritual Writings: Correspondence and Thoughts*, 710.

34 Coste and de Paul, *Saint Vincent de Paul: Correspondence, Conferences, Documents*, 1:265.

35 Ann Doyle, "Nursing by Religious Orders in the United States: Part 1, 1809–1840," *American Journal of Nursing* 29, no. 7 (1929): 781.

36 Ibid.

37 Sullivan, ed. and trans., *Louise de Marillac Spiritual Writings: Correspondence and Thoughts*, 515.

38 Stability refers to the vow not to leave and join another religious order.

39 Sullivan, *Louise de Marillac Spiritual Writings: Correspondence and Thoughts*, 782.

40 Ibid., 292.

41 Ibid., 524.

42 Ibid., 689.

43 A.44B "Formula of the Vows," in ibid., 782.

44 Ibid.

45 Ibid., 781.

46 "Papers from the Conference on the Age of Gold: The Roots of Our Tradition," *Vincentian Heritage* XI, no. 1 (1990).

47   Margaret John Kelly, "The Relationship of Saint Vincent and Saint Louise from Her Perspective," *Vincentian Heritage* XI, no. 1 (1990): 92.

48   Ibid., 110.

49   198. "Report on the State of the Works," in Coste and de Paul, *Regulations for the Sisters of the Angers Hospital*, 13b:432. A Hôtel-Dieu in addition to functioning as a hospital frequently houses the poor, those considered socially deviant, and the mentally ill.

50   149a. "Common Rules of the Company of Sisters of Charity Called Servants of the Sick Poor which They Must Keep to Perform their Duty Well by the Grace of God," in ibid., 13b:147.

51   McNeil, *The Vincentian Family Tree*, 21.

52   24. Love of Vocation and Assistance to the Poor, in Coste and de Paul, *Saint Vincent de Paul: Correspondence, Conferences, Documents*, 9:194.

53   Charism, a gift of the Holy Spirit to the founders of a religious community, is at the heart of congregational identity. It provides a defining touchstone. Charism both embodies and expresses mission and spirituality, providing a frame of reference for community living, service, relationship to God, and formation. Vincent de Paul and Louise de Marillac oriented the Daughters of Charity to "serve Jesus Christ in the person of the poor." That mission is the driving force from which all else flows. This orientation for persons who are poor is the founding charism and has focused the ministry of the Daughters of Charity since 1633. The spirituality of Sisters and Daughters of Charity is expressed as faith-filled responsiveness to persons who are poor within the world of today. The world view of Vincentian-Louisian women is one of solidarity with those who suffer.

54   McNeil, *The Vincentian Family Tree*, 16.

55   114. "Rules for Sisters in Parishes: Care of the Sick; Virtues of Barbe Angiboust," in Coste and de Paul, *Rules for Sisters in Parishes*, 537.

56   Amelia W. Sieveking and Catherine Winkworth, *Life of Amelia Wilhelmina Sieveking from the German Edited with the Author's Sanction* (London: Longman, Green, Longman, Roberts, & Green, 1863), 182. Google Books.

57   Florence Nightingale, Martha Vicinus, and Bea Nergaard, *Ever Yours, Florence Nightingale Selected Letters* (Cambridge, MA: Harvard University Press, 1990), 59.

58   Florence Nightingale. Writings. 1851–1853. British Library #43402, Florence Nightingale Papers, vol. X.124. Although the Nightingale papers do not specifically state that she is recording her memories of DC documents, she did lodge with the DC in 1853 when she recorded the papers with the title, "Maison de Santé," that are now archived in the British Library. She wrote of "novices" learning from "novice mistresses" and of private readings and "Conferences" given by "Superiors" upon one of the rules. These are words typically used by the DC to refer to the teachings of spiritual directors such as Vincent de Paul. The language she used to describe her experience as well as her description of the daily life of the nurse is also very reminiscent of

sections of the *Common Rules*. See also *Florence Nightingale's Theology: Essays, Letters, and Journal Notes,* ed. Lynn McDonald, vol. 3, *The Collected Works of Florence Nightingale* (www.wlupress.wlu.ca: Wilfrid Laurier University Press, 2002), 300–02. McDonald's analysis of the Maison de Santé notes concurs. Nightingale, McDonald records in footnote 94, page 300, "evidently at one time had the Manual of the Sisters of Charity, for she sent it to Mary Clare Moore, along with three other manuals not named." Mary Clare Moore was the Reverend Mother of the Convent of Mercy in Bermondsey, Ireland.

59 Cecil Woodham Smith, *Florence Nightingale, 1820–1910* (New York: McGraw-Hill, 1951), 64.

60 Secularization is used throughout this book to mean the presence or absence of religion. A synonym is laicization.

61 Sisters of Charity, *The Rule of 1812: Regulations for the Society of Sisters of Charity in the United States of America* (1812). Archives of the Daughters of Charity, St. Joseph's Provincial House, Emmitsburg, MD.

62 Sullivan, ed. and trans., *Louise de Marillac Spiritual Writings: Correspondence and Thoughts*, 510.

63 Ibid., 713.

64 143. "Regulations for the Sisters of the Angers Hospital," in Coste and de Paul, *Regulations for the Sisters of the Angers Hospital*, 13b:111.

65 L. 160 to Sister Élisabeth Martin at Nantes. In Sullivan, ed. and trans., *Louise de Marillac Spiritual Writings: Correspondence and Thoughts*, 182.

66 L. 290B Louise de Marillac to Sister Cécile Angiboust at Angers, in ibid., 329–30.

67 126. Charity of Women (Châtillon-les-Dombes), in Coste and de Paul, *Regulations for the Sisters of the Angers Hospital*, 13b:13.

68 149b. "Particular Rules for the Daughters of Charity. Particular Rules for the Sisters of the Hôtel-Dieu of Paris," in Coste and de Paul, *Saint Vincent de Paul: Correspondence, Conferences, Documents*, 207.

69 Dinan, *Women and Poor Relief in Seventeenth-Century France: The Early History of the Daughters of Charity*, 94.

70 Biographical Sketch of Father Andrew White, in Catholic Church of the United States, *The United States Catholic Almanac*, (1840): 63. University of Notre Dame Library.

71 Ibid.: 1840, 47.

72 *The American Vincentians: A Popular History of the Congregation of the Mission in the United States, 1815–1987*, ed. John Rybolt (New York: New City Press, 1988), 38.

73 Catholic Church of the United States: 1822, 79.

74 Elizabeth Ann Seton was canonized in 1975. She is the first canonized saint born in the United States.

75 6.93 Elizabeth Ann Seton to Robert Goodloe Harper, in Bechtle, Metz, and Kelly, eds., *Elizabeth Bayley Seton: Collected Writings*, 2:206.

76 Daughters of Charity. Act of Incorporation. Archives of the Daughters of Charity, St. Joseph's Provincial House, Emmitsburg, MD.

77 Bechtle and Metz, eds., and Kelly, mss. ed., *Elizabeth Bayley Seton: Collected Writings*, 1:3.

78 Elizabeth Ann Seton to Julia Sitgreaves Scott, 23rd March 1809 in ibid., vol. 2: 61.

79 1537. Vincent de Paul to a Coadjutor Brother in the Genoa House, in Coste and de Paul, *Saint Vincent de Paul: Correspondence, Conferences, Documents*, 4:440.

80 Sulpicians and Vincentians had many similarities; however, the Sulpicians were exclusively involved in seminary work and the Vincentians more involved in missions and parish work. The Sulpicians opened the first seminary in Baltimore in 1791. According to *The American Vincentians,* the Vincentians acclimated to American life much faster than the Sulpicians while still following European Vincentian practice closely.

81 Daniel Hannefin, *Daughters of the Church: A Popular History of the Daughters of Charity in the United States, 1809–1987* (New York: New City, 1989), 27.

82 A-12.4 Chapter I, Article 1, "Constitutions of the Sisters of Charity in the United States of America," in Bechtle, Metz, and Kelly, eds., *Elizabeth Bayley Seton: Collected Writings*, 13b:541.

83 Hannefin, *Daughters of the Church: A Popular History of the Daughters of Charity in the United States, 1809–1987*, 14.

84 John Dubois to Antoine Garnier, April 18, 1816, in John Dubois. Les Sulpician Français En Maryland Avec Elizabeth Seton. Archives of the Daughters of Charity, St. Joseph's Provincial House, Emmitsburg, MD.

85 Author's Note: The SC who joined the French DC in 1850 were only the SC based at Emmitsburg.

86 20. "Observance of the Rule," in Coste and de Paul, *Saint Vincent de Paul: Correspondence, Conferences, Documents*, 9:190–92.

87 1. Explanation of the Regulations," ibid., 4.

88 L. 353 Louise de Marillac to Barbe Angiboust, In Sullivan, ed. and trans., *Louise de Marillac Spiritual Writings: Correspondence and Thoughts*, 396.

Chapter 2 – Endnotes

1 Louise Sullivan, DC, ed. and trans., *Louise de Marillac Spiritual Writings: Correspondence and Thoughts.* (New York: New City Press, 1991), 735.

2 Ibid., 736.

3 Today, the word "formal" as it relates to education connotes that a person receives his or her education in an institution such as a public school, college, or university. The phrase as it is used here refers to structured and organized education as opposed to informal education that in the nineteenth century would have been such as reading an advice book or attending an educational meeting for ladies. Many college and university programs were not open

to women in the early and mid-nineteenth century. There were no nursing schools, and medical schools did not admit women. The sisters did receive structured, organized (i.e., formal) education to prepare them for their work and ministry as nurses.

4   Examples include Mother Seton's translations of the *Life of Louise de Marillac* and the *Life of Sister Francoise Bony, DC*, an eighteenth-century Infirmarian and hospital administrator. Regina Bechtle, SC, Judith Metz, SC, eds., and Ellin Kelly, ms. ed., *Elizabeth Bayley Seton: Collected Writings*, 3 vols. (Hyde Park, New York: New City Press, 2000–2006), Vol. 3b: 355–411 and Vol. 13:3, 4.

5   Merriam-Webster, Inc. *Merriam-Webster's Collegiate Dictionary*, 10th ed. (Springfield, MA: Merriam-Webster, 1999).

6   Sullivan, ed. and trans., *Louise de Marillac Spiritual Writings: Correspondence and Thoughts*, 744.

7   "Holistic nursing" was not a phrase used by the DC or the SC; however, they were instructed in educating the "whole" person. See Note 19. Holistic nursing is a contemporary phrase adopted for this history to succinctly describe the SC's focus of care. Holistic nursing is defined by the American Holistic Nurses Association as "all nursing that has the enhancement of healing the whole person from birth to death—and all age groups from infant to elder— as its goal. Holistic nursing recognizes that there are two views regarding holism: that holism involves identifying the interrelationships of the bio-psycho-social-spiritual dimensions of the person, recognizing that the whole is greater than the sum of its parts; and that holism involves understanding the individual as a unitary whole in mutual process with the environment." American Holistic Nurses Association, *Holistic Nursing: Scope & Standards of Practice* (Silver Spring, MD: Nursesbooks.org, 2007), 1.

8   Sullivan, ed. and trans., *Louise de Marillac Spiritual Writings: Correspondence and Thoughts*.

9   Francis de Sales, *Introduction to the Devout Life* (New York: Vintage Books, 2002 [Originally published 1609]). The earliest copy of this text is an 1802 French edition believed to have been used by Sisters of Charity because it was found at Emmitsburg in the collection of books at the White House. It is #111 in Rare Book collection at the Archives of the Daughters of Charity St. Joseph's Provincial House.

10   Catholic Church of the United States, *The United States Catholic Almanac, or, Laity's Directory for the Year*. University of Notre Dame Library, Microfilm Collection.

11   Hugh O'Donnell, *Vincent de Paul: His Life and Way* in F. Ryan and J. Rybolt, *Vincent de Paul and Louise de Marillac: Rules, Conferences, and Writings* (Mahwah, NJ: Paulist Press, 1995), 31.

12   Ibid., 33.

13   Ibid.

14   Ibid.

15   Ibid., 34.

16 Daughters of Charity, *Manual of the Daughters of Charity Servants of the Sick Poor in the Hospital and in the Homes of the Poor* (Emmitsburg, MD: Daughters of Charity, 1936), 60. Archives of the Daughters of Charity, St. Joseph's Provincial House, Emmitsburg, MD.

17 Ryan and Rybolt, *Vincent de Paul and Louise de Marillac: Rules, Conferences, and Writings*, 24.

18 Vincent de Paul as cited in ibid., 46.

19 Ibid., 56.

20 Ibid.

21 Ibid.

22 119. "The Virtues of Louise de Marillac," in Pierre Coste, CM, and Vincent de Paul, *Saint Vincent de Paul: Correspondence, Conferences, Documents*, Jacqueline Kilar, DC, and Marie Poole, DC, eds. and trans., 14 vols. (New York: New City Press, 1985–2008), 10:585. Archives of the Daughters of Charity, St. Joseph's Provincial House, Emmitsburg, MD.

23 Sister Bridget Farrell began her novitiate at age 47 in 1812. One of the first three SC sent to the kitchen and infirmary at Mount St. Mary's.

24 Sister Joanna Smith entered the Community in 1812. She became first Sister Servant of the Baltimore Infirmary.

25 Cabbage-leaf plasters are still used in nursing today. Chilled green cabbage leaves are used in the care of postpartum patients who suffer from breast engorgement.

26 Blistering was a common medical therapeutic used in the nineteenth century. A blister was caused by a plant or chemical substance placed on the skin. The purpose was to draw circulation to the area. The skin required care due to the toxic nature of the cantharides used in raising the blister.

27 Daughters of Charity, *Mother Seton—Notes by Rev. Simon Gabriel Bruté Bishop of Vincennes from Original Papers in the Possession of the Community* (1884), 282–86. Archives of the Daughters of Charity, St. Joseph's Provincial House, Emmitsburg, MD.

28 Daughters of Charity, *Articles of Constitution*, Article 29. Archives of the Daughters of Charity, St. Joseph's Provincial House, Emmitsburg, MD.

29 The term "Mistress of Novices" was used in the early American community, but it was not the term used by the DC because it was the language used by nuns of religious orders. The DC was a confraternity or community rather than a religious order. After the merger with France in 1850, the American SC became "Daughters of Charity," and they adopted the terms "Visitatrix" for that of "Mother" and the term "Seminary Directress" in place of Mistress of Novices.

30 Daughters of Charity, *Mother Augustine and Mother Xavier* (Saint Joseph's Provincial House–Emmitsburg, MD: Daughters of Charity, 1938), 127.

31 Ibid., 97.

32 Ibid., 104.

33 Ibid., 114.

34 Ibid., 127.

35 Ibid., 168.

36 Simon Gabriel Bruté de Remur and Sister Loyola Law, *Rev. Simon Gabriel Bruté Bishop of Vincennes in His Connection with the Community, 1812-1839* (Emmitsburg, MD: Daughters of Charity, 1886), 157. Archives of the Daughters of Charity, St. Joseph's Provincial House, Emmitsburg, MD.

37 Daughters of Charity, *Mother Augustine and Mother Xavier*, 134.

38 Mother Mary Xavier Clark, *Instruction on the Care of the Sick*, Archives of Daughters of Charity of St. Vincent de Paul—West Central Province, St. Louis, MO. (1846), 3–4.

39 Ibid., 4.

40 Ibid., 8.

41 Ibid., 10.

42 Ibid., 22.

43 Ibid., 28.

44 Mother Mary Xavier's instruction echoes that of Mother Seton: "and our Charity, does it extend to all." Cf. 9.15 "[Retreat meditations] The Sisters of Charity Meditate on the Service of God," in Bechtle and Metz, eds., and Kelly, ms. ed., *Elizabeth Bayley Seton: Collected Writings*, 3a: 332.

45 Clark, *Instruction on the Care of the Sick*, 32–36. Used with permission, Daughters of Charity of St. Vincent de Paul—West Central Province, Marillac Provincialate, St. Louis, MO.

47 Ibid., 75–78.

48 Ibid., 86.

49 Ibid., 68.

50 Ibid., 69.

51 Ibid., 41–42.

52 Ibid., 45.

53 Ibid., 135.

54 Daughters of Charity, *Mother Augustine and Mother Xavier*, 128.

55 Ibid., 129.

56 Nancy F. Cott, *The Bonds of Womanhood: "Woman's Sphere" in New England, 1780-1835* (New Haven: Yale University Press, 1977), 177.

57 Ibid., 178.

58 Ibid., 181.

59 Ibid.

60 Ladies Physiological Institute, *Records of the Meeting of the Ladies Physiological Institute of Boston and Vicinity* (1850). Schlesinger Library, Radcliffe Institute for Advanced Study.

61 Martha Libster, *Herbal Diplomats: The Contribution of Early American Nurses (1830–1860) to Nineteenth-Century Healthcare Reform and the Botanical Medical Movement* (www.GoldenApplePublications.com: Golden Apple Publications, 2004), 92.

62 Jane Lewis, *Women and Social Action in Victorian and Edwardian England* (Stanford, CA: Stanford University Press, 1991), 8.

63 Catholic Church of the United States: 1833, 115.

64 State of Maryland, *Maryland State Archives Early State Records Online, Vol. 3173, 1531–1532.* ([cited July 18, 2006]); available from http://www.mdarchives.state.md.us. Vol. 3173, 1531–1532.

65 Bruce Dorsey, *Reforming Men and Women: Gender in the Antebellum City* (Ithaca, NY: Cornell University Press, 2002), 216.

66 Ibid., 6.

67 Daughters of Charity. Provincial Annals. Archives of the Daughters of Charity, Saint Joseph's Provincial House, Emmitsburg, MD. #7-8. File-Sister Joanna (Miss Jane) Smith.

68 Eugene Cordell, *University of Maryland 1807–1907*, vol. 1 (New York: Lewis Publishing Company, 1907), 157. University of Maryland Health Sciences and Human Services Library.

69 Arthur Lomas, "As It Was in the Beginning: A History of the University Hospital," *Bulletin of the School of Medicine, University of Maryland* 23, no. 4 (1939): 190. Archives of the University of Maryland Health Sciences & Human Services Library.

70 Annabelle M. Melville, *Elizabeth Bayley Seton, 1774–1821* (New York: Scribner, 1951), 165.

71 Ibid., 164.

72 As cited in Lomas, "As It Was in the Beginning: A History of the University Hospital," 191.

73 Ibid.

74 As cited in ibid.

75 As cited in ibid.

76 Ibid., 192: Transcript of Letter from John Dubois to Mrs. M. Pattison dated May 16, 1822.

77 Ibid., 193.

78 Gedding's Baltimore Journal as cited in Ann Doyle, "Nursing by Religious Orders in the United States: Part 1, 1809–1840," *American Journal of Nursing* 29, no. 7 (1929): 781.

79 Regulations of the Baltimore Infirmary. n.d. Archives of the Daughters of Charity, Saint Joseph's Provincial House, Emmitsburg, MD 11-2-20.

80 University of Maryland, Annual Circular of the Faculty of Physic of the University of Maryland. Session 1844–5, 5. As cited in Nancy Bramucci,

Medicine in Maryland, 1752–1920, http://www.mdhistoryonline.net (Maryland State Archives, 2000– [cited 2006–2007]).

81 As transcribed in Lomas, "As It Was in the Beginning: A History of the University Hospital," 198.

82 Daughters of Charity. Provincial Annals. For the Year 1841.

83 Ibid.,1841: 298–299.

84 A description of Sister Adele Salva appears in Bruté de Remur and Law, *Rev. Simon Gabriel Bruté Bishop of Vincennes in His Connection with the Community, 1812–1839,* 123. Rev. William Dubourg brought two novices from Martinique, Louise Roger and Adele Salva. He described Adele as "about twenty-seven" and "everything good you can imagine; lively as a lark, simple and innocent as a dove, full of ardor for God, and His service, of activity in the performance of her external duties. She will be a treasure in your community."

85 Daughters of Charity. Provincial Annals. Vol III: 241–42a.

86 Sister Ambrosia's mother was a Collins, and her sister Josephine, also a Sister of Charity, went by the name of Collins. Ambrosia, it seems, went by both surnames, Magner and Collins.

87 Catholic Church of the United States: 1842, Obituary of Sr. Ambrosia Collins.

88 Daughters of Charity. Provincial Annals.

89 Lomas, "As It Was in the Beginning: A History of the University Hospital," 193: Copy of the Articles of Agreement.

90 Refers to Sisters of Charity of Nazareth. See chapter 2: Spalding Spirit.

91 Bruté de Remur and Law, *Rev. Simon Gabriel Bruté Bishop of Vincennes in His Connection with the Community, 1812–1839,* 360.

92 Sister Francis Xavier Love (Mary Ann) entered the Community as Sister Servant in 1820. She was the adopted daughter of a physician and is recorded (in ibid., 372) to have been one of the "holiest" and "zealous," who was always "calm, undisturbed and self-possessed." Sister Francis Xavier once accepted a rose from an Indian chief who was "struck by her grave and graceful manner." Sister did not realize that it was an offering of marriage, and Bishop Rosati had to explain diplomatically that Sister was already "espoused to the "Great Spirit."

93 In 1828 the Mother was Mary Augustine Decount.

94 Bruté de Remur and Law, *Rev. Simon Gabriel Bruté Bishop of Vincennes in His Connection with the Community, 1812–1839,* 368.

95 Bramucci, *Medicine in Maryland, 1752–1920,* http://www.mdhistoryonline. net. Medicine in Maryland 1752–1920. Accessed July 9, 2007.

96 Ibid.

97 William E. A. Aiken. Letter to Rev. John B. Purcell, February 5, 1833. 1833. Archives at Mount St. Mary's College, Emmitsburg, MD.

98 Daughters of Charity. Chronological Table, 1766–1891. DeAndreis-Rosati Memorial Archives, DePaul University, III A Souvay Collection.

99 Bramucci, *Medicine in Maryland, 1752–1920*, http://www.mdhistoryonline.net.

100 Winston Babb, "French Refugees from Saint-Domingue to the Southern United States: 1791–1810." http://freepages.genealogy.rootsweb.com/~Saintdomingue/Babb%20index.htm (University of Virginia).

101 Ibid.

102 James Bayley, *Memoirs of the Right Reverend Simon Wm. Gabriel Bruté* (New York: D. & J. Sadlier & Co., 1861). Archives of the Daughters of Charity, St. Joseph's Provincial House, Emmitsburg, MD.

103 Sister Mary Salesia Godecker, *Bishop Simon Gabriel Bruté De Remur, First Bishop of Vincennes* (St. Meinrad, IN: St. Meinrad Historical Essays, 1931). Archives of the Daughters of Charity, St. Joseph's Provincial House, Emmitsburg, MD, # 7-8-2-3: 263.

104 Rev. John Schipp, "Bishop Simon Bruté de Remur–Wall Case Exhibits" (Old Cathedral Library and Museum, Vincennes, IN).

105 Personal communication Rev. Albert Ledoux–Bruté scholar. Mount St. Mary's College, Emmitsburg, MD. June 16, 2002.

106 Daughters of Charity, *Mother Seton–Notes by Rev. Simon Gabriel Bruté Bishop of Vincennes from Original Papers in the Possession of the Community*, 307.

107 Bruté de Remur and Law, *Rev. Simon Gabriel Bruté Bishop of Vincennes in His Connection with the Community, 1812–1839*, 388.

108 Salesia Godecker, *Bishop Simon Gabriel Bruté de Remur, First Bishop of Vincennes*.

109 Mary Meline and Edward McSweeny, *The Story of the Mountain* (Emmitsburg, MD: Emmitsburg Chronicle, 1911), ch. 19. Emmitsburg Area Historical Society: http://www.emmitsburg.net/history/index.htm.

110 Refers to Sister Benedicta "Bene" Parsons (1797–1876).

111 Bruté de Remur and Law, *Rev. Simon Gabriel Bruté Bishop of Vincennes in His Connection with the Community, 1812–1839*.

112 Daniel Hannefin, *Daughters of the Church: A Popular History of the Daughters of Charity in the United States, 1809–1987* (New York: New City, 1989), 24. Mother Seton and a number of SC entered the Community after they had borne children or were widowed. Bec was the youngest of Mother Seton's five children.

113 Henry Cauthorn, *History of St. Francis Xavier Cathedral* (Indianapolis: 1892). The Old Cathedral Library and Museum, Vincennes, IN.

114 Ibid.

115 Charles E. Rosenberg, *The Cholera Years: The United States in 1832, 1849, and 1866* (Chicago: University of Chicago Press, 1962), 5.

116 Probably refers to Alexius J. Elder. Both Rev. Deluol and Rev. Elder were Sulpician priests of Saint Mary's Seminary.

117 T. Sheppard, Jacob Deems, and Peter Foy. Report of the Commissioners of Health, Baltimore City Health Department, 1815–1849. 1832. Maryland State Archives, Baltimore, MD. Appendix.

118 Ibid.

119 Augustus Warner. Account of the Cholera in Baltimore: A Journal of Admissions at Hospital No. 3. 1832. Archives of the Daughters of Charity, St. Joseph's Provincial House, Emmitsburg, MD. #7-7-1-1.

120 Ibid.

121 According to Sheppard, Deems, and Foy. Report of the Commissioners of Health, Baltimore City Health Department, 1815–1849.

122 Coste and de Paul, *Saint Vincent de Paul: Correspondence, Conferences, Documents*, 10:103. As chaplain at *Les Petites-Maisons* of the Daughters of Charity on rue de Sèvres (1787–1791), Rev. John Dubois became familiar with the Vincentian spirit of the forty Daughters of Charity who ministered to 400 patients there. This experience later benefited the Sisters of Charity at Emmitsburg.

123 Ibid., 11:17.

124 Ibid., Roman 274, 11:331.

125 The Maryland Hospital for the Insane was located where the renowned Johns Hopkins Hospital presently stands.

126 Records for the Coskery family vault located in the New Cathedral Cemetery show the name of Sister Matilda Coskery's mother as Bathilda Clementina Spalding, although sometimes the name "Matilda" appears instead of "Bathilda."

127 "Obituary Rev. Fr. Henry Benedictus Coskery," *Catholic Mirror*, March 2, 1872.

128 Henry Benedict was ordained a priest for the Archdiocese of Baltimore. He was the vicar-general successively under archbishops Samuel Eccleston (1834–1851), Francis Patrick Kenrick (1851–1863), and Martin J. Spalding (1864–1872) and was twice administrator of the archdiocese. He was appointed bishop of Portland in 1854 but declined the honor.

129 Mary Ellen Doyle, *Pioneer Spirit: Catherine Spalding, Sister of Charity of Nazareth* (Lexington: University Press of Kentucky, 2006), 2.

130 Margaret Maria Coon, *Her Spirit Lives: A Sketch of the Life of Catherine Spalding* (Louisville, KY: Sisters of Charity of Nazareth, 2007), 16.

131 Anna McGill, *The Sisters of Charity of Nazareth Kentucky* (New York: The Encyclopedia Press, 1917), 55. Later called the St. Joseph's Infirmary.

132 Remarks on Sister Matilda Coskery in Daughters of Charity, *Lives of Deceased Sisters* (Emmitsburg, MD: 1870–1879), 1870, 11. Archives of the Daughters of Charity, St. Joseph's Provincial House, Emmitsburg, MD.

133 Daughters of Charity, *Articles of Constitution*.

134 A seminary is the name for the period of initial formation or preparation that the novice Sister undergoes so that she and the Daughters of Charity can discern if she is truly called to religious life.

135 The candidates and novices of the Sisters of Charity of Saint Joseph's wore a dress and cape of dark linsey with a brown cap until they left the seminary. At that time they assumed the black habit of the Sisters of Charity based on

widows' "weeds" worn by Mother Seton, after the attire of Tuscan widows. This included a simple black dress, cape, and cap. See Daughters of Charity. Council Minutes. Archives of the Daughters of Charity, St. Joseph's Provincial House, Emmitsburg, MD, #3-3-5. August 1814, 17.

136 See Appendix D for a chronological list of Sister Matilda's missions.

137 In the Vincentian-Louisian tradition, a local superior is the "Sister Servant," a term that indicates that her role of authority and leadership is one of service. Vincent de Paul explained to the Sisters his rationale for asking them to accept the term "Servant." He told them that the nuns of the Annunciation Order referred to their Superioress as "Ancelle," which comes from the Latin *ancilla*, meaning handmaiden or servant. The title of handmaiden was "assumed by the Blessed Virgin when she told the angel she consented that the will of God should be fulfilled in her in the mystery of the Incarnation of His Son." #11. Obedience in Pierre Coste, CM, and Vincent de Paul, Saint Vincent De Paul: Correspondence, Conferences, Documents, ed. Jacqueline Kilar, DC, Marie Poole, DC, et al., 14 vols. (New York: New City Press, 1985–2008), 9:58. Archives of the Daughters of Charity, St. Joseph's Provincial House, Emmitsburg, MD. The SC and DC, in referring to their Superioress as Sister Servant, would reverence her devotion to the will of God.

138 Throughout the year, holy days commemorating the lives of saints are celebrated as "feasts." Although vows for the first time are made on significant feasts throughout the year, Sisters renew their vows annually on the date that the Church celebrates as the feast of the Annunciation of the birth of Jesus Christ to Mary, usually on or about March 25.

139 Sister Valentine replaced Sister Mary Xavier as Novice Mistress when the latter was elected assistant to Mother Mary Augustine.

140 Daughters of Charity. Provincial Annals. 1867–71, 7–8.

141 Daughters of Charity, *Lives of the Deceased Sisters* (Saint Joseph's Provincial House, Emmitsburg, MD: Daughters of Charity 1870), 1889: 43. Sister Martha Daddisman attended Saint Joseph's Academy during Mother Seton's lifetime. When she died in 1889, she was the last survivor of the companions of Mother Seton.

142 Daughters of Charity. Chronological Table, 1766–1891. June 1826.

143 Sullivan, ed. and trans., *Louise de Marillac Spiritual Writings: Correspondence and Thoughts*, 763.

144 Sisters of Charity, *The Rule of 1812: Regulations for the Society of Sisters of Charity in the United States of America* (1812, Archive's of St. Joseph Provincial House), On Obedience #IV: 250.

145 Simon Gabriel Bruté de Remur, "Bruté's Conferences with the Sisters of Charity," in *Translations of the Conferences 7-3-1-3:B268*, ed. Rev. Albert Ledoux (1831).

146 Remarks on Sister Matilda Coskery in Daughters of Charity, *Lives of Deceased Sisters*, 1870, 11.

147 Daughters of Charity. Vow Requests. Archives Daughters of Charity, Saint Joseph's Provincial House, Emmitsburg, MD.

148 The Maryland Hospital stood on land where the Johns Hopkins Hospital would be built in 1877. Its history dates back to 1794, when some citizens of Baltimore created a shelter for insane seamen. In 1798 the Maryland General Assembly appropriated monies to build a hospital for the pauper sick and insane, which they leased to Drs. Alexander MacKenzie and James Smyth. In 1828, in response to public concern about the conditions of the hospital, the state incorporated the hospital and appointed a president and board of visitors. Dr. MacKenzie stayed at the hospital as a physician until his lease ran out in 1834, the time that the SC were brought in.

149 R. M. Beam. Report of the Committee on the Maryland Hospital to the Legislature of Maryland. 1837. M61-70 December, General Assembly, 2.

150 Ibid., 4.

151 Maryland Hospital for the Insane. Patient Register. 1834–1872. Maryland State Archives, Annapolis, MD, S184.1.

152 In the early and mid-nineteenth century, "regular physician" was a term used to refer to a doctor who used "heroic treatment" such as bloodletting, calomel, and blistering, as opposed to a botanic physician or homeopath. Regulars were often university trained.

153 Daughters of Charity. Rules and Regulations for the Maryland Hospital, Appendix A. 1833. Archives of the Daughters of Charity, St. Joseph's Provincial House, Emmitsburg, MD. See Appendix A of this book.

154 Ibid.

155 Medical Case Book, Baltimore Infirmary. Maryland State Archives, MSA SC 4070.1832, 255.

156 James Russell Lowell, "A Virginian in New England Thirty-Five Years Ago, Written on the Basis of Papers Left by Mr. Lucian Minor, (1802–1858) Professor of Law at College of William and Mary, Who Visited Baltimore in 1834," *Atlantic Monthly*, no. October (1870).

157 Maryland Hospital for the Insane. Patient Register. Joshua Cohen, MD, one of the attending physicians, who signs another note written on page 2 of the same ledger.

158 Richard Sprigg Steuart's career was spent caring for the insane. The Medical Annals of Baltimore state that the Maryland Hospital would "prove an ever-enduring monument to his benevolence and humanity." Steuart served as Superintendent of the hospital from 1828 to 1842 and 1869 to 1876.

159 As cited in Ambrose Byrne, "History of The Seton Institute, Baltimore, Maryland and Its Affiliate School of Nursing Conducted by the Daughters of Charity of St. Vincent de Paul in the Eastern Province of the United States" (The Catholic University of America, 1950), 7. Archives of the Daughters of Charity, St. Joseph's Provincial House.

160 Steuart as cited in ibid., 8.

161 Steuart as cited in ibid.

162 Richard S. Steuart Biographical Sketch. Maryland State Archives, SC 5522-1-29.492.

163 Olympia McTaggert. Correspondence from Sister Olympia McTaggert to Rev. Deluol. Archives of the Daughters of Charity, St. Joseph's Provincial House, Emmitsburg, MD. As cited in Ambrose Byrne, *History of The Seton Institute*, 7.

164 Herbert Bradshaw, *History of Hampden-Sydney College*, vol. 1: From the beginnings to the year 1856 (Durham, NC: by Author, 1976), 292–93.

165 Ibid., 290. Body snatching for purposes of medical dissection was still common and of great concern to the public.

166 Later called the Medical College of Virginia. The Sisters referred to it as the "Richmond Medical College."

167 Jessie Faris, "Two Hundred Years of Nursing in Richmond," *American Journal of Nursing* 37, no. 8 (1937): 848.

168 Bradshaw, *History of Hampden-Sydney College*.

169 Ibid., 296–97.

170 Catholic Church of the United States: 1840.

171 Sister Josephine Collins was the younger sister of Sister Ambrosia Magner, second Sister Servant at the Baltimore Infirmary.

172 Sister Josephine Collins. Correspondence to Sister Margaret. October 13, 1840. Archives Daughters of Charity, St. Joseph's Provincial House, Emmitsburg, MD 7-10-2 #76.

173 Ibid.

174 Sister Josephine Collins. Correspondence to Sister Margaret. November 11, 1840. Archives of the Daughters of Charity, St. Joseph's Provincial House, Emmitsburg, MD 7-10-2 #78.

175 Collins. Correspondence to Sister Margaret.

Chapter 3 - Endnotes

1 The Maryland Hospital, the second psychiatric hospital in the United States, was formally founded in 1797 as "The Retreat." When the SC arrived, it was referred to as the Maryland Hospital and ultimately called Spring Grove Hospital Center. See www.springgrove.com/history.html.

2 Daughters of Charity, Council Minutes, Archives of the Daughters of Charity, St. Joseph's Provincial House, Emmitsburg, MD, #3-3-5, August 26, 1840.

3 Daughters of Charity, Corporation Minutes, Archives of the Daughters of Charity, St. Joseph's Provincial House, Emmitsburg, MD, July 20, 1840.

4 Daughters of Charity, Council Minutes, January 27, 1841.

5 Daughters of Charity, Provincial Annals, Archives of the Daughters of Charity, Saint Joseph's Provincial House, Emmitsburg, MD, 7–8.

6   Sister Matilda Coskery, *Cradle of Mount Hope: Historical Account of Mt. St. Vincent Hospital/Mount Hope Retreat,* n.d., Archives of the Daughters of Charity, St. Joseph's Provincial House, Emmitsburg, MD, #11-2-39.5.

7   Ibid. The document is written in both first and third person, suggesting that Sister Matilda may have dictated some of the history to another Sister or her notes may have been used by another to construct the present document. Sister Thecla Murphy (1809–1880) may be the Sister who consolidated the history of Mount Hope. She was missioned to the Central House in Emmitsburg from 1858 until her death in 1880 and would have known Sister Matilda since 1834, when she entered the Community. A 1947 thesis by Sister Bernadette Armiger, "The History of the Hospital Work of the Daughters of Charity of St. Vincent de Paul in the Eastern Province of the United States 1823–1860" (The Catholic University of America, 1947), Archives of the Daughters of Charity, St. Joseph's Provincial House, Emmitsburg, Maryland, states that Sister Thecla wrote the history based on "notes drawn from Sister Matilda Coskery's 'Account of the Beginning of Mount Hope' is a document that is no longer extant." The detail found in the historical account is vivid and clearly demonstrates that the Sister Servant who cofounded Mount Hope with Dr. Stokes was the author. For example, on page 59 she refers to herself as "the writer" of the history. The historical account that covers the period of 1840 to 1863 is not dated; however, based upon content in the document, it was written some time after 1852.

8   Coskery, *Cradle of Mount Hope: Historical Account of Mt. St. Vincent Hospital/ Mount Hope Retreat,* 2.

9   Ibid., 3. Note: emphasis in original document.

10 Ibid.

11 Ibid., 5.

12 Ibid., 23.

13 Ibid., 24.

14 Ibid.

15 Ibid.

16 Ibid. The Sisters prayed the Seven Dolours of our Queen of Martyrs.

17 Remarks on Sister Matilda Coskery in Daughters of Charity, *Lives of the Deceased Sisters* (Emmitsburg, MD, 1870), 15. Archives of the Daughters of Charity, St. Joseph's Provincial House, Emmitsburg, MD.

18 Coskery, *Cradle of Mount Hope: Historical Account of Mt. St. Vincent Hospital/ Mount Hope Retreat,* 25.

19 Daughters of Charity, Deed to Mount Hope College, 1844, Archives of the Daughters of Charity, St. Joseph's Provincial House, Emmitsburg, MD, #7-9-3, 413.

20 Remarks on Sister Matilda Coskery in Daughters of Charity, *Lives of the Deceased Sisters,* 15.

21 Coskery, *Cradle of Mount Hope: Historical Account of Mt. St. Vincent Hospital/ Mount Hope Retreat*, 51.

22 Ibid., 55.

23 Gerald Grob, *The Mad Among Us: A History of the Care of America's Mentally Ill* (Cambridge, MA: Harvard University Press, 1994), 102.

24 *Coskery, Cradle of Mount Hope: Historical Account of Mt. St. Vincent Hospital/ Mount Hope Retreat*, 33. The physician would have been Dr. Samuel B. Woodward (1787–1850).

25 Ibid., 27.

26 Ibid., 40.

27 Laignel-Lavastine and Vié as cited in Margaret Flinton, *Louise de Marillac, Social Aspect of Her Work* (New York: New City Press, 1992), 136.

28 Ibid., 135.

29 *Louise de Marillac Spiritual Writings: Correspondence and Thoughts*, trans. and ed. Louise Sullivan, DC (New York: New City Press, 1991), 472.

30 Vincent de Paul as cited in Flinton, *Louise de Marillac, Social Aspect of Her Work*, 136.

31 Louis Abelly, *The Life of the Venerable Servant of God Vincent de Paul*, 3 vols. (New Rochelle, New York: New City Press, 1993, originally published 1664 in French), 2:296.

32 Daughters of Charity, "Remarks on Sister Nicole Lequin," *Circulars and Notices* 2 (April 17, 1703), Archives of the Daughters of Charity, St. Joseph's Provincial House, Emmitsburg, MD.

33 Colin Jones, "The Treatment of the Insane in Eighteenth and Early Nineteenth-Century Montpellier: A Contribution to the Prehistory of the Lunatic Asylum in Provincial France," *Medical History* 24 (1980), 378. For more about the herbal tradition of the DC, see Martha Libster, *Herbal Diplomats: The Contribution of Early American Nurses (1830–1860) to Nineteenth-Century Healthcare Reform and the Botanical Medical Movement* (www.GoldenApplePublications.com: Golden Apple Publications, 2004). The herbal tradition was continued by American SC such as Sister Matilda and is described in chapter 5 of this book.

34 Jones, "The Treatment of the Insane in Eighteenth and Early Nineteenth-Century Montpellier: A Contribution to the Prehistory of the Lunatic Asylum in Provincial France," 380.

35 Ibid., 386.

36 Ibid.

37 Anne Digby, "Moral Treatment at the Retreat, 1796–1846," in *The Anatomy of Madness*, ed. W. F. Bynum, Roy Porter, and Michael Shepherd (London: Tavistock Publications, 1985), 57.

38 Anne Digby, *Madness, Morality, and Medicine: A Study of the York Retreat, 1796–1914* (New York: Cambridge University Press, 1985), 13.

39   As cited in ibid., 113.

40   Daughters of Charity, Mt. Hope Receipt Book, 1847–1851, Archives of the Daughters of Charity, St. Joseph's Provincial House, Emmitsburg, MD, #11-2-39, 4.

41   Our growth and progress in forty years, William Stokes, *38th Annual Report of the Mount Hope Retreat*. 1880, Archives of the Daughters of Charity, St. Joseph's Provincial House, Emmitsburg, MD, 18.

42   William Stokes, *The Eleventh Annual Report of the Mount Hope Institution near Baltimore*, 1853, Archives of the Daughters of Charity, St. Joseph's Provincial House, Emmitsburg, MD, 22.

43   Ibid., 23.

44   William Stokes, *Second Annual Report of the Physician of Mount Hope Hospital (Late Mount St. Vincent's) for 1844*; 1845, Archives of the Daughters of Charity, St. Joseph's Provincial House, Emmitsburg, Maryland, #11-2-39, 17.

45   Camilla Haw, "John Conolly's Attendants at the Hanwell Asylum, 1839–1852," *History of Nursing Society Journal* 3, no. 1 (1990): 44.

46   Mother Mary Xavier Clark, *Instruction on the Care of the Sick*, Archives of Daughters of Charity of St. Vincent De Paul—West Central Province, St. Louis, Mo. (1846), 55.

47   Ibid., 58.

48   Ibid., 56–57.

49   Jones, "The Treatment of the Insane in Eighteenth and Early Nineteenth-Century Montpellier: A Contribution to the Prehistory of the Lunatic Asylum in Provincial France," 389.

50   Sisters of Charity, *The Rule of 1812: Regulations for the Society of Sisters of Charity in the United States of America* (1812). Archives of the Daughters of Charity, St. Joseph's Provincial House, Emmitsburg, MD.

51   #156 in Pierre Coste, CM, and Vincent de Paul, *Saint Vincent De Paul: Correspondence, Conferences, Documents*, ed. and trans. Jacqueline Kilar, DC, and Marie Poole, DC., 14 vols. (New York: New City Press, 1985–2008), 13a:245, Archives of the Daughters of Charity, St. Joseph's Provincial House, Emmitsburg, MD.

52   Abelly as cited in Flinton, *Louise de Marillac, Social Aspect of Her Work*, 143.

53   Amariah Brigham, "Definition of Insanity—Nature of the Disease," *American Journal of Insanity* 1 (October 1844): 97, Archives of the American Psychiatric Association.

54   Thomas Andrew, *A Cyclopedia of Domestic Medicine and Surgery* (Glasgow, Scotland: Blackie and Son, 1842), 358, accessed Google Books.com.

55   Pliny Earle, "On the Causes of Insanity," *American Journal of Insanity* 4, no. 3 (1848), 193, Archives of the American Psychiatric Association.

56   James Cassedy, *American Medicine and Statistical Thinking, 1800–1860* (Cambridge, MA: Harvard University Press, 1984).

57 W. F. Bynum, *Science and the Practice of Medicine in the Nineteenth Century* (Cambridge: Cambridge University Press, 1994), 17.

58 Amariah Brigham, *Remarks on the Influence of Mental Cultivation Upon Health* (Boston: Marsh, Capen & Lyon, 1833), 77. Google Books.

59 George Makari, "Educated Insane: A Nineteenth-Century Psychiatric Paradigm," *Journal of the History of the Behavioral Sciences* 29 (1993): 10. The concept of "natural" was in the early and mid-nineteenth century construed as meaning healthy and that of the unnatural unhealthy. People avoided artificial practices, "any activity contrary to physical nature or moral principle," such as taking manufactured medicines and processed foods. Martha H Verbrugge, *Able-Bodied Womanhood: Personal Health and Social Change in Nineteenth-Century Boston* (New York: Oxford University Press, 1988), 35.

60 Amariah Brigham, "The Moral Treatment of Insanity," *American Journal of Insanity* 4, no. 1 (1847): 1, Archives of the American Psychiatric Association.

61 Digby, "Moral Treatment at the Retreat, 1796–1846," 58.

62 William Smith, "Facts and Arguments in Support of 'the Humane System of Non-Restraint in the Treatment of the Insane,'" *Lancet* 1166 (January 3, 1846), Wellcome Trust Library, London.

63 Digby, "Moral Treatment at the Retreat, 1796–1846," 61.

64 Stokes, *38th Annual Report of the Mount Hope Retreat*, 19.

65 Ibid.

66 Ibid., 20.

67 Ibid., 23.

68 Stokes, *The Eleventh Annual Report of the Mount Hope Institution near Baltimore*, 29.

69 Ibid.

70 William Stokes, *Report of the Mount Hope Institution for the Year 1845*; 1846, Archives of the Daughters of Charity, St. Joseph's Provincial House, Emmitsburg, MD, 25.

71 William Stokes, *First Annual Report of the Physician of the Mount Saint Vincent's Hospital for 1843*; 1844, Archives of the Daughters of Charity, St. Joseph's Provincial House, Emmitsburg, MD, #11-2-39, 15–16.

72 W. G. Read as cited in Stokes, *First Annual Report of the Physician of the Mount Saint Vincent's Hospital for 1843*, 16.

73 Coskery, *Cradle of Mount Hope: Historical Account of Mt. St. Vincent Hospital/ Mount Hope Retreat*, 15–16.

74 Stokes, *The Eleventh Annual Report of the Mount Hope Institution near Baltimore*, 28.

75 Ibid.

76 Ibid.

77   Charles E. Rosenberg, *The Care of Strangers: The Rise of America's Hospital System* (New York: Basic Books, 1987), 37.

78   Coskery, *Cradle of Mount Hope: Historical Account of Mt. St. Vincent Hospital/ Mount Hope Retreat*, 29–30.

79   Ibid.

80   See discussion of "nature cure" in Martha Libster, "Elements of Care: Nursing Environmental Theory in Historical Context," *Holistic Nursing Practice* 22, no. 3 (2008).

81   Gerald Grob, *Edward Jarvis and the Medical World of Nineteenth-Century America* (Knoxville: University of Tennessee Press, 1978), 60–61.

82   Coskery, *Cradle of Mount Hope: Historical Account of Mt. St. Vincent Hospital/ Mount Hope Retreat*, 32.

83   Ibid., 32–33.

84   Paula Baker, "The Domestication of Politics: Women and American Political Society, 1780–1920," *American Historical Review* 89, no. 3 (1984), 625.

85   H. Buttolph, "Modern Asylums," *American Journal of Insanity* 3, no. 4 (1847): 369, Archives of the American Psychiatric Association.

86   Baker, "The Domestication of Politics: Women and American Political Society, 1780–1920," 633.

87   Heroics included calomel (purgative), bloodletting, blistering, tartar emetic, and sweating.

88   The name of the medical sect of followers of Samuel Thomson's philosophy of treatment and users of his patented botanical remedies.

89   Phrenology postulated that the brain was an aggregate of organs constituting the mind, that the mind possesses a number of faculties that are proportionate to the size of the brain, and that the skull can be examined to determine the development of the thirty-seven potential faculties.

90   Colin Jones, "Sisters of Charity and the Ailing Poor," *Social History of Medicine* 2, no. 3 (1989), 340.

91   Mother Seton's father, Dr. Richard Bayley (1744–1801) was the owner of an anatomical laboratory after the Revolutionary War. One of Bayley's students instigated the New York Doctor's Riot of 1788 by shaking the arm of a cadaver at a group of boys playing in the street, saying that it belonged to the mother of one of the boys. A mob descended upon the lab and would have gone to the Bayley home had it not been for the intercession of city leaders.

92   Jane Sewall, *Medicine in Maryland: The Practice and the Profession, 1799–1999* (Baltimore: The Johns Hopkins University Press, 1999), 71.

93   Ibid.

94   William Rothstein in *Other Healers: Unorthodox Medicine in America*, ed. Norman Gevitz (Baltimore, MD: Johns Hopkins University Press, 1988), 41. Overtreatment or overprescribing is still an issue today, raised by physicians

themselves. See discussion of the diagnostic process associated with breast cancer in women in Christiane Northrup, *Women's Bodies, Women's Wisdom: Creating Physical and Emotional Health and Healing* (New York: Bantam Books, 1994), 301.

95 Sisters of Charity, *The Rule of 1812: Regulations for the Society of Sisters of Charity in the United States of America*, Chapter III, Article I, Number V. Archives of the Daughters of Charity, St. Joseph's Provincial House, Emmitsburg, MD.

96 Sylvester Graham's system of medicine comprised lifestyle and dietary changes including the use of unbolted wheat bread (now known as graham crackers). He encouraged a diet of fruits and vegetables in their natural state, chewing food thoroughly and slowly, and no stimulants such as coffee, tea, alcohol, or tobacco. He recommended daily bathing, walking, horseback riding, and sleeping seven hours on a hard mattress as part of his health-promotion regime.

97 Regina Morantz-Sanchez in Guenter Risse, Ronald Numbers, and Judith Leavitt, *Medicine without Doctors: Home Health Care in American History* (New York: Science History Publications, 1977), 77.

98 Regina Morantz-Sanchez in ibid., 76.

99 Thomas Brown, *Dorothea Dix: A New England Reformer* (Cambridge, MA: Harvard University Press, 1998), 106.

100 Dorothea Dix, *Memorial of Miss D. L. Dix to the Hon. General Assembly in Behalf of the Insane of Maryland*, Archives of the State of Maryland (1852), Archives of the State of Maryland Web site, http://www.msa.md.gov/.

101 Alex Robinson, "Report of the Lunatic Department of the Baltimore Alms-House" (J. Robinson, 1841).

102 Ibid., 19–21.

103 Coskery, *Cradle of Mount Hope: Historical Account of Mt. St. Vincent Hospital/ Mount Hope Retreat*, 52.

104 Daughters of Charity, Mt. Hope Receipt Book.

105 Coskery, *Cradle of Mount Hope: Historical Account of Mt. St. Vincent Hospital/ Mount Hope Retreat*, 52.

106 Ibid.

107 Refers to Rev. Deluol.

108 Coskery, *Cradle of Mount Hope: Historical Account of Mt. St. Vincent Hospital/ Mount Hope Retreat*, 52–53.

109 Clark, *Instruction on the Care of the Sick*, 36–37.

110 Ibid., 67.

111 Daughters of Charity, *Lives of the Deceased Sisters*.

112 Paul Applebaum and Kathleen Kemp, "The Evolution of Commitment Law in the Nineteenth Century," *Law and Human Behavior* 6, no. 3/4 (1982).

113 Known today as the American Psychiatric Association.

114 Gerald Grob, "The State Mental Hospital in Mid-Nineteenth Century America: A Social Analysis," *American Psychologist* 21, no. 6 (1966), 513.

115 Gerald Grob, *Rediscovering Asylums* in Morris J. Vogel and Charles E. Rosenberg, *The Therapeutic Revolution: Essays in the Social History of American Medicine* (Philadelphia: University of Pennsylvania Press, 1979), 140.

116 Daughters of Charity, Annals of the Community, 1846, Souvay IIIA Documents Sisters of Charity I, DeAndreis-Rosati Memorial Archives, DePaul University, 2.

117 There are no extant records of what occurred in Sister Matilda's discussions in New York.

118 Coskery, *Cradle of Mount Hope: Historical Account of Mt. St. Vincent Hospital/ Mount Hope Retreat*, 18–23.

119 Sister Josephine Collins, Correspondence to Sister Margaret, October 13, 1840, Archives of the Daughters of Charity, St. Joseph's Provincial House, Emmitsburg, MD, 7-10-2 #76.61; Sister Josephine Collins, Correspondence to Sister Margaret, November 1, 1840, Archives of the Daughters of Charity, St. Joseph's Provincial House, Emmitsburg, MD, 7-10-2 #77.

120 Coste and de Paul, *Saint Vincent de Paul: Correspondence, Conferences, Documents*, 9:5.

121 Ibid., February 24, 1653, vol. 9:474.

122 Ibid.

123 Ibid., 11:35.

124 Ibid., 11:216.

125 Ibid., 12:307–08.

126 Stokes, *38th Annual Report of the Mount Hope Retreat*, 27.

127 Catholic Church of the United States, *The United States Catholic Almanac, or, Laity's Directory for the Year*: May 15, 1849, 130–131, University of Notre Dame Library, Microfilm Collection. 1817, 1822, 1833–ongoing.

128 Remarks on Matilda Coskery in Daughters of Charity, *Lives of the Deceased Sisters*, 16.

129 The hospital was renamed Mullanphy Hospital in 1874 when it was rebuilt at a new location. The name was changed in 1930 to DePaul.

130 Daniel Hannefin, *Daughters of the Church: A Popular History of the Daughters of Charity in the United States, 1809-1987* (New York: New City Press, 1989), 44. Original Contract held in Archives of the Marillac Provincialate in St. Louis, MO.

131 Ibid. Records in DePaul Hospital Archives.

132 Coste and de Paul, *Saint Vincent de Paul: Correspondence, Conferences, Documents*, 11:32.

133 *Louise de Marillac Spiritual Writings: Correspondence and Thoughts*, 600.

134 II Cor 5:14

135 Ibid., 55.

136 Coskery, *Cradle of Mount Hope: Historical Account of Mt. St. Vincent Hospital/ Mount Hope Retreat*, 11–13.

137 Remarks on Sister Matilda Coskery in Daughters of Charity, *Lives of the Deceased Sisters*, 14.

138 Remarks on Sister Matilda Coskery in ibid., 17.

139 Ibid., 13.

140 Ibid., 12.

141 Ibid., 16.

142 Ibid., 14.

143 Ibid.

144 Ibid., 13.

145 Ibid., 18.

146 Ibid., 19.

147 Coskery, *Cradle of Mount Hope: Historical Account of Mt. St. Vincent Hospital/ Mount Hope Retreat*, 45.

148 Ibid., 41.

149 Remarks on Sister Matilda Coskery in Daughters of Charity, *Lives of the Deceased Sisters*, 18.

150 Coskery, *Cradle of Mount Hope: Historical Account of Mt. St. Vincent Hospital/ Mount Hope Retreat*, 35–36.

Chapter 4 – Endnotes

1 Now the American Psychiatric Association.

2 H. Buttolph, "Modern Asylums," *American Journal of Insanity* 3, no. 4 (1847): 367, Archives of the American Psychiatric Association.

3 Ibid., 368.

4 Ibid., 369.

5 Amariah Brigham, "Dr. William Stokes, of the Mount Hope Institution, near Baltimore, Md. and the *American Journal of Insanity*," *American Journal of Insanity* 5, no. 3 (1849): 279, Archives of the American Psychiatric Association.

6 Colin Jones, "Sisters of Charity and the Ailing Poor," *Social History of Medicine* 2, no. 3 (1989): 345.

7 Ibid., 347.

8 Leonard Stein, David Watts, and Timothy Howell, "The Doctor-Nurse Game Revisited," *New England Journal of Medicine* 322, no. 8 (1990): 264.

9 Adele Pillitteri and Michael Ackerman, "The 'Doctor-Nurse Game': A Comparison of 100 Years—1888–1990," *Nursing Outlook* 41, no. 3 (1993).

10 Ibid., 116.

11 As cited in ibid., 113.

12 S. J. Closs, "Interdisciplinary Research and the Doctor-Nurse Game," *Clinical Effectiveness in Nursing* 5 (2001): 103.

13 Sarah Sweet and Ian Norman, "The Nurse-Doctor Relationship: A Selective Literature Review," *Journal of Advanced Nursing* 22 (1995).

14 Dorothea Dix challenged the pope in Rome in 1856. She wrote in a letter to Dr. Buttolph and his wife, "In Naples, I did nothing for hospitals; indeed strange as it is, I found a better institution there for the insane than has been founded in all southern and central Italy. In Rome, things were quite different. 6,000 priests, 300 monks, and 3,000 nuns, and a spiritual sovereignty joined with the temporal powers had not assured for the miserable insane a decent much less intelligent care. . . . Since coming to Florence five days ago, I find a bad hospital here and mountains of difficulty in the way of remedy for serious ills. I have the idea of removing these mountains and seeing if Protestant energy cannot work what Catholic powers fail to undertake." In Francis Tiffany, *The Life of Dorothea Lynde Dix* (Boston: Houghton, Mifflin & Co., 1891), 286. Google Books.

15 Amariah Brigham, "Editorial Correspondence," *American Journal of Insanity* 5, no. 1 (1848), Archives of the American Psychiatric Association.

16 Ibid.

17 Ibid., 67.

18 Brigham, "Dr. William Stokes, of the Mount Hope Institution, near Baltimore, Md. and the *American Journal of Insanity*," 263.

19 Ibid.

20 Ibid., 265.

21 Ibid., 266.

22 Ibid., 269.

23 Ibid., 279.

24 Ibid., 272.

25 Ibid., 274.

26 Eugene Didier. Report of the Trial of Dr. Wm. H. Stokes and Mary Blenkinsop, Physician and Sister Superior of Mount Hope Institution before the Circuit Court from Baltimore Co., Md. 1866. Maryland State Archives, Annapolis, MD. The indictment brought against Dr. Stokes, Sister Euphemia (1816–1887), and the DC by fifteen psychiatric patients stated that Dr. Stokes and Sr. Euphemia had conspired by false pretenses and representations to entice caretakers of those patients to place them at Mount Hope in order to cheat and defraud those persons of the moneys they paid for board. The trial, which lasted a year, ended in a verdict of not guilty.

27 Patricia D'Antonio, *Founding Friends: Families, Staff, and Patients at the Friends Asylum in Early Nineteenth-Century Philadelphia* (Bethlehem, PA: Lehigh University Press, 2006), 30.

28 Unknown, "Obituary, Dr. Amariah Brigham," *American Journal of Insanity* 6, no. 2 (1849): 191, Archives of the American Psychiatric Association.

29   Ibid.

30   John Galt, "Report on the Organization of Asylums for the Insane," *American Journal of Insanity* 7, no. 1 (1850): 52, Archives of the American Psychiatric Association.

31   J. M. Higgins, "On the Necessity of a Resident Medical Superintendent in an Institution for the Insane," *American Journal of Insanity* 7, no. 1 (1850): 64, Archives of the American Psychiatric Association.

32   Romeyn Beck, "Proceedings of the Sixth Annual Meeting of Medical Superintendents of American Institutions for the Insane," *American Journal of Insanity* 8, no. 1 (1851): 84, Archives of the American Psychiatric Association.

33   Romeyn Beck, "Proceedings of the Eighth Annual Meeting of the Association of Medical Superintendents of American Institutions for the Insane," *American Journal of Insanity* 10, no. 1 (1853): 80, Archives of the American Psychiatric Association.

34   The Sisters of Charity at Cincinnati did not join the French Daughters.

35   See the large white headdress worn by the Sisters on the cover of the book.

36   Sister Matilda Coskery, *Cradle of Mount Hope: Historical Account of Mt. St. Vincent Hospital/Mount Hope Retreat*, n.d., Archives of the Daughters of Charity, St. Joseph's Provincial House, Emmitsburg, MD, #11-2-39.56.

37   Ibid.

38   Ibid., 59.

39   Sister Rosaline Brown, Sister Rosaline Brown's Narrative of the First Mission in Detroit, 1844–1854. Daughters of Charity Archives, Mater Dei Provincialate, Evansville, IN, 3–4.

40   The name was later changed to St. Mary's Hospital.

41   Brown, Sister Rosaline Brown's Narrative of the First Mission in Detroit, 7.

42   Ibid., 7–10

43   Ibid., 9.

44   Ibid.

45   Ibid.

46   John Finegan, How a Patient Remembers, a Letter to a Sister at St. Mary's Hospital Detroit, 1878, Daughters of Charity Archives, Mater Dei Provincialate, Evansville, IN.

47   Ibid.

48   Ibid.

49   Sister Ann Aloysia Reed, An Incident in the Hospital Life of Sr. Rebecca Delone [*sic*] as Related by Her Companion and Eye Witness, Sister Felicia Fenwick, n.d., Daughters of Charity Archives, Mater Dei Provincialate, Evansville, IN.

50   Ibid.

51   Ibid.

52 Edward G. Martin, *Early Detroit: St. Mary's Hospital 1845–1945* (Detroit: St. Mary's Hospital, 1945), 49.

53 Providence Hospital and Medical Centers and St. Vincent and Sarah Fisher Center, *Caritas Christi: 1844–1994 (The Daughters of Charity of St. Vincent de Paul—150 Years of Service to Detroit)* (Detroit: Providence Hospital and Medical Centers and St. Vincent and Sarah Fisher Center, 1994), 23.

54 Daughter of Charity, Name Unknown, Providence Retreat, Buffalo, New York, an Oral History, 1885, Archives of the Daughters of Charity of St. Vincent de Paul, Northeast Province, Albany, NY.

55 Ibid.

56 Ibid., 7.

57 Grover Cleveland was the 22nd and 24th president of the United States.

58 Daughter of Charity, Name Unknown, Providence Retreat, Buffalo, NY, an Oral History, 15.

59 Daughters of Charity, Council Minutes, Archives of the Daughters of Charity, St. Joseph's Provincial House, Emmitsburg, MD, #3-3-5, October 29, 1855.

60 Sister Matilda Coskery, *Advices Concerning the Sick* (Emmitsburg, MD: Archives of Daughters of Charity, St. Joseph's Provincial House, n.d., c. 1840).

61 Florence Nightingale, *Notes on Nursing: What It Is and What It Is Not* (Edinburgh, Scotland: Churchill Livingstone, 1980, Original publication, 1859).

62 Ibid., v.

63 Daughters of Charity, *Lives of the Deceased Sisters* (Emmitsburg, MD: 1870–1879), 21, Archives of the Daughters of Charity, St. Joseph's Provincial House, Emmitsburg, MD (emphasis added).

64 In nineteenth-century vernacular, the term "attendant" was not always interchangeable with the word "nurse." In general, nurse referred to females and attendant to males, as demonstrated in the *American Journal of Insanity* October 1852 article on the "Qualifications of attendants on the insane," by Dr. Francis Stribling. However, as demonstrated in some of the citations from the SC records, the Sisters also referred to themselves at times as "attendants," and in one case Sister Matilda referred in her history, *Cradle of Mount Hope*, to a "male nurse." (p. 34). She could have been referring to the SC Nurse who worked in the "gentlemen's department," or she could have meant that the nurse was male. It is not exactly clear from the text or the document which interpretation is correct.

65 Camilla Haw, "John Conolly's Attendants at the Hanwell Asylum, 1839–1852," *History of Nursing Society Journal* 3, no. 1 (1990): 35.

66 Remarks on Sister Matilda Coskery in Daughters of Charity, *Lives of the Deceased Sisters* (Emmitsburg, MD: 1870), Archives of the Daughters of Charity, St. Joseph's Provincial House, Emmitsburg, MD.

67 Coskery, *Cradle of Mount Hope: Historical Account of Mt. St. Vincent Hospital/ Mount Hope Retreat*, 26.

Chapter 5 – Endnotes

1 Florence Nightingale, *Notes on Nursing: What It Is and What It Is Not* (Edinburgh, Scotland: Churchill Livingstone, 1980. Originally published 1859), 2.

2 C. Cleaveland, "Nurses," *The Eclectic Medical Journal* 4, no. 8 (1852): 371.

3 For example, see Englishman William Buchan, *Domestic Medicine; or, the Family Physician: Being an Attempt to Render the Medical Art More Generally Useful, by Shewing People What Is in Their Own Power Both with Respect to the Prevention and Cure of Diseases. Chiefly Calculated to Recommend a Proper Attention to Regimen and Simple Medicines* (Edinburgh: Printed by Balfour, Auld, and Smellie, 1769). Wellcome Trust Library, London, or American John C. Gunn, *Gunn's Domestic Medicine or Poor Man's Friend in the Hours of Affliction, Pain and Sickness.* (Philadelphia: G. V. Raymond, 1839). Countway Library at Harvard University, Cambridge, MA.

4 Catharine E. Beecher, *Miss Beecher's Domestic Receipt-Book* (New York: Dover Publications, 2001. Originally published 1858). Beecher was the Martha Stewart of her day.

5 Lydia Maria Child, *The Family Nurse* (Bedford, MA: Applewood Books, 1997. Originally published 1837).

6 The D-R Bible is a translation of the Bible from the Latin Vulgate into English. The New Testament was published in one volume with extensive commentary and notes in 1582. The Old Testament followed in 1609–10 in two volumes, also extensively annotated. The notes took up the bulk of the volumes and had a strong polemical and patristic character. They also offered insights on issues of translation and on the Hebrew and Greek source texts of the Vulgate. The purpose of the version, both the text and notes, was an effort by English Catholics to uphold Catholic tradition in the face of the Protestant Reformation, which was heavily influencing England. Although the New Jerusalem Bible and New American Bible are commonly used in English-speaking Catholic churches, the Challoner revision of the Douay-Rheims is still often the Bible of choice of traditional Catholics today.

7 W. G. Read in William Stokes, *First Annual Report of the Physician of the Mount Saint Vincent's Hospital for 1843*, 1844, Archives of the Daughters of Charity, St. Joseph's Provincial House, Emmitsburg, MD, #11-2-39.15.

8 Catholic Church of the United States, *The United States Catholic Almanac, or, Laity's Directory for the Year*. University of Notre Dame Library, Microfilm Collection. 1817, 1822, 1833-ongoing.

9 Sister Matilda Coskery. Correspondence: Letter to Rev. Henry B. Coskery. Rochester, NY, April 18,1849. Archives of the Archdiocese of Baltimore, Coskery Collection, Sister Matilda Coskery. Correspondence: Letter to Rev. Henry B. Coskery on the Death of Archbishop Samuel Eccleston of Baltimore. Detroit, MI, April 28, 1851. Archives of Archdiocese, St. Mary's Seminary and University.

10 Sister Matilda Coskery. *Cradle of Mount Hope: Historical Account of Mt. St. Vincent Hospital / Mount Hope Retreat.* n.d. Archives of the Daughters of Charity, St. Joseph's Provincial House, Emmitsburg, MD, #11-2-39.15.

11 Ibid.

12 Ambrose Byrne, "History of The Seton Institute, Baltimore, Maryland and Its Affiliate School of Nursing Conducted by the Daughters of Charity of St. Vincent de Paul in the Eastern Province of the United States" (The Catholic University of America, 1950).

13 Bernadette Armiger, "The History of the Hospital Work of the Daughters of Charity of St. Vincent de Paul in the Eastern Province of the United States 1823–1860." (The Catholic University of America, 1947). Archives of the Daughters of Charity, St. Joseph's Provincial House, Emmitsburg, MD.

14 For example, see Byrne, "History of The Seton Institute, Baltimore, Maryland and Its Affiliate School of Nursing Conducted by the Daughters of Charity of St. Vincent de Paul in the Eastern Province of the United States," 16.

15 Daniel Hannefin, *Daughters of the Church: A Popular History of the Daughters of Charity in the United States, 1809–1987* (New York: New City Press, 1989), 58. Sister Daniel may have been made aware of the document by Sister Aloysia Dugan, DC Nurse and the archivist at Emmitsburg.

16 *Louise de Marillac Spiritual Writings: Correspondence and Thoughts,* trans. and ed. Louise Sullivan, DC (New York: New City Press, 1991), 726.

17 Ibid., 746.

18 Infusions refer to the medicinal teas given to patients. Infusions are made by steeping herbs in boiled water.

19 *Louise de Marillac Spiritual Writings: Correspondence and Thoughts,* 726.

20 Ibid., 742.

21 Stokes, *First Annual Report of the Physician of the Mount Saint Vincent's Hospital for 1843,* 3–6.

22 Ibid., 3.

23 Patients left when they chose to leave, and this was at times a concern for Dr. Stokes and the sisters. In his eighth *Annual Report,* Dr. Stokes wrote about the problem. "Of the sixty-five patients discharged from the insane department twenty-six were prematurely removed, and in opposition to the wishes and counsel of the physician. . . . In private establishments for the insane, like this, it being impossible to establish any compulsory regulations, obliging the friends of those committed to our charge to avoid all interference for a reasonable period, or to continue them until the disease is fully eradicated, we are often obliged to lament the infatuation of friends in taking their own course, without regard to the opinion of the medical officer of the institution. When a patient is admitted into the Asylum, the friends immediately, without considering the previous duration of the disease, become impatient for the results . . . they become weary of the charge." William Stokes, *The Eighth Annual Report of the Mount Hope Institution, near Baltimore, for the*

Year 1850. 1851. Archives of the Daughters of Charity, St. Joseph's Provincial House, Emmitsburg, MD.

24 *Louise de Marillac Spiritual Writings: Correspondence and Thoughts,* 128.

25 Ibid., 746.

26 Ibid., 709.

27 Document 149b in Pierre Coste, CM, and Vincent de Paul, *Saint Vincent de Paul: Correspondence, Conferences, Documents,* trans. and ed. Jacqueline Kilar, DC, and Marie Poole, DC. 14 vols. (New York: New City Press, 1985–2008), 13b:203.

28 *Louise de Marillac Spiritual Writings: Correspondence and Thoughts,* 808.

29 Martha Libster, *Herbal Diplomats: The Contribution of Early American Nurses (1830–1860) to Nineteenth-Century Healthcare Reform and the Botanical Medical Movement* (Thornton, CO: Golden Apple Publications, 2004), chapter 4.

30 Maria Eliza Rundell, *American Domestic Cookery Formed on Principles of Economy for the Use of Private Families* (New York: Evert Duyckince, 1823). Archives of the Daughters of Charity, St. Joseph's Provincial House, Emmitsburg, MD. File: Sister M. Felicita Dellone.

31 Ibid., 296–97.

32 Janet Theophano, *Eat My Words: Reading Women's Lives through the Cookbooks They Wrote* (New York: Palgrave, 2002), 25.

33 Child, *The Family Nurse,* 29.

34 Theophano, *Eat My Words: Reading Women's Lives through the Cookbooks They Wrote,* 86.

35 A "toddy" is a drink made from rum, brandy, or Scotch whiskey; spices such as nutmeg, cinnamon, cloves, lemon rind, and vanilla; and a small amount of butter. It is served hot.

36 Washing the feet demonstrated the compassionate response of those who followed the Vincentian-Louisian charitable tradition. Foot washing and footbaths will be discussed in detail later under the section of *Advices* titled "Foot-baths." Mustard and wood ash will also be discussed.

37 Camphor in the nineteenth century was derived from the Asian *Cinnamomum camphora* tree. To collect the spirits or essential oil of camphor, the Chinese "steep the chopped branches in water, then boil it, continuing the ebullition until a stick placed in the fluid will, when cooled, be covered with the camphor. The liquor is then strained, and by cooling, the camphor solidifies. This is then placed alternately in layers, with powdered dry earth, in a copper vessel, over which another one is placed, and the camphor, being sublimed by heat, attaches itself to the upper inverted vessel." Harvey Wickes Felter and John Uri Lloyd, *King's American Dispensatory,* 18th ed., 3d rev. ed. (Sandy, OR: Eclectic Medical Publications, 1983), 415. The crude camphor is a grey color. The essential oils of other aromatic plants such as lavender, rosemary, peppermint, and feverfew also contain camphor as one of their

constituents. Camphor was used medicinally in the nineteenth century as a sedative, antispasmodic, diaphoretic, and antiparasitic. Very small doses were considered stimulating and large doses depressing. It was used to calm the nervous system, relieve pain and bowel problems, and induce sleep and was sometimes effective in treatment of cholera. Felter and Lloyd, *King's American Dispensatory*, 418.

38 Bay rum was a popular distillate originally made from rum and the leaves and/or berries of the West Indian Bay tree, *Pimenta racemosa*. Citrus and spice oils may have also been used. Bay rum was used as aftershave and also used medicinally. A distillate is a hydrosol, or water solution, of essential oils obtained by steam processing aromatic plants. Distillates were so common that women in the nineteenth century often had their own stillery equipment in stillrooms or "stills" in or behind their kitchens. There is no record that the Daughters of Charity distilled their own products for use in nursing care; they most likely purchased them from local vendors and apothecaries, especially in facilities such as Mount Hope, where many patients suffered from alcoholism and the "spirits" would have needed to be controlled.

39 R. E. Griffith and Anthony Todd Thomson, *The Domestic Management of the Sick-Room Necessary, in Aid of Medical Treatment, for the Cure of Diseases*, 1st American from the second London ed. (Philadelphia: Lea and Blanchard, 1845), 94. Countway Library at Harvard Untiversity, Cambridge, MA.

40 Ibid.

41 Francis Gurney Smith, *Domestic Medicine, Surgery, and Materia Medica with Directions for the Diet and Management of the Sick Room* (Philadelphia: Lindsay and Blakiston, 1851), 337. Lloyd Library, Cincinnati, OH.

42 William Stokes, *Tenth Annual Report of the Mount Hope Institution for the Year 1852*, 1853, Archives of the Daughters of Charity, St. Joseph's Provincial House, Emmitsburg, MD, 22.

43 Nancy Stotts et al., "Nutrition Education in Schools of Nursing in the United States. Part 2: The Status of Nutrition Education in Schools of Nursing," *Journal of Parenteral and Enteral Nutrition* 11, no. 4 (1987). 406–11.

44 Neva Crogan and Bronwynne Evans, "Nutrition Assessment: Experience Is Not a Predictor of Knowledge," *Journal of Continuing Education in Nursing* 32, no. 5 (2001), 219–22.

45 Ague was a fever with symptoms like malaria. It was described in one 1845 text as a fever caused by decomposing vegetable substances. The patient feels intensely cold; he becomes sleepy, his flesh diminishes, and he trembles. The coldness leaves and is replaced by heat. The patient's face becomes red and swollen, and the fever stage is followed by excessive perspiration and tremendous fatigue. Cinchona bark (quinine) was the treatment of choice for curing ague; but white willow bark (which contains salicylates), drops of arsenic in the form of Fowler's solution, infusions of chamomile flowers, marsh trefoil, buck-bean, and calamus root were also used with success. Thomas Webster, Mrs. Parkes, and D. Meredith Reese, *An Encyclopedia*

of Domestic Economy: Comprising Such Subjects as Are Most Immediately Connected with Housekeeping; as, the Construction of Domestic Edifices, with the Modes of Warming, Ventilating, and Lighting Them; a Description of the Various Articles of Furniture; a General Account of the Animal and Vegetable Substances Used in Food, and the Methods of Preserving and Preparing Them by Cooking; Making Bread; Materials Employed in Dress and Toilet; Business of the Laundry; Description of the Various Wheel-Carriages; Preservation of Health; Domestic Medicines, &C. (New York: Harper & Brothers, 1845), 1207. Old Sturbridge Village Research Library, Sturbridge, MA.

46 The recipe for toast water is in a number of mid-nineteenth-century advice books. It was used for fever. Child suggests soaking a piece of toasted bread in West India molasses and water with a little lemon juice in it. The water from this was then drunk as a "nutritious and grateful beverage in fever." Child, *The Family Nurse*, 31. Catharine Beecher's recipe for toast water was one of her "simple drinks for the sick": "Pour boiling water on to bread toasted very brown, and boil it a minute, then strain it, and add a little cream and sugar." Beecher, *Miss Beecher's Domestic Receipt-Book*, 193.

47 Most likely refers to gum arabic water. Gum arabic is the hardened sap from the acacia tree that grows in India. It is used as a food stabilizer today, but in the nineteenth century Child states that the water from the gum arabic was "nourishing and demulcent with a tendency to allay inward inflammation. Excellent in fever, diarrheas, and other bowel complaints." The gum was dissolved in water, cooled, and sweetened with sugar. Child, *The Family Nurse*, 23.

48 Jelly water may have simply been jelly mixed in water. Beecher, however, describes only an "effervescing" jelly drink made from jellies that were too old for table use. She advised to "mix them with good vinegar, and then use them with soda or saleratus" (i.e., baking soda). Beecher, *Miss Beecher's Domestic Receipt-Book*, 185.

49 Tartar emetic is a chemical mixture of antimony and potassium tartrate. Antimony is toxic. Tartar emetic was a common emetic from the sixteenth century and into the early and mid-nineteenth century; a very small amount of the chemical compound was used to cause the patient to vomit. The use of emetics such as tartar emetic and calomel and, in the case of botanical treatments, lobelia (*Lobelia inflata*) or cayenne pepper (*Capsicum frutescens*) was thought to rid the stomach of inflammation and heat that were believed to be the cause of illness. Tartar emetic, like calomel, gradually fell out of favor in later nineteenth-century medicine. The presence of this remedy in *Advices* suggests that the text was written in the earlier part of the nineteenth century. In the middle and later years of the century, the Eclectic School of Medicine was founded to counter the abuse of tartar emetic by Regular physicians. Felter and Lloyd, *King's American Dispensatory*, 215.

Tartar emetic is not included in Child's or Beecher's domestic-medicine books. Some physicians, such as Thomas Cooper in his advice book in 1824, suggested to families that they have tartar emetic on hand along with other medicines such as calomel, castor oil, and Epsom salts. As cited by John Blake in Guenter Risse, Ronald Numbers, and Judith Leavitt, *Medicine without Doctors: Home Health Care in American History* (New York: Science History Publications, 1977), 17. Child, in *The Family Nurse*, included suggestions for dealing with the effects of overdoses of mineral poisons such as tartar emetic. She wrote that yellow Peruvian bark "will prevent the fatal effects. Quarter of a gill of the strong infusion is said to neutralize the effect of twenty grains of tartar-emetic. Almost any vegetable bitter will have the same effect; therefore it is very improper to give chamomile tea, when you wish to vomit with *antimony*." Child, *The Family Nurse*, 134.

50   Child refers to the drink as apple water and suggests steeping for two to three hours. Child, *The Family Nurse*, 29. Beecher's recipe for apple "tea" is identical to Sister Matilda's. Beecher, *Miss Beecher's Domestic Receipt-Book*, 199.

51   Sister Matilda advises that a patient in the sinking state receive some brandy and a temple rub with camphor. This recommendation is a modification of a prescription suggested by a Dr. Andrew, who in the 1840s wrote that a patient "sinking" during treatment for cholera must receive "stimulants such as ether and laudanum, warm brandy and water, camphor mixture of double strength, and combined with sweet spirit of nitre." Thomas Andrew, *A Cyclopedia of Domestic Medicine and Surgery* (Glasgow, Scotland: Blackie and Son, 1842), 113. Accessed Google Books.com. Sister Matilda advises that the patient be given the brandy and that the camphor be applied topically, a milder approach using similar remedies.

52   The use of mustard is explained in the section of *Advices* on footbaths. A plaster is a topical application of a powdered plant material that has been mixed into a pastelike consistency.

53   Arrowroot, sago, and tapioca are all plants that are typically used as thickening agents because of the constituents in their roots. They are a starch produced from the root of the *Maranta arundinacea*, the sago palm (*Metroxylon sagu*), and the cassava bush (*Manihot esculenta*) respectively. The starch in the root is demulcent; it creates a thin, moistening coating on mucous membranes, thus relieving inflammation and pain.

54   Pap is a common remedy used in the care of the sick in the nineteenth century. It was a thin gruel made from grain.

55   Holy Bible, Matthew 25:45. Through faith, the Daughter-Nurses were able to nurse their patients as if they were Jesus the Christ. The DC saw Christ in poor persons and the poor in Christ. In so doing, the sisters' spiritual love for Christ was transferred to their patients.

56   Sister Matilda demonstrates some of the simple ways in which nurses work with the psychology of the patient to promote comfort during treatment. Physicians may have been critical of nurses' giving patients drinks and foods before the patient could tolerate them; but the caregiver who is with the patient every day has to learn to help each patient manage his or her illness,

which is particularly difficult when a patient is hungry and is told by the physician and nurses to fast or eat certain foods. Sister Matilda shows her ingenuity in creating a "bare bones" remedy that encourages the patient's desire for the "sloppy, watery things" he or she is allowed.

57 Gerald Burke, "Caring for the Medically Ill Psychiatric Patient on a Psychiatric Unit," *Psychiatric Annals* 13, no. 8 (1983): 627.

58 Romeyn Beck, "Proceedings of the Eighth Annual Meeting of the Association of Medical Superintendents of American Institutions for the Insane," *American Journal of Insanity* 10, no. 1 (1853): 85. Archives of the American Psychiatric Association.

59 Assessing the tongue fur or coating is an ancient practice. In traditional Chinese medicine it is believed that the health status of the inner organs of the body is reflected in the tongue and its coating. Giovanni Maciocia, *Tongue Diagnosis in Chinese Medicine* (Seattle, WA: Eastland Press, 1987). Nineteenth-century physician Thomas Andrew wrote that "the tongue is a sure index of the existence of debility in the digestive apparatus." Andrew, *A Cyclopedia of Domestic Medicine and Surgery*, 235.

60 National Marine Sanctuaries, "Our Whaling Pasts" (2005 [cited July, 2006]). http://sanctuaries.noaa.gov/maritime/whaling.html.

61 Cindy Munro and Mary Jo Grap, "Oral Health and Care in the Intensive Care Unit: State of the Science," *American Journal of Critical Care* 13, no. 1 (2004), 25–33.

62 Ibid.: 25.

63 Trent Outhouse, "Tongue Scraping for Treating Halitosis," *The Cochrane Database of Systematic Reviews* 1 (2006).

64 George White and Mirna Armaleh, "Tongue Scraping as a Means of Reducing Oral Mutans Streptococci," *The Journal of Clinical Pediatric Dentistry* 28, no. 2 (2004), 163–66.

65 Theresa Tetuan, "The Role of the Nurse in Oral Health," *The Kansas Nurse* 79, no. 10 (2004), 1–2.

66 Carol Rawlins and Ian Trueman, "Effective Mouth Care for Seriously Ill Patients," *Professional Nurse* 16, no. 4 (2001), 1025–28.

67 Oilcloth refers to any cloth that has been permeated with oil to render it waterproof. Whale or vegetable oil was probably used instead of animal oil, which would turn rancid more quickly. Silk fabric is nearly waterproof because it can be woven tightly and because of the natural properties of a filament produced by the silkworm.

68 The procedure described here is typical hydrotherapeutic practice used in cooling the body.

69 Following the patient's lead and preserving his or her energy for healing is an example of holistic nursing intervention.

70 Hygiene was important in the sickroom. Neatness and orderliness were believed to promote a sick person's sense of comfort; disorder and filth

produced annoyance. Catharine Esther Beecher and Harriet Beecher Stowe, *The American Woman's Home or, Principles of Domestic Science: Being a Guide to the Formation and Maintenance of Economical, Healthful, Beautiful, and Christian Homes* (Piscataway, NJ: Rutgers University Press, 2002. Originally published 1869).

71 William Stokes, *The Sixth Annual Report of the Mount Hope Institution near Baltimore, for the Year 1848*, 1849, Archives of the Daughters of Charity, St. Joseph's Provincial House, Emmitsburg, MD, 8–9.

72 Ventilation in and around a patient in the sickroom was a common topic in nineteenth-century advice books. The difference here would be that a nurse would need to know which diseases were increased by fresh air.

73 One of the outcomes sought in moral therapy was the successful calming of the insane patient.

74 Although Dr. Stokes and the sisters used purgatives in the treatment of the insane, the descriptions in *Advices* imply that purgatives, as well as other medicines, were prescribed in low doses. Stokes was clear that he disagreed with the series of popular treatments used earlier in the century, such as leeches, "drastic purgatives," and "large and frequent doses of tartarized antimony" (tartar emetic). William Stokes, *The Fortieth Annual Report of the Mount Hope Retreat, for the Year 1882*, 1883, Archives of the Daughters of Charity, St. Joseph's Provincial House, Emmitsburg, MD.

75 William Stokes, *The Forty-Second Annual Report of the Mount Hope Retreat, for the Year 1884*, 1885, Archives of the Daughters of Charity, St. Joseph's Provincial House, Emmitsburg, MD.

76 W. F. Bynum, *Science and the Practice of Medicine in the Nineteenth Century* (Cambridge: Cambridge University Press, 1994), 17.

77 Charles E. Rosenberg, *The Care of Strangers: The Rise of America's Hospital System* (New York: Basic Books, 1987), 76.

78 Samuel Woodward in Amariah Brigham, "Lunatic Asylums of the United States," *American Journal of Insanity* 2, no. July (1845): 59. Archives of the American Psychiatric Association.

79 Ibid.: 61.

80 Samuel Woodward, "Observations on the Medical Treatment of Insanity," *American Journal of Insanity* 7, no. 1 (1850): 6. Archives of the American Psychiatric Association.

81 Andrew, *A Cyclopedia of Domestic Medicine and Surgery*, 108.

82 Lydia Maria Child does include blistering in her advice book, *The Family Nurse.*

83 Amariah Brigham, "The Medical Treatment of Insanity," *American Journal of Insanity* 3, no. 4 (1847): 355. Archives of the American Psychiatric Association.

84 W. G. Read interview with Sister Matilda at Mount Hope in Stokes, *First Annual Report of the Physician of the Mount Saint Vincent's Hospital for 1843*, 17

85 William G. Rothstein, *American Physicians in the Nineteenth Century: From*

Sects to Science (Baltimore: Johns Hopkins University Press, 1972), 183.

86 Laudanum is an alcohol extraction of opium used to relieve pain and promote sleep. It was available to and used by the general public.

87 Also known as nitric acid or HNO_3 which is found in small amounts in rainwater falling during a thunderstorm. It was commonly used in the nineteenth century for such conditions as pneumonia, typhoid, dysentery, and chronic ague. Felter and Lloyd, *King's American Dispensatory*, 69.

88 Lydia Maria Child also recommended flaxseed tea (*Linum* spp.) for strangury as well as hard coughs, dysentery, piles, and inflammatory states of the lungs. When the seed is steeped in boiled water, a mucilaginous substance seeps into the water, causing it to become thick. Child recommended a "tumbler full sweetened with honey, molasses, or sugar." Child, *The Family Nurse*, 30.

89 Felter and Lloyd, *King's American Dispensatory*, 1759.

90 Ann Leighton, *Early American Gardens "for Meate or Medicine"* (Amherst: University of Massachusetts Press, 1986), 263.

91 Kathryn Roberts, "A Comparison of Chilled Cabbage Leaves and Chilled Gelpaks in Reducing Breast Engorgement," *Journal of Human Lactation* 11, no. 1 (1995), 17–20.

92 Sheila Humphrey, *The Nursing Mother's Herbal* (Minneapolis, MN: Fairview Press, 2003), 149.

93 George Wood and Franklin Bache, *The Dispensatory of the United States of America* (Philadelphia: Grigg & Elliot, 1839), 860. Lloyd Library, Cincinnati, OH.

94 M. Grieve, *A Modern Herbal* (New York: Dover Publications, 1971), 569.

95 Martha Libster, *Delmar's Integrative Herb Guide for Nurses* (Albany, NY: Delmar Thomson Learning, 2002), 175.

96 Here again, Sister Matilda demonstrates the requirements for intelligent, judicious nurses to do what today would be called "critical thinking."

97 Poultices, plasters, and compresses were still in use by nurses well into the twentieth century. See nurses' "materia medica" texts, such as B. Harmer, *Text-Book of the Principles and Practice of Nursing* (New York: Macmillan Co., 1924). Denison Library, University of Colorado, and B. Harmer and V. Henderson, *Textbook of the Principles and Practice of Nursing* (New York: Macmillan Co., 1955). All three therapeutic interventions involve the topical application of herbs. Also known as cataplasms, poultices are made with a slurry, or softened paste, of the plant material, which is placed in a cloth and then applied to the skin. Poultices are typically applied warm. A sticky plaster is made from the powder of a plant material that goes directly on the skin. A compress is a topical application in which the plant to be used is decocted or infused in water. A cloth is dipped into the herb water and placed on the skin. Compresses are often used to cool the body but can also be used to warm the body as in the case of a ginger (*Zingiber officinale*) compress.

98 Sister Matilda's reference to bedsores reveals that she wrote her text for those nurses taking care of chronically ill bedridden patients and the elderly.

Bedsores are an example of an ongoing challenge in nursing care.

99   Martha Libster, *Herbal Diplomats: The Contribution of Early American Nurses (1830–1860) to Nineteenth-Century Healthcare Reform and the Botanical Medical Movement*

100 Regina Bechtle, SC, and Judith Metz, SC, eds., and Ellin Kelly, mss. ed., *Elizabeth Bayley Seton: Collected Writings*, 3 vols. (Hyde Park, NY: New City Press, 2000–2006).

101 Mother Mary Xavier Clark, *Instruction on the Care of the Sick*, Archives of Daughters of Charity of St. Vincent de Paul - West Central Province, St. Louis, Mo. (1846), 50.

102 Holy Bible, John 13:1–30.

103 Herold Weiss, "Foot Washing in the Johannine Community," *Novum Testamentum* 21, no. Fasc. 4 (1979): 299.

104 *Louise de Marillac Spiritual Writings: Correspondence and Thoughts*, 291 and 751.

105 Woodward, "Observations on the Medical Treatment of Insanity," 21.

106 Brigham, "The Medical Treatment of Insanity," 353.

107 Child, *The Family Nurse*, 6.

108 Thomas Jefferson et al., *The Life and Selected Writings of Thomas Jefferson* (New York: The Modern library, 1944), 690.

109 Martha Libster, "Integrative Care—Product and Process: Considering the Three T's of Timing, Type and Tuning," *Complementary Therapies in Nursing and Midwifery.* 9, no. 1 (2003). 1–4.

110 Injections was the name used in the nineteenth century referring to enemas. Sister Matilda, like many women of her time, ascribed to the use of water in healing. Hydropathy or "water cure" was very popular in mid-century. Some of the health reformers who led the water-cure movement in America, most notably Mary Gove Nichols, were also associated with the free-love movement, something with which the sisters would not have been aligned. Jean L. Silver-Isenstadt, *Shameless: The Visionary Life of Mary Gove Nichols* (Baltimore: Johns Hopkins University Press, 2002).

111 Brigham, "The Medical Treatment of Insanity," 355.

112 Brittania metal is a silverlike alloy of tin, antimony, and copper first used in 1770.

113 John Barlow, "On Man's Power over Himself to Prevent or Control Insanity," *American Journal of Insanity* 1 (1845), 289–319.

114 Ibid.: 293.

115 Amariah Brigham, "Dr. William Stokes, of the Mount Hope Institution, near Baltimore, Md. And the American Journal of Insanity," *American Journal of Insanity* 5, no. 3 (1849): 276. Archives of the American Psychiatric Association.

116 Ibid.: 275.

117 *Coskery, Cradle of Mount Hope: Historical Account of Mt. St. Vincent Hospital / Mount Hope Retreat*, 13–14.

118 James Miller, Case Notes—Josiah Manty, 1833–1837. The Alms-House Medical Records, H. Furlong Baldwin Library, Maryland Historical Society, Baltimore, MD, MS# 2474.

119 Brigham, "Dr. William Stokes, of the Mount Hope Institution, near Baltimore, Md. and the American Journal of Insanity," 275.

120 William Stokes, *Fourth Annual Report of the Mount Hope Institution for the Year 1846*, 1847, Archives of the Daughters of Charity, St. Joseph's Provincial House, Emmitsburg, MD, 33.

121 Edward Brown, "What Shall We Do with the Inebriate?" Asylum Treatment and the Disease Concept of Alcoholism in the Late Nineteenth Century," *Journal of the History of the Behavioral Sciences* 21, no. January (1985), 48–59.

122 This is an example of the type of care that crossed gender boundaries in mid-nineteenth-century society. Sister Matilda expected the Daughter-Nurses to be present for the majority of the disrobing of the patient so that they could do a thorough safety inspection. The early DC Nurses did not typically delegate important tasks to their hired patient attendants.

123 E. K. Hunt, "Statistics of Suicides in the United States," *American Journal of Insanity* 1, no. January (1845): 229. Archives of the American Psychiatric Association.

124 Ruby Martinez and Dana Murphy-Parker, "Examining the Relationship of Addiction Education and Beliefs of Nursing Students toward Persons with Alcohol Problems," *Archives of Psychiatric Nursing* 17, no. 4 (2003), 156–64. Dana Murphy-Parker and Ruby Martinez, "Nursing Students' Personal Experiences Involving Alcohol Problems," *Archives of Psychiatric Nursing* 19, no. 3 (2005), 150–58.

125 This is the only reference in *Advices* to the "Daughters of Charity." Sister Matilda also uses the term "Sister of Charity" on page 34. Though the terms "Sister of Charity" and "Daughter of Charity" were often used interchangeably from the earliest Community documents until well into the twentieth century, this evidence could date the writing of the text to the post-1850 merger with France. Most of the evidence suggests otherwise.

126 Holy Bible, Matthew 12:20. "A bruised reed he will not break, a smoldering wick he will not quench, until he brings justice to victory."

127 *Imitation of Christ* by Thomas à Kempis was first published in the early fifteenth century and was widely read by many Catholics, as well as by the Sisters and Daughters of Charity, in the nineteenth century.

128 Francis Stribling, "Qualifications and Duties of Attendants on the Insane," *American Journal of Insanity* 9, no. 2 (1852): 97–103. Archives of the American Psychiatric Association.

129 Henri Falret, "On the Construction and Organization of Establishments for the Insane," *American Journal of Insanity* 10, no. 4 (1854): 405–35. Archives of the American Psychiatric Association.

130 See #11 Obedience in Coste and de Paul, *Saint Vincent de Paul: Correspondence,*

Conferences, Documents, 9:60.

131 Ibid., 9:56.

132 Sisters of Charity, *The Rule of 1812: Regulations for the Society of Sisters of Charity in the United States of America* (1812). Archives of the Daughters of Charity, St. Joseph's Provincial House, Emmitsburg, MD.

133 Article I in ibid.

134 Harmer, *Text-Book of the Principles and Practice of Nursing*, 207.

135 William Weaver, *Sauer's Herbal Cures: America's First Book of Botanical Healing, 1762–1778* (New York: Routledge, 2001), 170.

136 Felter and Lloyd, *King's American Dispensatory*, 1000.

137 Holy Bible, 1 Pt 5:8: "Be sober and vigilant. Your opponent the devil is prowling around like a roaring lion looking for (someone) to devour."

138 Holy Bible, Romans 8:28.

139 Holy Bible, Mark 6:13.

140 Holy Bible, Luke 10:25–37.

141 See chapter 3 for discussion about restraints.

142 This criterion is still used in current psychiatric care.

143 Holy Bible, Phil 1:8, "For God is my witness, how I long after you all in the bowels of Jesus Christ."

144 It was tradition for the Daughters to rejoice in the opportunity to nurse and minister to the sick poor and the insane. Vincent de Paul said to the DC in 1643, "What a happiness, Sisters, to serve the person of Our Lord in His poor members! He has told you that He will consider this service as done to himself." #15 "Explanation Of the Rule," In Coste and de Paul, *Saint Vincent de Paul: Correspondence, Conferences, Documents*, 9:96. Cf. 1 Corinthians 2:16.

145 Note that Sister Matilda added common language in parentheses next to the anatomical name for the "spine" and the medical instrument "scarificator." This will be discussed later, as she does this quite a bit in her section on nursing and sickroom management.

146 *Louise de Marillac Spiritual Writings: Correspondence and Thoughts*, 763.

147 Sally Hardy et al., "Re-Defining Nursing Expertise in the United Kingdom," *Nursing Science Quarterly* 19, no. 3 (2006), 260–64.

148 Ibid.: 262.

149 Ibid.

150 Ibid.

151 Stokes, *Fourth Annual Report of the Mount Hope Institution for the Year 1846*, 14.

152 W. G. Read in Stokes, *First Annual Report of the Physician of the Mount Saint Vincent's Hospital for 1843*.

153 Another example of early nursing theory can be found in the "Careful Nursing" of Irish nurse Catherine McAuley (1778–1841). See Therese

Meehan, "Careful Nursing: A Model for Contemporary Nursing Practice," *Journal of Advanced Nursing* 44, no. 1 (2003), 99–107.

154 Luther Christman, "Who Is a Nurse?" *Image: Journal of Nursing Scholarship* 30, no. 3 (1998), 211–14.

155 Sister Matilda's use of the term "Hospital" here may suggest that this part of or all of *Advices* was written when Mount Hope was first being established and was referred to as St. Vincent's Hospital.

156 Being disappointed in love is one of the common moral causes of insanity listed in the sisters' registers.

157 Sister Matilda is probably assessing for paranoia and psychosis.

158 Sister Matilda makes two assessments related to opiates: one for recreational use and one related to physician prescription.

159 Sister Matilda recounts an episode of a patient who committed suicide while in their care.

160 Diane Price Herndl, *Invalid Women: Figuring Feminine Illness in American Fiction and Culture, 1840–1940* (Chapel Hill: University of North Carolina Press, 1993), 85.

161 She was most likely referring to popular physician writers such as Philippe Pinel, Jean-Étienne Esquirol, William Tuke, and possibly American physician Samuel Woodward. She may also be referring to Saint Vincent de Paul, who wrote: "Then, Sisters, you should nurse those poor sick with great charity and gentleness so that they may see you are going to their assistance with a heart filled with compassion for them." #100 "To Four Sisters Who Were Sent To Calais," In Coste and de Paul, *Saint Vincent de Paul: Correspondence, Conferences, Documents*, 10:445.

162 This was the proper medical term used to describe those who were mentally retarded, especially from birth.

163 Sister Matilda again demonstrates *how and when* kindness should be used as a therapeutic intervention.

164 Holy Bible, Isaiah 42:1–4: "Not crying out, not shouting, not making his voice heard in the street. A bruised reed he shall not break, and a smoldering wick he shall not quench, until he establishes justice on the earth; the coastlands will wait for his teaching."

165 Holy Bible, Exodus 23:20, "See, I am sending an angel before you, to guard you on the way and bring you to the place I have prepared." Angels in the Catholic tradition are God's messengers to humankind. They are God's instruments who communicate the will of God.

166 Sister Matilda is most likely alluding to the parable of the Good Samaritan in which the evangelist describes what it means to be a good neighbor and render works of mercy to persons in need. Jesus instructs his disciples to "Go and do likewise." See Luke 10:29–37.

167 202. "De La Douceur," In Pierre Coste, *Saint Vincent de Paul: Correspondance, Entretiens, Documents.* (Paris: Lecoffre and Gabaldo, 1924), 12:192.

168 The term "friends" was used in the mid-nineteenth century to refer to significant others such as family and close friends.

169 Holy Bible, 1 Corinthians 3:16.

170 Holy Bible, Luke 6:31.

171 Bandler and Grinder, as cited in John Walter and Jane Peller, *Becoming Solution-Focused in Brief Therapy* (New York: Brunner/Mazel, 1992), 42.

172 Ibid., 204.

173 Rosemary (*Rosmarinus officinalis*) increases blood flow through the coronary artery. Mark Blumenthal, *Bundesinstitut für Arzneimittel und Medizinprodukte* (Germany), and Commission E, *Herbal Medicine Expanded Commission E Monographs* (Newton, MA: Integrative Medicine Communications, 2000).

174 Coffee (*Coffea arabica*) is a botanical example of a narcotic stimulant. Libster, *Delmar's Integrative Herb Guide for Nurses*, 531.

175 Chamomile (*Matricaria recutita*) is a botanical example. Ibid., 402.

176 Rose (*Rosa damascena*) is a botanical example. Ibid., 364.

177 Witch hazel (*Hamamelis virginiana*) is an example. Ibid., 374.

178 A botanical emetic is mustard (*Brassica alba*). Ibid., 169.

179 Elder (*Sambucus nigra*) is a botanical cathartic. Ibid., 278.

180 Coffee (*Coffea arabica*) is a botanical diuretic. Ibid., 528.

181 Horseradish (*Armoracia rusticana*) is a botanical antilithic. Ibid., 482.

182 Yarrow (*Achillea millefolium*) is a diaphoretic. Ibid., 359.

183 Garlic (*Allium sativum*) is a botanical expectorant. Ibid., 287.

184 Libster, *Herbal Diplomats: The Contribution of Early American Nurses (1830–1860) to Nineteenth-Century Healthcare Reform and the Botanical Medical Movement*, 255–261.

185 Ibid.

186 Jacob Bigelow, "Discourse on Self-Limited Diseases," in *Nature in Disease: Illustrated in Various Discourses and Essays* (Boston: Phillips, Sampson, and Company, 1835), 48. Lloyd Library, Cincinnati, OH.

187 Wooster Beach, *The Family Physician, or, the Reformed System of Medicine on Vegetable or Botanic Principles Being a Compendium of the "American Practice" Designed for All Classes*, 4th ed. (New York: Published by the author, 1843), 188. Lloyd Library, Cincinnati, OH.

188 Child, *The Family Nurse*, 12.

189 Martha. Libster, "Elements of Care: Nursing Environmental Theory in Historical Context," *Holistic Nursing Practice* 22, no. 3 (2008), 160–70.

190 Nightingale, *Notes on Nursing: What It Is and What It Is Not*, 110.

191 Buchan, *Domestic Medicine; or, the Family Physician Being an Attempt to Render the Medical Art More Generally Useful, by Shewing People What Is in Their Own Power Both with Respect to the Prevention and Cure of Diseases.*

Chiefly Calculated to Recommend a Proper Attention to Regimen and Simple Medicines.

192 Gunn, *Gunn's Domestic Medicine or Poor Man's Friend in the Hours of Affliction, Pain and Sickness.*

193 Editors, "Critical Review of Dewees' *A Practice of Physic,*" London Medical and Surgical Journal, 5, no. 26 (1830): 91. Google Books.

194 John Scudder, *Domestic Medicine or Home Book of Health: A Popular Treatise on Anatomy, Physiology, Hygiene, Materia Medica, Surgery, Practice of Medicine, and Nursing,* vol. 1 (Cincinnati: J. R. Hawley & Co., 1865), 471–580, Lloyd Library, Cincinnati, OH.

195 William Dewees, *A Practice of Physic: Comprising Most of the Diseases Not Treated in "Diseases of Females" and "Diseases of Children"* (Philadelphia: Carey, Lea & Blanchard, 1833), 22. Laupus Library—History Collection, East Carolina University.

196 Ibid.

197 Ibid.

198 Elizabeth Mott, *The Ladies Medical Oracle; or, Mrs. Mott's Advice to Young Females, Wives, and Mothers Being a Non-Medical Commentary on the Cause, Prevention, and Cure of Diseases of the Female Frame Together with an Explanation of Her System of European Vegetable Medicine for the Cure of Diseases and the Patent Medicated Champoo Baths* (Boston: Samuel N. Dickinson, 1834). Schlesinger Library, Cambridge, MA.

199 Ruth J. Abram, *Send Us a Lady Physician: Women Doctors in America, 1835–1920* (New York: Norton, 1985), 75.

200 Dewees, *A Practice of Physic: Comprising Most of the Diseases Not Treated in "Diseases of Females" and "Diseases of Children,"* 26.

201 Ibid.

202 Ibid., 27.

203 Ibid.

204 Sisters of Charity, *The Rule of 1812: Regulations for the Society of Sisters of Charity in the United States of America.*

205 Dewees, *A Practice of Physic: Comprising Most of the Diseases Not Treated in "Diseases of Females" and "Diseases of Children,"* 28.

206 Ibid., 35.

207 These are Dewees' exact words.

208 Dewees, *A Practice of Physic: Comprising Most of the Diseases Not Treated in "Diseases of Females" and "Diseases of Children,"* 31.

209 Sister Matilda substitutes the word "vomited" for Dewees' words, "regurgitate the superabundant draughts."

210 Dewees, *A Practice of Physic: Comprising Most of the Diseases Not Treated in "Diseases of Females" and "Diseases of Children,"* 32.

211 Libster, *Herbal Diplomats: The Contribution of Early American Nurses (1830–*

1860) to Nineteenth-Century Healthcare Reform and the Botanical Medical Movement.

212 *Louise de Marillac Spiritual Writings: Correspondence and Thoughts.*

213 Libster, *Herbal Diplomats: The Contribution of Early American Nurses (1830–1860) to Nineteenth-Century Healthcare Reform and the Botanical Medical Movement.*

214 Dewees, *A Practice of Physic: Comprising Most of the Diseases Not Treated in "Diseases of Females" and "Diseases of Children,"* 32.

215 Ibid., 33.

216 Ibid.

217 Ibid.

218 Dewees wrote "tenacious" slime, not sticky.

219 Dewees, *A Practice of Physic: Comprising Most of the Diseases Not Treated in "Diseases of Females" and "Diseases of Children,"* 34.

220 Ibid.

221 Ibid., 38.

222 Ibid., 39.

223 Ibid., 40.

224 Ibid., 42.

225 Dorothea Orem, *Nursing Concepts of Practice*, 6th ed. (St. Louis, MO: Mosby, 2001). Dorothea Orem (1914–2007), an American nurse scholar, was inspired by her aunts, who were Daughters of Charity, one a nurse and the other a pharmacist. Susan Taylor, "The Development of Self-Care Deficit Nursing Theory: An Historical Analysis," *Self Care and Dependent-Care Nursing* 15, no. 1 (2007), 22–25.

226 Dewees, *A Practice of Physic: Comprising Most of the Diseases Not Treated in "Diseases of Females" and "Diseases of Children,"* 45.

227 Spirits of hartshorn is a volatile alkali originally prepared from the horns of a stag or hart, but later prepared from other substances. It is now referred to as spirits of ammonia. Beecher and Stowe, *The American Woman's Home or, Principles of Domestic Science: Being a Guide to the Formation and Maintenance of Economical, Healthful, Beautiful, and Christian Homes*, 352.

228 According to the Dewees section on blistering, the substitution of adhesive plasters for bandages was a new improvement in 1833 when the book was written.

229 This is one rule and deviation that Sister Matilda and Dr. Dewees agreed upon.

230 Basilicon ointment was made of fresh lard, pine resin, and yellow wax. Child, *The Family Nurse*, 129.

231 Simple cerate was made from fresh lard, white wax, and spermaceti. Ibid. Spermaceti is the wax from the head of a sperm whale.

232 Slippery elm (*Ulmus fulva*) is a mucilaginous plant whose bark has been used topically and internally for centuries especially by First Nation peoples such as the Mohawk and Cherokee.

233 Vinegar's properties as an antiseptic have been well known for centuries. One young scientist in a 2006 state fair in California found that all vinegars are good disinfectants but apple cider vinegar worked best to prevent bacterial growth. See http://www.usc.edu/CSSF/History/2006/Projects/J1435.pdf . Web site accessed April 2006. Louise de Marillac recommended that the early Daughters use it when they went into homes of the sick. She said the sisters should rub it on their noses and temples. *Louise de Marillac Spiritual Writings: Correspondence and Thoughts*, 640. Apple cider vinegar is still used in folk medicine and self-care practices in the United States.

234 Child, *The Family Nurse*, 28.

235 Dewees, *A Practice of Physic: Comprising Most of the Diseases Not Treated in "Diseases of Females" and "Diseases of Children,"* 87.

236 Coskery, Correspondence: Letter to Rev. Henry B. Coskery on the Death of Archbishop Samuel Eccleston of Baltimore.

237 Felix Coskery, "Fever" (University of Maryland, 1836). Health Sciences and Human Services Library, University of Maryland.

238 Daughters of Charity, *Lives of the Deceased Sisters* (Emmitsburg, MD: 1870), 12. Archives of the Daughters of Charity, St. Joseph's Provincial House, Emmitsburg, MD.

Chapter 6 – Endnotes

1 Daughters of Charity, *Lives of Deceased Sisters* (Emmitsburg, Maryland: 1870–1879), 22. Archives of the Daughters of Charity, St. Joseph's Provincial House, Emmitsburg, MD.

2 Ibid.

3 Daughters of Charity. Provincial Annals. Archives of the Daughters of Charity, Saint Joseph's Provincial House, Emmitsburg, MD 7–8. 1867:8.

4 Ibid.

5 Remarks on Sister Matilda Coskery in Daughters of Charity, *Lives of Deceased Sisters*, 12.

6 Ibid.

7 Ibid., 14.

8 Daughters of Charity, *Lives of the Deceased Sisters* (Emmitsburg, MD: Daughters of Charity, 1870). Archives of the Daughters of Charity, St. Joseph's Provincial House, Emmitsburg, MD.

9 The earliest religious women's orders in America were comprised of white women, according to the *Catholic Almanac*, a journal that served as a central public record for the activities of the Catholic Church. They were the

Carmelites of Port Tobacco, Maryland; the Ladies of the Visitation; and the Sisters of Charity at Emmitsburg (Catholic Church of the United States, *The United States Catholic Almanac, or, Laity's Directory for the Year*. University of Notre Dame Library, Microfilm Collection. 1817, 1822, 1833-ongoing). The Sisters of Providence, a community of "colored women," was established in Baltimore in 1829 (Catholic Church of the United States: 1840, 94). Earlier in the century the Congregation of the Mission (called the Vincentian priests and brothers, who began their work in St. Louis), and especially one of the original American missionaries, Felix de Andreis, had determined not to become slave holders. The priests had actually wanted to recruit free blacks as brothers but realized that the prejudice in American society was too great for a white man to associate with or work beside a black man. (*The American Vincentians: A Popular History of the Congregation of the Mission in the United States, 1815–1987*, ed. John Rybolt [New York: New City Press, 1988], 37.) De Andreis, before dying in 1820, evangelized both free and slave blacks despite the views of locals. He was succeeded by Joseph Rosati, who purchased slaves, as did brothers in other orders for work in the seminaries.

10 Daughters of Charity. *Mother Ann Simeon* (Louisa A. Norris) #5 Provincial Superior. Archives of the Daughters of Charity, St. Joseph's Provincial House, Emmitsburg, MD.

11 Ibid.

12 Sister Matilda Coskery. *Civil War Notes*. 1866. Archives of the Daughters of Charity, St. Joseph's Provincial House, Emmitsburg, MD.63

13 Ibid.

14 Pere Louis-Hippolyte Gache and Cornelius Buckley (trans.), *A Frenchman, a Chaplain, a Rebel* (Chicago: Loyola University Press, 1981), 148.

15 Ibid., 147.

16 Kate Cumming, *A Journal of Hospital Life in the Confederate Army of Tennessee*, 1866, as cited in Mary Denis Maher, *To Bind Up the Wounds: Catholic Sister Nurses in the U.S. Civil War* (New York: Greenwood Press, 1989).

17 Pest House Medical Museum, Old City Cemetery, Lynchburg, VA. http://www.gravegarden.org/

18 Mary Ashton Rice Livermore, *My Story of the War: A Woman's Narrative of Four Years Personal Experience as Nurse in the Union Army, and in Relief Work at Home, in Hospitals, Camps, and at the Front During the War of the Rebellion. With Anecdotes, Pathetic Incidents, and Thrilling Reminiscences Portraying the Lights and Shadows of Hospital Life and the Sanitary Service of the War* (Hartford, CT: A. D. Worthington and Company, 1889), 247.

19 Jane Hoge, *The Boys in Blue: Heroes of the "Rank and File"* (New York: E. B. Treat & Co., 1867), 280. Google Books.

20 Daughters of Charity. Provincial Annals. 1867–71, 7–8.

21 Ibid.. 1867–71, 7.

22 Ibid.1867–71, 8.

23 Madge Preston and Virginia Beauchamp, *A Private War: Letters and Diaries of Madge Preston, 1862–1867* (New Brunswick, NJ: Rutgers University Press, 1987), 243.

24 Ibid., 240.

25 Sister Bernard Boyle, Mother Ann Simeon's Death, 1866, Archives of the Daughters of Charity, St. Joseph's Provincial House, Emmitsburg, MD, 8.

26 Ibid.

27 "Notes on the Life of Our Beloved Mother Ann Simeon Norris," in Daughters of Charity, *Lives of Deceased Sisters Prior to 1969* (Emmitsburg, MD: 1866–1868), 11, Archives of the Daughters of Charity, St. Joseph's Provincial House, Emmitsburg, MD.

28 Ibid., 13.

29 Louis Abelly, *The Life of the Venerable Servant of God Vincent de Paul*, 3 vols. (New Rochelle, NY: New City Press, 1993; originally published 1664 in French), 3: 117.

30 Daughters of Charity, *Lives of the Deceased Sisters.*

31 Remarks on Sister Matilda Coskery in ibid.

32 Henri Ramiere, *The Apostleship of Prayer: A Holy League of Christian Hearts United with the Heart of Jesus* (Baltimore, MD: John Murphy, 1866).

33 Daughters of Charity, *Lives of the Deceased Sisters.*

34 Sister Matilda Coskery, *Cradle of Mount Hope: Historical Account of Mt. St. Vincent Hospital / Mount Hope Retreat*, n.d., Archives of the Daughters of Charity, St. Joseph's Provincial House, Emmitsburg, MD, #11-2-39.59.

35 The Catholic Health Association currently represents more than 2,000 Catholic healthcare organizations and 617 hospitals. Sister Carol Keehan, Daughter of Charity, currently serves as the CEO and president. She is the third religious woman to hold that position in the association's history.

36 Barbra Mann Wall, *Unlikely Entrepreneurs: Catholic Sisters and the Hospital Marketplace, 1865–1925, Women, Gender, and Health* (Columbus: Ohio State University Press, 2005), 189.

37 Ambrose Byrne, "History of The Seton Institute, Baltimore, Maryland and Its Affiliate School of Nursing Conducted by the Daughters of Charity of St. Vincent de Paul in the Eastern Province of the United States" (The Catholic University of America, 1950), 53.

38 Ibid., 57.

39 Sister Maureen Delahunt, DC, and Sister Annina Sharper, DC, July 3, 2007.

40 #85, "Conference on Serving the Sick and the Care of One's Health," in Pierre Coste, CM, and Vincent de Paul, *Saint Vincent de Paul: Correspondence, Conferences, Documents*, ed. and trans. Jacqueline Kilar, DC, and Marie Poole, DC. 14 vols. (New York: New City Press, 1985–2008), 10: 268. Archives of the Daughters of Charity, St. Joseph's Provincial House, Emmitsburg, MD.

41 The Daughters of Charity owned and administered hospitals until recently.

They are still involved in the sponsorship and governance of many hospitals and are part of the governance structure of Ascension Health, which they cofounded.

42 Catholic Almanac as cited in Ann Doyle, "Nursing by Religious Orders in the United States: Part 2, 1841–1870," *American Journal of Nursing* 29, no. 8 (1929): 963.

43 The Daughters of Charity also created hospital-based training programs. The first was the School of Nursing at Sisters' Hospital in Buffalo, New York, in 1889.

44 Kate Cumming, *Gleanings from Southland* (Birmingham, AL: Roberts & Son, 1895), 87.

45 Ibid., 88.

46 As cited in Maher, *To Bind Up the Wounds: Catholic Sister Nurses in the U.S. Civil War*, 135.

47 Catharine Esther Beecher and Harriet Beecher Stowe, *The American Woman's Home or, Principles of Domestic Science: Being a Guide to the Formation and Maintenance of Economical, Healthful, Beautiful, and Christian Homes* (Piscataway, NJ: Rutgers University Press, 2002; originally published in 1869); Livermore, *My Story of the War: A Woman's Narrative of Four Years Personal Experience as Nurse in the Union Army, and in Relief Work at Home, in Hospitals, Camps, and at the Front During the War of the Rebellion. With Anecdotes, Pathetic Incidents, and Thrilling Reminiscences Portraying the Lights and Shadows of Hospital Life and the Sanitary Service of the War.*

48 Editorial, "Sick Room Needs," *The Eclectic Medical Journal* LV, no. 10 (1895): 589. Lloyd Library, Cincinnati, OH.

49 Martha Libster, *Herbal Diplomats: The Contribution of Early American Nurses (1830–1860) to Nineteenth-Century Healthcare Reform and the Botanical Medical Movement* (Thornton, CO: Golden Apple Publications, 2004).

50 Arthur Lomas, "As It Was in the Beginning: A History of the University Hospital. Includes Reprints of the 1823 Original Correspondence between Rev. John Dubois on Behalf of the Sisters of Charity and Dr. Granville Pattison," *Bulletin of the School of Medicine University of Maryland* 23, no. 4 (1939): 182. University of Maryland Health Sciences and Human Services Library, Baltimore, MD.

51 *Pioneer Healers: The History of Women Religious in American Health Care*, ed. M. Ursula Stepsis and Dolores Ann Liptak (New York: Crossroad, 1989), 28.

52 Ibid., 148. Those Communities of Sisters of Charity that separated from Emmitsburg in 1846 and 1852 retained the name Sisters of Charity of Vincent de Paul.

53 Lavinia L. Dock and Isabel Maitland Stewart, *A Short History of Nursing from the Earliest Times to the Present Day*, 2nd ed. (New York, London: G. P. Putnam's Sons, 1925), 147.

54 Ibid., 148.

55 Patricia D'Antonio, "The Legacy of Domesticity," *Nursing History Review* 1

(1993): 233.

56 Anne Marie Rafferty, *The Politics of Nursing Knowledge* (London: Routledge, 1996), 9.

57 D'Antonio, "The Legacy of Domesticity," 239.

58 Eva MacDougall, "Review: A Short History of Nursing," *American Journal of Public Health* 22, no. 3 (1932).

59 Oliver Sacks, "Scotoma: Forgetting and Neglect in Science," in Robert B. Silvers, *Hidden Histories of Science*, 1st ed. (New York: New York Review of Books, 1995).

60 As cited in ibid., 160.

61 Ibid., 161.

62 Mary Poovey, *Uneven Developments: The Ideological Work of Gender in Mid-Victorian England, Women in Culture and Society* (Chicago: University of Chicago Press, 1988), 174.

63 S. Nelson and S. Gordon, "The Rhetoric of Rupture: Nursing as a Practice with a History?" *Nursing Outlook* 52, no. 5 (2004).

64 Anna Jameson, *Sisters of Charity and the Communion of Labour: A Lecture Delivered Privately February 14, 1855 and Printed by Desire* (London: Longman, Brown, Green, Longmans, and Roberts, 1859). Google Books.

65 Ibid., 56.

66 Ibid., 89.

67 Ibid., 90.

68 Ibid., 84.

69 Ibid., 61.

70 Ibid., 50.

71 Mary Adelaide Nutting and Lavinia L. Dock, *A History of Nursing; the Evolution of Nursing Systems from the Earliest Times to the Foundation of the First English and American Training Schools for Nurses* (New York and London: G. P. Putnam's Sons, 1907), 363.

72 Ibid., 329–34.

73 Ibid., 334.

74 Ibid., 367.

75 Samuel D. Gross, Report of the Committee on the Training of Nurses, 1869, American Medical Association Archives, Chicago, 163.

76 Ibid.

77 Ibid.

78 Ibid., 165.

79 Brian Abel-Smith as cited in Susan Reverby, *Ordered to Care: The Dilemma of American Nursing, 1850–1945* (Cambridge, NY: Cambridge University Press, 1987), 22.

80 Ibid., 23.

81 Sharon Radzyminski, "Legal Parameters of Alternative-Complementary Modalities in Nursing Practice," *Nursing Clinics of North America* 42, no. 2 (2007).

82 Nutting and Dock, *A History of Nursing; the Evolution of Nursing Systems from the Earliest Times to the Foundation of the First English and American Training Schools for Nurses*, 61.

83 Ibid., 100.

84 Ibid., 439.

85 Ibid., 168.

86 Lavinia L. Dock, "History of the Reform in Nursing at Bellevue Hospital," *American Journal of Nursing* 2, no. 2 (1901): 92.

87 Ibid., 97. This matron model was the same model that Dr. Buttolph had suggested for asylums in 1847. See Chapter 4.

88 Photo of Sister Helen in ibid.

89 See Chapter 1 Endnote 58

90 Florence Nightingale, "Nightingale Papers Vol X Autobiographical and Other Memoranda, 34–196," (British Library 43402: 1845–1860), 99–103.

91 Letter to her father, February 2, 1862, Florence Nightingale, "Nightingale Papers: Correspondence with Her Parents," (British Library 45790: 1850–1869).

92 Nightingale wrote, "The wound is too deep for the Ch. [church] of England to heal. I belong as little to the Ch. of England as to that of Rome—or rather my heart belongs as much to the Catholic Ch. as to that of England. The only difference is that the former insists peremptorily upon my believing what I cannot believe. . . ." See Letter to Rev. Henry Manning, 1982 in Florence Nightingale, Martha Vicinus, and Bea Nergaard, *Ever Yours, Florence Nightingale Selected Letters* (Cambridge, MA: Harvard University Press, 1990), 58.

93 Barbara Montgomery Dossey, *Florence Nightingale Mystic, Visionary, Healer* (Springhouse, PA: Springhouse Corp, 2000), Florence Nightingale, Michael D. Calabria, and Janet Macrae, *Suggestions for Thought* (Philadelphia: University of Pennsylvania Press, 1994).

94 Florence Nightingale, Writings, 1851–1853, British Library #43402, Florence Nightingale Papers, vol. X.

95 Correspondence of Florence Nightingale, British Library, 45796:ff 39–42 as cited in Nightingale, Vicinus, and Nergaard, *Ever Yours, Florence Nightingale Selected Letters*, 68.

96 Ibid., 70.

97 Nightingale, Writings, 81.

98 Florence Nightingale, *Notes on Nursing: What It Is and What It Is Not* (Edinburgh, Scotland: Churchill Livingstone, 1980; originally published 1859), 112.

99 Charles E. Rosenberg, *The Care of Strangers: The Rise of America's Hospital System* (New York: Basic Books, 1987), 222.

100 Paula Baker, "The Domestication of Politics: Women and American Political Society, 1780–1920," *American Historical Review* 89, no. 3 (1984): 644.

101 Ibid., 637.

102 Letter to Edwin Chadwick, July 9, 1866, in Nightingale, Vicinus, and Nergaard, *Ever Yours, Florence Nightingale Selected Letters*, 271.

103 Editor, "Wanted-Trained Nurses for the Middle Class," *Journal of the American Medical Association*, no. July 10 (1909).

104 Poovey, *Uneven Developments: The Ideological Work of Gender in Mid-Victorian England*, 169.

105 Nightingale, *Notes on Nursing: What It Is and What It Is Not*, 111.

106 Reverby, *Ordered to Care: The Dilemma of American Nursing, 1850–1945*, 65.

107 Barbara Melosh, *"The Physician's Hand": Work Culture and Conflict in American Nursing* (Philadelphia: Temple University Press, 1982), 19.

108 Lazar Greenfield, "Doctors and Nurses: A Troubled Partnership," *Annals of Surgery* 230, no. 3 (1999): 286.

109 Ibid.

110 C. Fay Raines, Correspondence from American Association of Colleges of Nursing to American Medical Association Representatives Dr. David Lichtman and Dr. Craig Anderson, June 11, 2008.

111 Adele Pike, "Moral Outrage and Moral Discourse in Nurse-Physician Collaboration," *Journal of Professional Nursing* 7, no. 6 (1991): 361.

112 Elaine Larson, "The Impact of Physician-Nurse Interaction on Patient Care," *Holistic Nursing Practice* 13, no. 2 (1999), Gina Rollins, "Medical Errors, Poor Communication Undermine Quality of Care, Patient Satisfaction," *Report on Medical Guidelines & Outcomes Research* 13, no. 10 (2002), Merrick Zwarenstein and Scott Reeves, "Working Together but Apart: Barriers and Routes to Nurse-Physician Collaboration," *Joint Commission Journal on Quality Improvement* 28, no. 5 (2002).

113 Arlene Wynbeek Keeling, *Nursing and the Privilege of Prescription, 1893–2000, Women, Gender, and Health* (Columbus: Ohio State University Press, 2007), 132.

114 Letter #3077 in Pierre Coste, CM, and Vincent de Paul, *Saint Vincent De Paul: Correspondence, Conferences, Documents*, ed. Jacqueline Kilar, DC, Marie Poole, DC, et al., 14 vols. (New York: New City Press, 1985–2008), 8:277. Archives of the Daughters of Charity, St. Joseph's Provincial House, Emmitsburg, MD.

115 In seeking support for their human services, the Daughters also forged new legal ground. See *Providence Hospital* Law Suit; 175 US, 295; 20 Sup. Ct.. The Honorable Thaddeus Stevens was a friend of the Daughters of Charity at Providence Hospital during its early days. Appropriations in 1866 ($19,700) and again in 1868 ($30,000) were passed by Congress with his help and influence. Stevens was also responsible for the annual receipt of additional appropriations for the hospital for the care of transient medical indigents.

Those not in sympathy with such governmental support to Providence challenged the constitutionality of the congressional appropriations by bringing suit to prevent the expenditure of federal funds by the Daughters of Charity. The case was finally settled by the Supreme Court in 1898, which ruled in favor of the Daughters of Charity. This is a landmark decision that paved the way for federal funds to be received by faith-based organizations with religious sponsorship for the provision of human services rather than promotion of religion. (See Archives of the Daughters of Charity, St. Joseph's Provincial House, Emmitsburg, MD, 11-23-3-8, *1861–1961. Providence Hospital*, "Building Programs—Congressional Help").

116 Therese Meehan, "Careful Nursing: A Model for Contemporary Nursing Practice," *Journal of Advanced Nursing* 44, no. 1 (2003): 100.

117 Ibid.

118 See Rosemarie Rizzo Parse, *Man-Living-Health: A Theory of Nursing* (New York: Wiley, 1981), Jean Watson, *Caring Science as Sacred Science* (Philadelphia: F. A. Davis Co., 2005).

119 Joan Miller, Timothy McConnell, and Troy Klinger, "Religiosity and Spirituality: Influence on Quality of Life and Perceived Patient Self-Efficacy among Cardiac Patients and Their Spouses," *Journal of Religion and Health Online*, no. September (2006).

120 Meredith Wallace et al., "Integrating Spirituality into Undergraduate Nursing Curricula," *International Journal of Nursing Scholarship* 5, no. 1 (2008).

121 Dalai Lama, *Ethics for the New Millennium* (New York: Riverhead Books, 1999), 22.

122 Marie Manthey, "The Timeless Values of Nursing," *Creative Nursing* 6, no. 1 (2000).

123 Isabel Hampton (1860–1910) was a graduate of the Bellevue School in 1883. She was superintendent of the Illinois Training School associated with Cook County Hospital in Chicago before her position at Johns Hopkins. In 1994 Hampton married Dr. Hunter Robb and followed him to Case Western Reserve, where she continued her work in nursing education. She was president of what is now the National League for Nursing and the American Nurses Association and was one of those who founded the *American Journal of Nursing*.

124 Janet Wilson James, "Isabel Hampton and the Professionalization of Nursing in the 1890s," in Morris J. Vogel and Charles E. Rosenberg, *The Therapeutic Revolution: Essays in the Social History of American Medicine* (Philadelphia: University of Pennsylvania Press, 1979).

125 Ibid., 203.

126 Lavinia Dock (1858–1956) trained at Bellevue from 1884–1886. Adelaide Nutting was in the first class at Johns Hopkins training school. She was Isabel Hampton's successor as superintendent at Johns Hopkins.

127 Students studied nursing skills, anatomy, and food chemistry, as well as sick diet and Swedish massage.

128 James, in Vogel and Rosenberg, *The Therapeutic Revolution: Essays in the Social History of American Medicine*, 219.

129 Ibid., 238.

130 Libster, *Herbal Diplomats: The Contribution of Early American Nurses (1830–1860) to Nineteenth-Century Healthcare Reform and the Botanical Medical Movement*, 218.

131 Ibid., 256.

132 Elliot Freidson, *Professionalism: The Third Logic* (Chicago: University of Chicago Press, 2001), 12.

133 Ibid., 95.

134 Editor, "Graduating Exercises," *Michigan Catholic*, October 15 1895, Daughters of Charity Archives, Mater Dei Provincialate, Evansville, IN.

Epilogue – Endnotes

1 Francis de Sales, *Introduction to the Devout Life* (New York: Vintage Books, 2002. Originally published 1609), 4.

2 David Snowdon, *Aging with Grace: What the Nun Study Teaches Us About Leading Longer, Healthier, and More Meaningful Lives* (New York: Bantam Books, 2001).

3 Ibid., 202.

4 M. Scott Peck, *The Different Drum: Community Making and Peace* (New York: Touchstone, 1987).

5 Rosemary Donley, "Nursing at the Crossroads," *Nursing Economics* 14, no. 6 (1996); Marilyn Ray et al., "The Edge of Chaos: Caring and the Bottom Line," *Nursing Management* 26, no. 9 (1995).

6 Simon Gabriel Bruté de Remur and Sister Loyola Law, *Rev. Simon Gabriel Bruté Bishop of Vincennes in His Connection with the Community, 1812–1839* (Emmitsburg, MD: Daughters of Charity, 1886), 86. Archives of the Daughters of Charity, St. Joseph's Provincial House, Emmitsburg, MD.

7 Esther Lucille Brown, *Newer Dimensions of Patient Care: Part 1, The Use of the Physical Environment of the General Hospital for Therapeutic Purposes* (New York: Russell Sage Foundation, 1961), 127.

8 Michael DeSisto et al., "The Maine and Vermont Three-Decade Studies of Serious Mental Illness. Ii. Longitudinal Course Comparisons," *British Journal of Psychiatry* 167, no. 3 (1995).

9 Ralph Waldo Emerson, "Circles," in *Selected Essays, Lectures, and Poems* (New York: Bantam Books, 1990), 200.

10 Vincent de Paul said, "If love of God is the fire, zeal is its flame. If love is the sun, then zeal is its ray. Zeal is what is most pure in the love of God." See Pierre Coste, *Saint Vincent De Paul: Correspondance, Entretiens, Documents* (Paris: Lecoffre and Gabaldo, 1924), 12:307.

Appendix E – Endnotes

1   Web site of the National League for Nursing. http://www.nln.org/aboutnln/PositionStatements/innovation082203.pdf.

2   Bunny McBride, *Women of the Dawn* (Lincoln: University of Nebraska Press, 1999).

3   Ibid.

4   Anna Jameson, *Sisters of Charity and the Communion of Labour: A Lecture Delivered Privately February 14, 1855 and Printed by Desire* (London: Longman, Brown, Green, Longmans, and Roberts, 1859). Google Books.

5   Rebecca J. Tannenbaum, *The Healer's Calling: Women and Medicine in Early New England* (Ithaca, NY: Cornell University Press, 2002).

6   Martha Libster, *Herbal Diplomats: The Contribution of Early American Nurses (1830–1860) to Nineteenth-Century Health Care Reform and the Botanical Medical Movement* (www.GoldenApplePublications.com, 2004).

7   Leavitt, Judith Walzer, and Ronald L. Numbers, eds. *Sickness and Health in America: Readings in the History of Medicine and Public Health*, 3rd ed. (Madison: University of Wisconsin Press, 1997).

8   Margarete Sandelowski, *Devices and Desires: Gender, Technology, and American Nursing* (Chapel Hill: University of North Carolina Press, 2000).

Bibliography

Preface – Bibliography

Carr, Edward Hallett. *What Is History?* New York: Vintage Books, 1961.

Libster, Martha. *Herbal Diplomats: The Contribution of Early American Nurses (1830–1860) to 19th Century Healthcare Reform and the Botanical Medical Movement.* www.GoldenApplePublications.com: Golden Apple Publications, 2004.

Sullivan, Louise, DC. , ed. and trans. *Louise de Marillac Spiritual Writings: Correspondence and Thoughts.* New York: New City Press, 1991.

Introduction – Bibliography

Barmby, Catherine. "On Forbearance, 1839." In *Women and Radicalism in the Nineteenth Century*, edited by Mike Sanders, 312-15. London: Routledge, 2001.

Beecher, Catharine Esther, and Harriet Beecher Stowe. *The American Woman's Home or, Principles of Domestic Science: Being a Guide to the Formation and Maintenance of Economical, Healthful, Beautiful, and Christian Homes.* Piscataway, NJ: Rutgers University Press, 2002.

Catholic Church of the United States. *The United States Catholic Almanac, or, Laity's Directory for the Year.* University of Notre Dame Library, Microfilm Collection. 1817, 1822, 1833–ongoing.

Coskery, Sister Matilda. *Advices Concerning the Sick.* Emmitsburg, MD: Archives of Daughters of Charity, St. Joseph's Provincial House, n.d., c. 1840.

———. *Cradle of Mount Hope: Historical Account of Mt. St. Vincent Hospital/Mount Hope Retreat.* n.d. Archives of the Daughters of Charity, St. Joseph's Provincial House, Emmitsburg, MD, #11-2-39.

Coste, Pierre, CM, and Vincent de Paul. *Regulations for the Sisters of the Angers Hospital.* Edited and translated by Jacqueline Kilar, DC, and Marie Poole, DC. Vol. 13b, *In Correspondence, Conferences, Documents.* New York: New City Press, 1985–2008. Archives of the Daughters of Charity, St. Joseph's Provincial House, Emmitsburg, MD.

Dix, Dorothea. Memorial of Miss D. L. Dix to the Hon. General Assembly in Behalf of the Insane of Maryland. March 5, 1852. Archives of the State of Maryland Web site: http://www.msa.md.gov/.

Gross, Samuel D. *Report of the Committee on the Training of Nurses.* 1869. American Medical Association Archives, Chicago, IL.

Jameson, Anna. *Sisters of Charity and the Communion of Labour: A Lecture Delivered Privately February 14, 1855 and Printed by Desire*. London: Longman, Brown, Green, Longmans, and Roberts, 1859. Google Books.

Lomas, Arthur. "As It Was in the Beginning: A History of the University Hospital." *Bulletin of the School of Medicine, University of Maryland* 23, no. 4 (1939): 182–209. Archives of the University of Maryland Health Sciences & Human Services Library.

Porter, Roy. *The Enlightenment*. 2nd ed. London: Palgrave, 2001.

Ramsey, Matthew. *Medical Fringe & Medical Orthodoxy, 1750–1850*. Edited by W. F. Bynum and Roy Porter. London: Croom Helm, 1987.

Rese, Rt. Rev. Frederick. Correspondence to Mother Rose White at Emmitsburg. November 2, 1834. Daughters of Charity Archives, Mater Dei Provincialate, Evansville, IN.

Stokes, William. *First Annual Report of the Physician of the Mount Saint Vincent's Hospital for 1843*. 1844. Archives of the Daughters of Charity, St. Joseph's Provincial House, Emmitsburg, MD, #11-2-39.

———. *Report of the Mount Hope Institution near Baltimore*. 1846-1888. Archives of the Daughters of Charity, St. Joseph's Provincial House, Emmitsburg, MD, #11-2-39.

Webster, Thomas, Mrs. Parkes, and D. Meredith Reese. *An Encyclopaedia of Domestic Economy: Comprising Such Subjects as Are Most Immediately Connected with Housekeeping; as, the Construction of Domestic Edifices, with the Modes of Warming, Ventilating, and Lighting Them; a Description of the Various Articles of Furniture; a General Account of the Animal and Vegetable Substances Used in Food, and the Methods of Preserving and Preparing Them by Cooking; Making Bread; Materials Employed in Dress and Toilet; Business of the Laundry; Description of the Various Wheel-Carriages; Preservation of Health; Domestic Medicines, &C*. New York: Harper & Brothers, 1845. Old Sturbridge Village Research Library, Sturbridge, MA.

Chapter 1 – Bibliography

The American Vincentians: A Popular History of the Congregation of the Mission in the United States, 1815–1987. Edited by John Rybolt. New York: New City Press, 1988.

Barmby, Catherine. "On Forbearance, 1839." In *Women and Radicalism in the Nineteenth Century*, edited by Mike Sanders, 312–15. London: Routledge, 2001.

Bechtle, Regina, SC, and Judith Metz, SC, eds., and Ellin Kelly, mss. ed. *Elizabeth Bayley Seton: Collected Writings*. 3 vols. Hyde Park, New York: New City Press, 2000–2006.

Beecher, Catharine Esther, and Harriet Beecher Stowe. *The American Woman's Home or, Principles of Domestic Science: Being a Guide to the Formation and Maintenance of Economical, Healthful, Beautiful, and Christian Homes*. Piscataway, NJ: Rutgers University Press, 2002.

Catholic Church of the United States. *The United States Catholic Almanac, or, Laity's Directory for the Year*. University of Notre Dame Library, Microfilm Collection. 1817, 1822, 1833–ongoing.

Coskery, Sister Matilda. *Advices Concerning the Sick.* Emmitsburg, MD: Archives of Daughters of Charity, St. Joseph's Provincial House, n.d., c. 1840.

———. *Cradle of Mount Hope: Historical Account of Mt. St. Vincent Hospital / Mount Hope Retreat.* n.d. Archives of the Daughters of Charity, St. Joseph's Provincial House, Emmitsburg, MD, #11-2-39.

Coste, Pierre, CM, and Vincent de Paul. *Regulations for the Sisters of the Angers Hospital.* Edited and translated by Jacqueline Kilar, DC, and Marie Poole, DC. Vol. 13b, In Correspondence, Conferences, Documents. New York: New City Press, 1985–2008. Archives of the Daughters of Charity, St. Joseph's Provincial House, Emmitsburg, MD.

———. *Rules for Sisters in Parishes.* Edited by Jacqueline Kilar, DC, and Marie Poole, DC. Vol. 10, In Correspondence, Conferences, Documents. New York: New City Press, 1985–2008. Archives of the Daughters of Charity, St. Joseph's Provincial House, Emmitsburg, MD.

———. Saint Vincent de Paul: *Correspondence, Conferences, Documents.* Edited by Jacqueline Kilar, DC, Marie Poole, DC, et al. 14 vols. New York: New City Press, 1985–2008. Archives of the Daughters of Charity, St. Joseph's Provincial House, Emmitsburg, MD.

Daughters of Charity. Act of Incorporation. Archives of the Daughters of Charity, St. Joseph's Provincial House, Emmitsburg, MD.

———. Origins of the Company. 2004. Archives of the Daughters of Charity, St. Joseph's Provincial House, Emmitsburg, MD.

Deville, Raymond. *"Saint Vincent and Saint Louise in Relation to the French School of Spirituality."* Vincentian Heritage 11, no. 1 (1990): 29–44.

Dinan, Susan. *Women and Poor Relief in Seventeenth-Century France: The Early History of the Daughters of Charity.* Burlington, VT: Ashgate, 2006.

Dix, Dorothea. *Memorial of Miss D. L. Dix to the Hon. General Assembly in Behalf of the Insane of Maryland.* March 5, 1852. Archives of the State of Maryland Web site.

Doyle, Ann. "Nursing by Religious Orders in the United States: Part 1, 1809–1840." *American Journal of Nursing* 29, no. 7 (1929): 775–86.

Dubois, John. *Les Sulpician Français En Maryland Avec Elizabeth Seton.* Archives of the Daughters of Charity, St. Joseph's Provincial House, Emmitsburg, MD.

Florence Nightingale's Theology: Essays, Letters, and Journal Notes. Edited by Lynn McDonald. Vol. 3, *The Collected Works of Florence Nightingale.* www.wlupress.wlu.ca: Wilfrid Laurier University Press, 2002.

Gross, Samuel D. *Report of the Committee on the Training of Nurses.* 1869. American Medical Association Archives, Chicago, Illinois.

Hannefin, Daniel. *Daughters of the Church: A Popular History of the Daughters of Charity in the United States, 1809–1987.* New York: New City, 1989.

Jameson, Anna. *Sisters of Charity and the Communion of Labour: A Lecture Delivered Privately February 14, 1855, and Printed by Desire.* London: Longman, Brown, Green, Longmans, and Roberts, 1859. Google Books.

Kelly, Margaret John. "The Relationship of Saint Vincent and Saint Louise from Her Perspective." *Vincentian Heritage* XI, no. 1 (1990): 77–114.

Lomas, Arthur. "As It Was in the Beginning: A History of the University Hospital." *Bulletin of the School of Medicine, University of Maryland* 23, no. 4 (1939): 182–209. Archives of the University of Maryland Health Sciences & Human Services Library.

McNeil, Betty Ann. *The Vincentian Family Tree.* Chicago: Vincentian Studies Institute, 1996.

Nightingale, Florence. Writings. 1851–1853. British Library #43402, Florence Nightingale Papers, vol. X.

Nightingale, Florence, Martha Vicinus, and Bea Nergaard. *Ever Yours, Florence Nightingale Selected Letters.* Cambridge, MA: Harvard University Press, 1990.

"Papers from the Conference on the Age of Gold: The Roots of Our Tradition." *Vincentian Heritage* XI, no. 1 (1990).

Porter, Roy. *The Enlightenment.* 2nd ed. London: Palgrave, 2001.

Ramsey, Matthew. *Medical Fringe & Medical Orthodoxy, 1750–1850.* Edited by W. F. Bynum and Roy Porter. London: Croom Helm, 1987.

Rese, Rt. Rev. Frederick. Correspondence to Mother Rose White at Emmitsburg. November 2, 1834. Daughters of Charity Archives, Mater Dei Provincialate, Evansville, IN.

Sieveking, Amelia W., and Catherine Winkworth. *Life of Amelia Wilhelmina Sieveking from the German Edited with the Author's Sanction.* London: Longman, Green, Longman, Roberts, & Green, 1863. Google Books.

Sisters of Charity. *The Rule of 1812: Regulations for the Society of Sisters of Charity in the United States of America, 1812.* Archives of the Daughters of Charity, St. Joseph's Provincial House, Emmitsburg, MD.

Stokes, William. *First Annual Report of the Physician of the Mount Saint Vincent's Hospital for 1843.* 1844. Archives of the Daughters of Charity, St. Joseph's Provincial House, Emmitsburg, MD, # 11-2-39.

———. *Report of the Mount Hope Institution near Baltimore.* 1846–1888. Archives of the Daughters of Charity, St. Joseph's Provincial House, Emmitsburg, MD, #11-2-39.

Sullivan, Louise, DC. , ed. and trans. *Louise de Marillac Spiritual Writings: Correspondence and Thoughts.* New York: New City Press, 1991.

Udovic, Edward, CM. "Caritas Christi Urget Nos': The Urgent Challenges of Charity in Seventeenth Century France." *Vincentian Heritage* 12, no. 2 (1991): 84–104.

Webster, Thomas, Mrs. Parkes, and D. Meredith Reese. *An Encyclopaedia of Domestic Economy: Comprising Such Subjects as Are Most Immediately Connected with Housekeeping; as, the Construction of Domestic Edifices, with the Modes of Warming, Ventilating, and Lighting Them; a Description of the Various Articles of Furniture; a General Account of the Animal and Vegetable Substances Used in Food, and the Methods of Preserving and Preparing Them by Cooking; Making Bread; Materials Employed in Dress and Toilet;*

Business of the Laundry; Description of the Various Wheel-Carriages; Preservation of Health; Domestic Medicines, &C. New York: Harper & Brothers, 1845. Old Sturbridge Village Research Library, Sturbridge, MA.

Woodham Smith, Cecil. *Florence Nightingale, 1820–1910.* New York: McGraw-Hill, 1951.

Wright, Wendy. "Hearts Have a Secret Language": The Spiritual Friendship of Francis de Sales and Jane de Chantal." *Vincentian Heritage* XI, no. 1 (1990): 45–58.

Chapter 2 – Bibliography

Aiken, William E. A. Letter to Rev. John B. Purcell, February 5, 1833. 1833. Archives at Mount St. Mary's College, Emmitsburg, MD.

American Holistic Nurses Association. *Holistic Nursing: Scope & Standards of Practice.* Silver Spring, MD: Nursesbooks.org, 2007.

Babb, Winston. "French Refugees from Saint-Domingue to the Southern United States: 1791-1810. http://freepages.genealogy.rootsweb.com/~Saintdomingue/Babb%20index.Htm." University of Virginia.

Bayley, James. *Memoirs of the Right Reverend Simon Wm. Gabriel Bruté.* New York: D. & J. Sadlier & Co., 1861. Archives of the Daughters of Charity, St. Joseph's Provincial House, Emmitsburg, MD.

Beam, R. M. Report of the Committee on the Maryland Hospital to the Legislature of Maryland. 1837. M61-70 December, General Assembly.

Bechtle, Regina, SC, and Judith Metz, SC, eds., and Ellin Kelly, mss. ed. *Elizabeth Bayley Seton: Collected Writings.* 3 vols. Hyde Park, NY: New City Press, 2000–2006.

Bradshaw, Herbert. *History of Hampden-Sydney College.* Vol. 1: From the beginnings to the year 1856. Durham, NC: by Author, 1976.

Bramucci, Nancy. 2000–. *Medicine in Maryland, 1752–1920,* http://www.mdhistoryonline. net. In Maryland State Archives. (accessed, 2006–2007).

Bruté de Remur, Simon Gabriel. "Bruté's Conferences with the Sisters of Charity." In *Translations of the Conferences 7-3-1-3:B268,* edited by Rev. Albert Ledoux, 1831. Archives of the Daughters of Charity, St Joseph's Provincial House, Emmitsburg, MD.

Bruté de Remur, Simon Gabriel, and Sister Loyola Law. *Rev. Simon Gabriel Bruté Bishop of Vincennes in His Connection with the Community, 1812–1839.* Emmitsburg, MD: Daughters of Charity, 1886. Archives of the Daughters of Charity, St. Joseph's Provincial House, Emmitsburg, MD.

Byrne, Ambrose. "History of The Seton Institute, Baltimore, Maryland and Its Affiliate School of Nursing Conducted by the Daughters of Charity of St. Vincent de Paul in the Eastern Province of the United States." The Catholic University of America, 1950.

Catholic Church of the United States. *The United States Catholic Almanac, or, Laity's Directory for the Year.* University of Notre Dame Library, Microfilm Collection.

Cauthorn, Henry. *History of St. Francis Xavier Cathedral.* Indianapolis, 1892. The Old Cathedral Library and Museum, Vincennes, IN.

Charity, Daughters of. *Lives of the Deceased Sisters.* Saint Joseph's Provincial House. Emmitsburg, MD: Daughters of Charity, 1870.

Clark, Mother Mary Xavier. *Instruction on the Care of the Sick*, Archives of Daughters of Charity of St. Vincent de Paul—West Central Province, St. Louis, MO., 1846.

Collins, Sister Josephine. Correspondence to Sister Margaret. October 13, 1840. Archives Daughters of Charity, St. Joseph's Provincial House, Emmitsburg, MD 7-10-2 #76.

———. Correspondence to Sister Margaret. November 11, 1840. Archives of the Daughters of Charity, St. Joseph's Provincial House, Emmitsburg, MD 7-10-2 #78.

Coon, Margaret Maria. *Her Spirit Lives: A Sketch of the Life of Catherine Spalding.* Louisville, KY: Sisters of Charity of Nazareth, 2007.

Cordell, Eugene. *University of Maryland 1807–1907.* Vol. 1. New York: Lewis Publishing Company, 1907. University of Maryland Health Sciences and Human Services Library.

Coste, Pierre, CM, and Vincent de Paul. *Saint Vincent de Paul: Correspondence, Conferences, Documents.* Jacqueline Kilar, DC, and Marie Poole, DC, eds. and trans. 14 vols. New York: New City Press, 1985–2008. Archives of the Daughters of Charity, St. Joseph's Provincial House, Emmitsburg, MD.

Cott, Nancy F. *The Bonds of Womanhood: "Woman's Sphere" in New England, 1780–1835.* New Haven, CT: Yale University Press, 1977.

Daughters of Charity. *Articles of Constitution.* Archives of the Daughters of Charity, St. Joseph's Provincial House, Emmitsburg, MD.

———. Chronological Table, 1766–1891. Souvay Collection-III A. DeAndreis-Rosati Memorial Archives, DePaul University, Chicago, IL.

———. Council Minutes. Archives of the Daughters of Charity, St. Joseph's Provincial House, Emmitsburg, MD, #3-3-5.

———. *Lives of Deceased Sisters.* Emmitsburg, Maryland, 1870–1879. Archives of the Daughters of Charity, St. Joseph's Provincial House, Emmitsburg, MD.

———. *Manual of the Daughters of Charity Servants of the Sick Poor in the Hospital and in the Homes of the Poor.* Emmitsburg, MD: Daughters of Charity, 1936. Archives of the Daughters of Charity, St. Joseph's Provincial House, Emmitsburg, MD.

———. *Mother Augustine and Mother Xavier.* Saint Joseph's Provincial House. Emmitsburg, MD: Daughters of Charity, 1938.

———. *Mother Seton—Notes by Rev. Simon Gabriel Bruté Bishop of Vincennes from Original Papers in the Possession of the Community.* 1884. Archives of the Daughters of Charity, St. Joseph's Provincial House, Emmitsburg, MD.

———. Provincial Annals. Archives of the Daughters of Charity, Saint Joseph's Provincial House, Emmitsburg, MD 7-8.

———. Rules and Regulations for the Maryland Hospital, Appendix A. 1833. Archives of the Daughters of Charity, St. Joseph's Provincial House, Emmitsburg, MD.

———. Vow Requests. Archives Daughters of Charity, Saint Joseph's Provincial House, Emmitsburg, MD.

De Sales, Francis. *Introduction to the Devout Life*. New York: Vintage Books, 2002 (Originally published 1609).

Dorsey, Bruce. *Reforming Men and Women: Gender in the Antebellum City*. Ithaca, NY: Cornell University Press, 2002.

Doyle, Ann. "Nursing by Religious Orders in the United States: Part 1, 1809–1840." *American Journal of Nursing* 29, no. 7 (1929): 775–86.

Doyle, Mary Ellen. *Pioneer Spirit: Catherine Spalding, Sister of Charity of Nazareth*. Lexington: University Press of Kentucky, 2006.

Faris, Jessie. "Two Hundred Years of Nursing in Richmond." *American Journal of Nursing* 37, no. 8 (1937): 847–49.

Hannefin, Daniel. *Daughters of the Church: A Popular History of the Daughters of Charity in the United States, 1809–1987*. New York: New City, 1989.

Ladies Physiological Institute. *Records of the Meeting of the Ladies Physiological Institute of Boston and Vicinity*, 1850. Schlesinger Library, Radcliffe Institute for Advanced Study.

Lewis, Jane. *Women and Social Action in Victorian and Edwardian England*. Stanford, CA: Stanford University Press, 1991.

Libster, Martha. *Herbal Diplomats: The Contribution of Early American Nurses (1830–1860) to 19th Century Healthcare Reform and the Botanical Medical Movement*. www. GoldenApplePublications.com: Golden Apple Publications, 2004.

Lomas, Arthur. "As It Was in the Beginning: A History of the University Hospital." *Bulletin of the School of Medicine, University of Maryland* 23, no. 4 (1939): 182–209. Archives of the University of Maryland Health Sciences & Human Services Library.

Lowell, James Russell. "A Virginian in New England Thirty-Five Years Ago, Written on the Basis of Papers Left by Mr. Lucian Minor, (1802–1858) Professor of Law at College of William and Mary, Who Visited Baltimore in 1834." *Atlantic Monthly*, no. October (1870): 482–92.

Maryland Hospital for the Insane. Patient Register. 1834–1872. Maryland State Archives, Annapolis, MD, S184.

Maryland, State of. Maryland State Archives Early State Records Online, Vol. 3173, P. 1531–1532. In *Early State Records Online*, http://www.mdarchives.state.md.us. (accessed July 18, 2006). Vol. 3173, p. 1531–1532.

McGill, Anna. *The Sisters of Charity of Nazareth Kentucky*. New York: The Encyclopedia Press, 1917.

McTaggert, Olympia. Correspondence from Sister Olympia McTaggert to Father Deluol. Archives of the Daughters of Charity, St. Joseph's Provincial House, Emmitsburg, MD.

Medical Case Book, Baltimore Infirmary. Maryland State Archives, MSA SC 4070.

Meline, Mary, and Edward McSweeny. *The Story of the Mountain*. Emmitsburg, MD: Emmitsburg, Chronicle, 1911. Emmitsburg Area Historical Society: http://www.emmitsburg.net/history/index.htm.

Melville, Annabelle M. *Elizabeth Bayley Seton, 1774–1821*. New York: Scribner, 1951.

Merriam-Webster, Inc. *Merriam-Webster's Collegiate Dictionary*. 10th ed. Springfield, MA: Merriam-Webster, 1999.

"Obituary Rev. Fr. Henry Benedictus Coskery." *Catholic Mirror*, March 2, 1872.

Regulations of the Baltimore Infirmary. n.d. Archives of the Daughters of Charity, Saint Joseph's Provincial House, Emmitsburg, MD 11-2-20.

Richard S. Steuart Biographical Sketch. Maryland State Archives, SC 5522-1-29.

Rosenberg, Charles E. *The Cholera Years: The United States in 1832, 1849, and 1866*. Chicago: University of Chicago Press, 1962.

Ryan, F., and J. Rybolt. *Vincent de Paul and Louise de Marillac: Rules, Conferences, and Writings*. Mahwah, NJ: Paulist Press, 1995.

Salesia Godecker, Sister Mary. *Bishop Simon Gabriel Bruté de Remur, First Bishop of Vincennes*. St. Meinrad, IN: St. Meinrad Historical Essays, 1931. Archives of the Daughters of Charity, St. Joseph's Provincial House, Emmitsburg, MD, # 7-8-2-3:263.

Schipp, Rev. John. "Bishop Simon Bruté de Remur—Wall Case Exhibits." Old Cathedral Library and Museum, Vincennes, IN.

Sheppard, T., Jacob Deems, and Peter Foy. Report of the Commissioners of Health, Baltimore City Health Department, 1815–1849. 1832. Maryland State Archives, Baltimore, MD.

Sisters of Charity. *The Rule of 1812: Regulations for the Society of Sisters of Charity in the United States of America*, 1812. Archives of St. Joseph's Provincial House.

Sullivan, Louise, DC. , ed. and trans. *Louise de Marillac Spiritual Writings: Correspondence and Thoughts*. New York: New City Press, 1991.

Warner, Augustus. Account of the Cholera in Baltimore: A Journal of Admissions at Hospital No. 3. 1832. Archives of the Daughters of Charity, St. Joseph's Provincial House, Emmitsburg, MD. #7-7-1-1.

Chapter 3 – Bibliography

Abelly, Louis. *The Life of the Venerable Servant of God Vincent de Paul*. 3 vols. New Rochelle, NY: New City Press, 1993. Originally published 1664 in French.

Andrew, Thomas. *A Cyclopedia of Domestic Medicine and Surgery*. Glasgow, Scotland: Blackie and Son, 1842. Accessed Google Books.com.

Applebaum, Paul, and Kathleen Kemp. "The Evolution of Commitment Law in the Nineteenth Century." *Law and Human Behavior* 6, no. 3/4 (1982): 343–54.

Armiger, Bernadette. "The History of the Hospital Work of the Daughters of Charity of St. Vincent de Paul in the Eastern Province of the United States 1823–1860." The Catholic University of America, 1947. Archives of the Daughters of Charity, St. Joseph's Provincial House, Emmitsburg, MD.

Baker, Paula. "The Domestication of Politics: Women and American Political Society, 1780–1920." *American Historical Review* 89, no. 3 (1984): 620–47.

Brigham, Amariah. "Definition of Insanity–Nature of the Disease." *American Journal of Insanity* 1 (October 1844): 97–116. Archives of the American Psychiatric Association.

———. "The Moral Treatment of Insanity." *American Journal of Insanity* 4, no. 1 (1847): 1–15. Archives of the American Psychiatric Association.

———. *Remarks on the Influence of Mental Cultivation Upon Health*. Boston: Marsh, Capen & Lyon, 1833. Google Books.

Brown, Thomas. *Dorothea Dix: A New England Reformer*. Cambridge, MA: Harvard University Press, 1998.

Buttolph, H. "Modern Asylums." *American Journal of Insanity* 3, no. 4 (1847): 364–78. Archives of the American Psychiatric Association.

Bynum, W. F. *Science and the Practice of Medicine in the Nineteenth Century*. Cambridge: Cambridge University Press, 1994.

Cassedy, James. *American Medicine and Statistical Thinking, 1800–1860*. Cambridge, MA: Harvard University Press, 1984.

Catholic Church of the United States. *The United States Catholic Almanac, or, Laity's Directory for the Year*. University of Notre Dame Library, Microfilm Collection. 1817, 1822, 1833–ongoing.

Clark, Mother Mary Xavier. *Instruction on the Care of the Sick*, Archives of Daughters of Charity of St. Vincent de Paul—West Central Province, St. Louis, MO., 1846.

Collins, Sister Josephine. Correspondence to Sister Margaret. October 13, 1840. Archives of the Daughters of Charity, St. Joseph's Provincial House, Emmitsburg, MD, 7-10-2 #76.

———. Correspondence to Sister Margaret. November 1, 1840. Archives of the Daughters of Charity, St. Joseph's Provincial House, Emmitsburg, MD, 7-10-2 #77.

Coskery, Sister Matilda. *Cradle of Mount Hope: Historical Account of Mt. St. Vincent Hospital / Mount Hope Retreat*. n.d. Archives of the Daughters of Charity, St. Joseph's Provincial House, Emmitsburg, MD, #11-2-39.

Coste, Pierre. *Saint Vincent de Paul: Correspondance, Entretiens, Documents*. Paris: Lecoffre and Gabaldo, 1924. Archives of the Daughters of Charity, St. Joseph's Provincial House, Emmitsburg, MD.

Coste, Pierre, CM, and Vincent de Paul. *Saint Vincent de Paul: Correspondence, Conferences, Documents*. Edited and translated by Jacqueline Kilar, DC, and Marie Poole, DC. 14 vols. New York: New City Press, 1985–2008. Archives of the Daughters of Charity, St. Joseph's Provincial House, Emmitsburg, MD.

Daughters of Charity. Annals of the Community. 1846. Souvay Collection-III A. DeAndreis-Rosati Memorial Archives, DePaul University, Chicago, IL.

———. Corporation Minutes. Archives of the Daughters of Charity, St. Joseph's Provincial House, Emmitsburg, MD.

———. Council Minutes. Archives of the Daughters of Charity, St. Joseph's Provincial House, Emmitsburg, MD, #3-3-5.

———. Deed to Mount Hope College. 1844. Archives of the Daughters of Charity, St. Joseph's Provincial House, Emmitsburg, MD, #7-9-3, 413.

———. *Lives of the Deceased Sisters*. Emmitsburg, MD, 1870. Archives of the Daughters of Charity, St. Joseph's Provincial House, Emmitsburg, MD.

———. Mt. Hope Receipt Book. 1847–1851. Archives of the Daughters of Charity, St. Joseph's Provincial House, Emmitsburg, MD, #11-2-39:4.

———. Provincial Annals. Archives of the Daughters of Charity, Saint Joseph's Provincial House, Emmitsburg, MD, 7–8.

———. "Remarks on Sister Nicole Lequin." *Circulars and Notices* 2 (April 17, 1703): 554. Archives of the Daughters of Charity, St. Joseph's Provincial House, Emmitsburg, MD.

Digby, Anne. *Madness, Morality, and Medicine: A Study of the York Retreat, 1796–1914*. New York: Cambridge University Press, 1985.

———. "Moral Treatment at the Retreat, 1796–1846." In *The Anatomy of Madness*, edited by W. F. Bynum, Roy Porter, and Michael Shepherd, 52–72. London: Tavistock Publications, 1985.

Dix, Dorothea. *Memorial of Miss D. L. Dix to the Hon. General Assembly in Behalf of the Insane of Maryland, Archives of the State of Maryland*, 1852. Archives of the State of Maryland Web site: http://www.msa.md.gov/

Earle, Pliny. "On the Causes of Insanity." *American Journal of Insanity* 4, no. 3 (1848): 185–211. Archives of the American Psychiatric Association.

Flinton, Margaret. *Louise de Marillac, Social Aspect of Her Work*. New York: New City Press, 1992.

Grob, Gerald. *Edward Jarvis and the Medical World of Nineteenth-Century America*. Knoxville: University of Tennessee Press, 1978.

———. *The Mad Among Us: A History of the Care of America's Mentally Ill*. Cambridge, MA: Harvard University Press, 1994.

———. "The State Mental Hospital in Mid-Nineteenth Century America: A Social Analysis." *American Psychologist* 21, no. 6 (1966): 510–23.

Hannefin, Daniel. *Daughters of the Church: A Popular History of the Daughters of Charity in the United States, 1809–1987*. New York: New City Press, 1989.

Haw, Camilla. "John Conolly's Attendants at the Hanwell Asylum, 1839–1852." *History of Nursing Society Journal* 3, no. 1 (1990): 26–58.

Jones, Colin. "Sisters of Charity and the Ailing Poor." *Social History of Medicine* 2, no. 3 (1989): 339–48.

———. "The Treatment of the Insane in Eighteenth and Early Nineteenth-Century Montpellier: A Contribution to the Prehistory of the Lunatic Asylum in Provincial France." *Medical History* 24 (1980): 371–90.

Libster, Martha. "Elements of Care: Nursing Environmental Theory in Historical Context." *Holistic Nursing Practice* 22, no. 3 (2008): 160–70.

———. *Herbal Diplomats: The Contribution of Early American Nurses (1830–1860) to 19ᵗʰ Century Healthcare Reform and the Botanical Medical Movement*. www.GoldenApplePublications.com: Golden Apple Publications, 2004.

Louise de Marillac Spiritual Writings: Correspondence and Thoughts. Edited and translated by Louise Sullivan, DC. New York: New City Press, 1991.

Makari, George. "Educated Insane: A Nineteenth-Century Psychiatric Paradigm." *Journal of the History of the Behavioral Sciences* 29 (1993): 8–21.

Northrup, Christiane. *Women's Bodies, Women's Wisdom: Creating Physical and Emotional Health and Healing*. New York: Bantam Books, 1994.

Other Healers: Unorthodox Medicine in America. Edited by Norman Gevitz. Baltimore, MD: Johns Hopkins University Press, 1988.

Risse, Guenter, Ronald Numbers, and Judith Leavitt. *Medicine without Doctors: Home Health Care in American History*. New York: Science History Publications, 1977.

Robinson, Alex. "Report of the Lunatic Department of the Baltimore Alms-House." J. Robinson, 1841. Maryland State Archives.

Rosenberg, Charles E. *The Care of Strangers: The Rise of America's Hospital System*. New York: Basic Books, 1987.

Sewall, Jane. *Medicine in Maryland: The Practice and the Profession, 1799–1999*. Baltimore, MD: The Johns Hopkins University Press, 1999.

Sisters of Charity. *The Rule of 1812: Regulations for the Society of Sisters of Charity in the United States of America*, 1812. Archives of the Daughters of Charity, St. Joseph's Provincial House, Emmitsburg, MD.

Smith, William. "Facts and Arguments in Support of 'the Humane System of Non-Restraint in the Treatment of the Insane.'" *Lancet* 1166 (January 3, 1846): 13–15. Wellcome Trust Library, London.

Stokes, William. *38th Annual Report of the Mount Hope Retreat*. 1880. Archives of the Daughters of Charity, St. Joseph's Provincial House, Emmitsburg, MD.

———. *The Eleventh Annual Report of the Mount Hope Institution near Baltimore*. 1853. Archives of the Daughters of Charity, St. Joseph's Provincial House, Emmitsburg, MD.

———. *First Annual Report of the Physician of the Mount Saint Vincent's Hospital for 1843.* 1844. Archives of the Daughters of Charity, St. Joseph's Provincial House, Emmitsburg, MD, #11-2-39.

———. *Report of the Mount Hope Institution for the Year 1845.* 1846. Archives of the Daughters of Charity, St. Joseph's Provincial House, Emmitsburg, MD.

———. *Second Annual Report of the Physician of Mount Hope Hospital (Late Mount St. Vincent's) for 1844.* 1845. Archives of the Daughters of Charity, St. Joseph's Provincial House, Emmitsburg, MD, #11-2-39.

Verbrugge, Martha H. *Able-Bodied Womanhood: Personal Health and Social Change in Nineteenth-Century Boston.* New York: Oxford University Press, 1988.

Vogel, Morris J., and Charles E. Rosenberg. *The Therapeutic Revolution: Essays in the Social History of American Medicine.* Philadelphia: University of Pennsylvania Press, 1979.

Chapter 4 – Bibliography

Beck, Romeyn. "Proceedings of the Eighth Annual Meeting of the Association of Medical Superintendents of American Institutions for the Insane." *American Journal of Insanity* 10, no. 1 (1853): 70–89. Archives of the American Psychiatric Association.

———. "Proceedings of the Sixth Annual Meeting of Medical Superintendents of American Institutions for the Insane." *American Journal of Insanity* 8, no. 1 (1851): 82–93. Archives of the American Psychiatric Association.

Brigham, Amariah. "Dr. William Stokes, of the Mount Hope Institution, near Baltimore, Md., and the *American Journal of Insanity.*" *American Journal of Insanity* 5, no. 3 (1849): 262–80. Archives of the American Psychiatric Association.

———. "Editorial Correspondence." *American Journal of Insanity* 5, no. 1 (1848): 63–86. Archives of the American Psychiatric Association.

Brown, Sister Rosaline. *Sister Rosaline Brown's Narrative of the First Mission in Detroit.* 1844–1854. Daughters of Charity Archives, Mater Dei Provincialate, Evansville, IN.

Buttolph, H. "Modern Asylums." *American Journal of Insanity* 3, no. 4 (1847): 364–78. Archives of the American Psychiatric Association.

Closs, S. J. "Interdisciplinary Research and the Doctor-Nurse Game." *Clinical Effectiveness in Nursing* 5 (2001): 101–03.

Coskery, Sister Matilda. *Advices Concerning the Sick.* Emmitsburg, MD: Archives of Daughters of Charity, St. Joseph's Provincial House, n.d. c. 1840.

———. *Cradle of Mount Hope: Historical Account of Mt. St. Vincent Hospital/Mount Hope Retreat.* n.d. Archives of the Daughters of Charity, St. Joseph's Provincial House, Emmitsburg, MD, #11-2-39

D'Antonio, Patricia. *Founding Friends: Families, Staff, and Patients at the Friends Asylum in Early Nineteenth-Century Philadelphia.* Bethlehem, PA: Lehigh University Press, 2006.

Daughter of Charity, Name Unknown. Providence Retreat, Buffalo, New York, an Oral History. 1885. Archives of the Daughters of Charity of St. Vincent de Paul, Northeast Province, Albany, NY.

Daughters of Charity. Council Minutes. Archives of the Daughters of Charity, St. Joseph's Provincial House, Emmitsburg, MD, #3-3-5.

———. *Lives of the Deceased Sisters.* Emmitsburg, MD, 1870. Archives of the Daughters of Charity, St. Joseph's Provincial House, Emmitsburg, MD.

———. *Lives of the Deceased Sisters.* Emmitsburg, Maryland, 1870–1879. Archives of the Daughters of Charity, St. Joseph's Provincial House, Emmitsburg, MD.

Didier, Eugene. Report of the Trial of Dr. Wm. H. Stokes and Mary Blenkinsop, Physician and Sister Superior of Mount Hope Institution before the Circuit Court from Baltimore Co., Md. 1866. Maryland State Archives, Annapolis, MD.

Finegan, John. How a Patient Remembers, a Letter to a Sister at St. Mary's Hospital Detroit. 1878. Daughters of Charity Archives, Mater Dei Provincialate, Evansville, IN.

Galt, John. "Report on the Organization of Asylums for the Insane." *American Journal of Insanity* 7, no. 1 (1850): 45–53. Archives of the American Psychiatric Association.

Haw, Camilla. "John Conolly's Attendants at the Hanwell Asylum, 1839–1852." *History of Nursing Society Journal* 3, no. 1 (1990): 26–58.

Higgins, J. M. "On the Necessity of a Resident Medical Superintendent in an Institution for the Insane." *American Journal of Insanity* 7, no. 1 (1850): 64–69. Archives of the American Psychiatric Association.

Jones, Colin. "Sisters of Charity and the Ailing Poor." *Social History of Medicine* 2, no. 3 (1989): 339–48.

Martin, Edward G. *Early Detroit: St. Mary's Hospital 1845–1945.* Detroit, MI: St. Mary's Hospital, 1945.

Nightingale, Florence. *Notes on Nursing: What It Is and What It Is Not.* Edinburgh, Scotland: Churchill Livingstone, 1980. Original publication, 1859.

Pillitteri, Adele, and Michael Ackerman. "The 'Doctor-Nurse Game': A Comparison of 100 Years—1888–1990." *Nursing Outlook* 41, no. 3 (1993): 113–16.

Providence Hospital and Medical Centers, and St. Vincent and Sarah Fisher Center. *Caritas Christi: 1844–1994 (The Daughters of Charity of St. Vincent De Paul—150 Years of Service to Detroit).* Detroit, MI: Providence Hospital and Medical Centers and St. Vincent and Sarah Fisher Center, 1994.

Reed, Sister Ann Aloysia. An Incident in the Hospital Life of Sr. Rebecca Delone [*sic*] as Related by Her Companion and Eye Witness, Sister Felicia Fenwick. n.d. Daughters of Charity Archives, Mater Dei Provincialate, Evansville, IN.

Stein, Leonard, David Watts, and Timothy Howell. "The Doctor-Nurse Game Revisited." *New England Journal of Medicine* 322, no. 8 (1990): 546–49.

Sweet, Sarah, and Ian Norman. "The Nurse-Doctor Relationship: A Selective Literature Review." *Journal of Advanced Nursing* 22 (1995): 165–70.

Tiffany, Francis. *The Life of Dorothea Lynde Dix.* Boston: Houghton, Mifflin & Co., 1891. Google Books.

Unknown. "Obituary, Dr. Amariah Brigham." *American Journal of Insanity* 6, no. 2 (1849): 185–92. Archives of the American Psychiatric Association.

Chapter 5 – Bibliography

Abram, Ruth J. *Send Us a Lady Physician: Women Doctors in America, 1835–1920.* New York: Norton, 1985.

Andrew, Thomas. *A Cyclopedia of Domestic Medicine and Surgery.* Glasgow, Scotland: Blackie and Son, 1842. Accessed Google Books.com.

Armiger, Bernadette. "The History of the Hospital Work of the Daughters of Charity of St. Vincent de Paul in the Eastern Province of the United States 1823–1860." The Catholic University of America, 1947. Archives of the Daughters of Charity, St. Joseph's Provincial House, Emmitsburg, MD.

Barlow, John. "On Man's Power over Himself to Prevent or Control Insanity." *American Journal of Insanity* 1 (1845): 289–319.

Beach, Wooster. *The Family Physician, or, the Reformed System of Medicine on Vegetable or Botanic Principles Being a Compendium of the "American Practice" Designed for All Classes.* 4th ed. New York: Published by the author, 1843. Lloyd Library, Cincinnati, OH.

Bechtle, Regina, S.C., and Judith Metz, S.C., eds., and Ellin Kelly, mss. ed. *Elizabeth Bayley Seton: Collected Writings.* 3 vols. Hyde Park, NY: New City Press, 2000–2006.

Beck, Romeyn. "Proceedings of the Eighth Annual Meeting of the Association of Medical Superintendents of American Institutions for the Insane." *American Journal of Insanity* 10, no. 1 (1853): 70–89. Archives of the American Psychiatric Association.

Beecher, Catharine E. *Miss Beecher's Domestic Receipt-Book.* New York: Dover Publications, 2001. Originally published 1858.

Beecher, Catharine Esther, and Harriet Beecher Stowe. *The American Woman's Home or, Principles of Domestic Science: Being a Guide to the Formation and Maintenance of Economical, Healthful, Beautiful, and Christian Homes.* Piscataway, NJ: Rutgers University Press, 2002. Originally published 1869.

Bigelow, Jacob. "Discourse on Self-Limited Diseases." In *Nature in Disease: Illustrated in Various Discourses and Essays.* Boston: Phillips, Sampson, and Company, 1835. Medical Communications of the Massachusetts Medical Society, Lloyd Library, Cincinnati, OH.

Blumenthal, Mark, Bundesinstitut für Arzneimittel und Medizinprodukte (Germany), and Commission E. *Herbal Medicine Expanded Commission E Monographs.* Newton, MA: Integrative Medicine Communications, 2000.

Brigham, Amariah. "Dr. William Stokes, of the Mount Hope Institution, near Baltimore, MD. And the American Journal of Insanity." *American Journal of Insanity* 5, no. 3 (1849): 262–80. Archives of the American Psychiatric Association.

———. "Lunatic Asylums of the United States." *American Journal of Insanity* 2, no. July (1845): 46–68.

———. "The Medical Treatment of Insanity." *American Journal of Insanity* 3, no. 4 (1847): 353–58. Archives of the American Psychiatric Association.

Brown, Edward. "'What Shall We Do with the Inebriate?' Asylum Treatment and the Disease Concept of Alcoholism in the Late Nineteenth Century." *Journal of the History of the Behavioral Sciences* 21, no. January (1985): 48–59.

Buchan, William. *Domestic Medicine; or, the Family Physician: Being an Attempt to Render the Medical Art More Generally Useful, by Shewing People What Is in Their Own Power Both with Respect to the Prevention and Cure of Diseases. Chiefly Calculated to Recommend a Proper Attention to Regimen and Simple Medicines.* Edinburgh, Scotland: Printed by Balfour, Auld, and Smellie, 1769. Wellcome Trust Library, London.

Burke, Gerald. "Caring for the Medically Ill Psychiatric Patient on a Psychiatric Unit." *Psychiatric Annals* 13, no. 8 (1983): 627–34.

Bynum, W. F. *Science and the Practice of Medicine in the Nineteenth Century.* Cambridge: Cambridge University Press, 1994.

Byrne, Ambrose. "History of The Seton Institute, Baltimore, Maryland and Its Affiliate School of Nursing Conducted by the Daughters of Charity of St. Vincent de Paul in the Eastern Province of the United States." The Catholic University of America, 1950.

Catholic Church of the United States. *The United States Catholic Almanac, or, Laity's Directory for the Year.* University of Notre Dame Library, Microfilm Collection. 1817, 1822, 1833–ongoing.

Child, Lydia Maria. *The Family Nurse.* Bedford, MA: Applewood Books, 1997. Originally published 1837.

Christman, Luther. "Who Is a Nurse?" *Image: Journal of Nursing Scholarship* 30, no. 3 (1998): 211–14.

Clark, Mother Mary Xavier. *Instruction on the Care of the Sick,* Archives of Daughters of Charity of St. Vincent de Paul - West Central Province, St. Louis, MO., 1846.

Cleaveland, C. "Nurses." *The Eclectic Medical Journal* 4, no. 8 (1852): 371–73.

Coskery, Felix. "Fever." University of Maryland, 1836. Health Sciences and Human Services Library, University of Maryland.

Coskery, Sister Matilda. Correspondence: Letter to Rev. Henry B. Coskery. Rochester, NY, April 18,1849. Archives of the Archdiocese of Baltimore, Coskery Collection.

———. Correspondence: Letter to Rev. Henry B. Coskery on the Death of Archbishop Samuel Eccleston of Baltimore. Detroit, MI, April 28, 1851. Archives of Archdiocese, St. Mary's Seminary and University.

———. *Cradle of Mount Hope: Historical Account of Mt. St. Vincent Hospital / Mount Hope Retreat*. n.d. Archives of the Daughters of Charity, St. Joseph's Provincial House, Emmitsburg, MD, #11-2-39.

Coste, Pierre. *Saint Vincent de Paul: Correspondance, Entretiens, Documents*. Paris: Lecoffre and Gabaldo, 1924.

Coste, Pierre, CM, and Vincent de Paul. *Saint Vincent de Paul: Correspondence, Conferences, Documents*. Edited and translated by Jacqueline Kilar, DC, and Marie Poole, DC. 14 vols. New York: New City Press, 1985–2008.

Crogan, Neva, and Bronwynne Evans. "Nutrition Assessment: Experience Is Not a Predictor of Knowledge." *Journal of Continuing Education in Nursing* 32, no. 5 (2001): 219–22.

Daughters of Charity. *Lives of the Deceased Sisters*. Emmitsburg, MD, 1870. Archives of the Daughters of Charity, St. Joseph's Provincial House, Emmitsburg, MD.

Dewees, William. *A Practice of Physic: Comprising Most of the Diseases Not Treated in "Diseases of Females" and "Diseases of Children."* Philadelphia: Carey, Lea & Blanchard, 1833. Laupus Library-History Collection, East Carolina University.

Editors. Critical Review of Dewees' "A Practice of Physic". *London Medical and Surgical Journal*, 5, no. 26 (1830): 91. Google Books.

Falret, Henri. "On the Construction and Organization of Establishments for the Insane." *American Journal of Insanity* 10, no. 4 (1854): 405–35. Archives of the American Psychiatric Association.

Felter, Harvey Wickes, and John Uri Lloyd. *King's American Dispensatory*. 18th ed., 3d rev. ed. Sandy, OR Eclectic Medical Publications, 1983.

Grieve, M. *A Modern Herbal*. New York: Dover Publications, 1971.

Griffith, R. E., and Anthony Todd Thomson. *The Domestic Management of the Sick-Room Necessary, in Aid of Medical Treatment, for the Cure of Diseases*. 1st American from the second London ed. Philadelphia: Lea and Blanchard, 1845. Countway Library at Harvard University, Cambridge, MA.

Gunn, John C. *Gunn's Domestic Medicine or Poor Man's Friend in the Hours of Affliction, Pain and Sickness*. Philadelphia, PA: G. V. Raymond, 1839. Countway Library at Harvard University, Cambridge, MA.

Hannefin, Daniel. *Daughters of the Church: A Popular History of the Daughters of Charity in the United States, 1809–1987*. New York: New City Press, 1989.

Hardy, Sally, Angie Titchen, Kim Manley, and Brendan McCormack. "Re-Defining Nursing Expertise in the United Kingdom." *Nursing Science Quarterly* 19, no. 3 (2006): 260–64.

Harmer, B. *Text-Book of the Principles and Practice of Nursing*. New York: Macmillan Co., 1924. Denison Library, University of Colorado.

Harmer, B., and V. Henderson. *Textbook of the Principles and Practice of Nursing*. New York: Macmillan Co.,1955.

Humphrey, Sheila. *The Nursing Mother's Herbal*. Minneapolis, MN: Fairview Press, 2003.

Hunt, E. K. "Statistics of Suicides in the United States." *American Journal of Insanity* 1, no. January (1845): 225–34. Archives of the American Psychiatric Association.

Jefferson, Thomas, Adrienne Koch, and William Harwood Peden. *The Life and Selected Writings of Thomas Jefferson*. New York: The Modern Library, 1944.

Leighton, Ann. *Early American Gardens "for Meate or Medicine."* Amherst: University of Massachusetts Press, 1986.

Libster, Martha. *Delmar's Integrative Herb Guide for Nurses*. Albany, NY: Delmar Thomson Learning, 2002.

———. "Elements of Care: Nursing Environmental Theory in Historical Context." *Holistic Nursing Practice* 22, no. 3 (2008): 160–70.

———. *Herbal Diplomats: The Contribution of Early American Nurses (1830-1860) to 19th Century Healthcare Reform and the Botanical Medical Movement*. www.GoldenApplePublications.com: Golden Apple Publications, 2004.

———. "Integrative Care—Product and Process: Considering the Three T's of Timing, Type and Tuning." *Complementary Therapies in Nursing and Midwifery*. 9, no. 1 (2003): 1–4.

Louise de Marillac Spiritual Writings: Correspondence and Thoughts. Translated and edited by Louise Sullivan, DC. New York: New City Press, 1991.

Maciocia, Giovanni. *Tongue Diagnosis in Chinese Medicine*. Seattle, WA: Eastland Press, 1987.

Martinez, Ruby, and Dana Murphy-Parker. "Examining the Relationship of Addiction Education and Beliefs of Nursing Students toward Persons with Alcohol Problems." *Archives of Psychiatric Nursing* 17, no. 4 (2003): 156–64.

Meehan, Therese. "Careful Nursing: A Model for Contemporary Nursing Practice." *Journal of Advanced Nursing* 44, no. 1 (2003): 99–107.

Miller, James. *Case Notes—Josiah Manty. 1833-1837*. The Alms-House Medical Records, H. Furlong Baldwin Library, Maryland Historical Society, Baltimore, MD, MS# 2474.

Mott, Elizabeth. *The Ladies Medical Oracle; or, Mrs. Mott's Advice to Young Females, Wives, and Mothers; Being a Non-Medical Commentary on the Cause, Prevention, and Cure of Diseases of the Female Frame Together with an Explanation of Her System of European Vegetable Medicine for the Cure of Diseases and the Patent Medicated Champoo Baths*. Boston: Samuel N. Dickinson, 1834. Schlesinger Library, Cambridge, MA.

Munro, Cindy, and Mary Jo Grap. "Oral Health and Care in the Intensive Care Unit: State of the Science." *American Journal of Critical Care* 13, no. 1 (2004): 25–33.

Murphy-Parker, Dana, and Ruby Martinez. "Nursing Students' Personal Experiences Involving Alcohol Problems." *Archives of Psychiatric Nursing* 19, no. 3 (2005): 150–58.

National Marine Sanctuaries. 2005. "Our Whaling Pasts." In http://sanctuaries.noaa.gov/maritime/whaling.html.

Nightingale, Florence. *Notes on Nursing: What It Is and What It Is Not*. Edinburgh, Scotland: Churchill Livingstone, 1980. Originally published 1859.

Orem, D. *Nursing Concepts of Practice*. 6th ed. St. Louis, MO: Mosby, 2001.

Outhouse, Trent. "Tongue Scraping for Treating Halitosis." The Cochrane Database of Systematic Reviews 1 (2006).

Price Herndl, Diane. *Invalid Women: Figuring Feminine Illness in American Fiction and Culture, 1840–1940*. Chapel Hill: University of North Carolina Press, 1993.

Rawlins, Carol, and Ian Trueman. "Effective Mouth Care for Seriously Ill Patients." *Professional Nurse* 16, no. 4 (2001): 1025–28.

Risse, Guenter, Ronald Numbers, and Judith Leavitt, eds. *Medicine without Doctors: Home Health Care in American History*. New York: Science History Publications, 1977.

Roberts, Kathryn. "A Comparison of Chilled Cabbage Leaves and Chilled Gelpaks in Reducing Breast Engorgement." *Journal of Human Lactation* 11, no. 1 (1995): 17–20.

Rosenberg, Charles E. *The Care of Strangers: The Rise of America's Hospital System*. New York: Basic Books, 1987.

Rothstein, William G. *American Physicians in the Nineteenth Century: From Sects to Science*. Baltimore, MD: Johns Hopkins University Press, 1972.

Rundell, Maria Eliza. *American Domestic Cookery Formed on Principles of Economy for the Use of Private Families*. New York: Evert Duyckince, 1823. Archives of the Daughters of Charity, St. Joseph's Provincial House, Emmitsburg, MD. File: Sister M. Felicita Dellone.

Scudder, John. *Domestic Medicine or Home Book of Health: A Popular Treatise on Anatomy, Physiology, Hygiene, Materia Medica, Surgery, Practice of Medicine, and Nursing*. Vol.1. Cincinnati, OH: J. R. Hawley & Co., 1865. Lloyd Library, Cincinnati, OH.

Silver-Isenstadt, Jean L. *Shameless: The Visionary Life of Mary Gove Nichols*. Baltimore, MD: Johns Hopkins University Press, 2002.

Sisters of Charity. *The Rule of 1812: Regulations for the Society of Sisters of Charity in the United States of America, 1812*. Archives of the Daughters of Charity, St. Joseph's Provincial House, Emmitsburg, MD.

Smith, Francis Gurney. *Domestic Medicine, Surgery, and Materia Medica with Directions for the Diet and Management of the Sick Room*. Philadelphia: Lindsay and Blakiston, 1851. Lloyd Library, Cincinnati, OH.

Stokes, William. *The Eighth Annual Report of the Mount Hope Institution, near Baltimore, for the Year 1850*. 1851. Archives of the Daughters of Charity, St. Joseph's Provincial House, Emmitsburg, MD.

———. *First Annual Report of the Physician of the Mount Saint Vincent's Hospital for 1843*. 1844. Archives of the Daughters of Charity, St. Joseph's Provincial House, Emmitsburg, MD # 11-2-39.

———. *The Fortieth Annual Report of the Mount Hope Retreat, for the Year 1884*. 1883. Archives of the Daughters of Charity, St. Joseph's Provincial House, Emmitsburg, MD.

———. *The Forty-Second Annual Report of the Mount Hope Retreat, for the Year 1884*. 1885. Archives of the Daughters of Charity, St. Joseph's Provincial House, Emmitsburg, MD.

———. *Fourth Annual Report of the Mount Hope Institution for the Year 1846*. 1847. Archives of the Daughters of Charity, St. Joseph's Provincial House, Emmitsburg, MD.

———. *The Sixth Annual Report of the Mount Hope Institution near Baltimore, for the Year 1848*. 1849. Archives of the Daughters of Charity, St. Joseph's Provincial House, Emmitsburg, MD.

———. *Tenth Annual Report of the Mount Hope Institution for the Year 1852*. 1853. Archives of the Daughters of Charity, St. Joseph's Provincial House, Emmitsburg, MD.

Stotts, Nancy, DeAnn Englert, Kathleen Crocker, Nancy Bennum, and Mary Hoppe. "Nutrition Education in Schools of Nursing in the United States. Part 2: The Status of Nutrition Education in Schools of Nursing." *Journal of Parenteral and Enteral Nutrition* 11, no. 4 (1987): 406–11.

Stribling, Francis. "Qualifications and Duties of Attendants on the Insane." *American Journal of Insanity* 9, no. 2 (1852): 97–103. Archives of the American Psychiatric Association.

Taylor, Susan. "The Development of Self-Care Deficit Nursing Theory: An Historical Analysis." *Self Care and Dependent-Care Nursing* 15, no. 1 (2007): 22–25.

Tetuan, Theresa. "The Role of the Nurse in Oral Health." *The Kansas Nurse* 79, no. 10 (2004): 1–2.

Theophano, Janet. *Eat My Words: Reading Women's Lives through the Cookbooks They Wrote*. New York: Palgrave, 2002.

Walter, John, and Jane Peller. *Becoming Solution-Focused in Brief Therapy*. New York: Brunner/Mazel, 1992.

Weaver, William. *Sauer's Herbal Cures: America's First Book of Botanical Healing, 1762–1778*. New York: Routledge, 2001.

Webster, Thomas, Mrs. Parkes, and D. Meredith Reese. *An Encyclopedia of Domestic Economy: Comprising Such Subjects as Are Most Immediately Connected with Housekeeping; as, the Construction of Domestic Edifices, with the Modes of Warming, Ventilating, and Lighting Them; a Description of the Various Articles of Furniture; a General Account of the Animal and Vegetable Substances Used in Food, and the Methods of Preserving and Preparing Them by Cooking; Making Bread; Materials Employed in Dress and Toilet; Business of the Laundry; Description of the Various Wheel-Carriages; Preservation of Health; Domestic Medicines, &C*. New York: Harper & Brothers, 1845. Old Sturbridge Village Research Library, Sturbridge, MA.

Weiss, Herold. "Foot Washing in the Johannine Community." *Novum Testamentum* 21, no. Fasc. 4 (1979): 298–325.

White, George, and Mirna Armaleh. "Tongue Scraping as a Means of Reducing Oral Mutans Streptococci." *The Journal of Clinical Pediatric Dentistry* 28, no. 2 (2004): 163–66.

Wood, George, and Franklin Bache. *The Dispensatory of the United States of America*. Philadelphia: Grigg & Elliot, 1839. Lloyd Library, Cincinnati, OH.

Woodward, Samuel. "Observations on the Medical Treatment of Insanity." *American Journal of Insanity* 7, no. 1 (1850): 1–34. Archives of the American Psychiatric Association.

Chapter 6 – Bibliography

Abelly, Louis. *The Life of the Venerable Servant of God Vincent de Paul.* 3 vols. New Rochelle, NY: New City Press, 1993. Originally published 1664 in French.

The American Vincentians: A Popular History of the Congregation of the Mission in the United States, 1815–1987. Edited by John Rybolt. NY: New City Press, 1988.

Baker, Paula. "The Domestication of Politics: Women and American Political Society, 1780–1920." *American Historical Review* 89, no. 3 (1984): 620–47.

Beecher, Catharine Esther, and Harriet Beecher Stowe. *The American Woman's Home or, Principles of Domestic Science: Being a Guide to the Formation and Maintenance of Economical, Healthful, Beautiful, and Christian Homes.* Piscataway, NJ: Rutgers University Press, 2002. Originally published in 1869.

Boyle, Bernard. Mother Ann Simeon's Death. 1866. Archives of the Daughters of Charity, St. Joseph's Provincial House, Emmitsburg, MD.

Byrne, Ambrose. "History of The Seton Institute, Baltimore, Maryland and Its Affiliate School of Nursing Conducted by the Daughters of Charity of St. Vincent de Paul in the Eastern Province of the United States." The Catholic University of America, 1950.

Catholic Church of the United States. *The United States Catholic Almanac, or, Laity's Directory for the Year.* University of Notre Dame Library, Microfilm Collection. 1817, 1822, 1833–ongoing.

Coskery, Sister Matilda. *Civil War Notes.* 1866. Archives of the Daughters of Charity, St. Joseph's Provincial House, Emmitsburg, MD.

———. *Cradle of Mount Hope: Historical Account of Mt. St. Vincent Hospital / Mount Hope Retreat.* n.d. Archives of the Daughters of Charity, St. Joseph's Provincial House, Emmitsburg, MD, #11-2-39.

Coste, Pierre. *Saint Vincent de Paul: Correspondance, Entretiens, Documents.* Paris: Lecoffre and Gabaldo, 1924.

Coste, Pierre, CM, and Vincent de Paul. *Saint Vincent de Paul: Correspondence, Conferences, Documents.* Edited and translated by Jacqueline Kilar, DC, and Marie Poole, DC. 14 vols. New York: New City Press, 1985–2008. Archives of the Daughters of Charity, St. Joseph's Provincial House, Emmitsburg, MD.

Cumming, Kate. *Gleanings from Southland.* Birmingham, AL: Roberts & Son, 1895.

Dalai Lama. *Ethics for the New Millennium.* New York: Riverhead Books, 1999.

D'Antonio, Patricia. "The Legacy of Domesticity." *Nursing History Review* 1 (1993): 229–46.

Daughters of Charity. *Lives of Deceased Sisters*. Emmitsburg, Maryland, 1870–1879. Archives of the Daughters of Charity, St. Joseph's Provincial House, Emmitsburg, MD.

―――. *Lives of Deceased Sisters Prior to 1969*. Emmitsburg, Maryland, 1866–1868. Archives of the Daughters of Charity, St. Joseph's Provincial House, Emmitsburg, MD.

―――. *Lives of the Deceased Sisters*. Emmitsburg, Maryland: Daughters of Charity, 1870. Archives of the Daughters of Charity, St. Joseph's Provincial House, Emmitsburg, MD.

―――. Louisa A. Norris (Mother Ann Simeon), Mission #5 Provincial Superior. Archives of the Daughters of Charity, St. Joseph's Provincial House, Emmitsburg, MD.

―――. Provincial Annals. Archives of the Daughters of Charity, Saint Joseph's Provincial House, Emmitsburg, MD, 7-8-2, 7-8-9.

Delahunt, Maureen, and Annina Sharper. July 3, 2007. Personal communication.

Dock, Lavinia L. "History of the Reform in Nursing at Bellevue Hospital." *American Journal of Nursing* 2, no. 2 (1901): 89–98.

Dock, Lavinia L., and Isabel Maitland Stewart. *A Short History of Nursing from the Earliest Times to the Present Day*. 2nd ed. New York, London: G. P. Putnam's Sons, 1925.

Dossey, Barbara Montgomery. *Florence Nightingale: Mystic, Visionary, Healer*. Springhouse, PA: Springhouse Corp, 2000.

Doyle, Ann. "Nursing by Religious Orders in the United States: Part 2, 1841–1870." *American Journal of Nursing* 29, no. 8 (1929): 959–69.

Editor. "Graduating Exercises." *Michigan Catholic*, October 15 1895. Daughters of Charity Archives, Mater Dei Provincialate, Evansville, IN.

―――. "Wanted-Trained Nurses for the Middle Class." *Journal of the American Medical Association*, no. July 10 (1909): 121–22.

Editorial. "Sick Room Needs." *The Eclectic Medical Journal* LV, no. 10 (1895): 589–90. Lloyd Library, Cincinnati, OH.

Freidson, Elliot. *Professionalism: The Third Logic*. Chicago: University of Chicago Press, 2001.

Gache, Pere Louis-Hippolyte, and Cornelius Buckley (trans.). *A Frenchman, a Chaplain, a Rebel*. Chicago: Loyola University Press, 1981.

Greenfield, Lazar. "Doctors and Nurses: A Troubled Partnership." *Annals of Surgery* 230, no. 3 (1999): 279–88.

Gross, Samuel D. *Report of the Committee on the Training of Nurses*. 1869. American Medical Association Archives, Chicago, IL.

Hoge, Jane. *The Boys in Blue: Heroes of the "Rank and File."* New York: E. B. Treat & Co., 1867. Google Books.

Jameson, Anna. *Sisters of Charity and the Communion of Labour: A Lecture Delivered Privately February 14, 1855 and Printed by Desire*. London: Longman, Brown, Green, Longmans, and Roberts, 1859. Google Books.

Keeling, Arlene Wynbeek. *Nursing and the Privilege of Prescription, 1893–2000, Women, Gender, and Health.* Columbus: Ohio State University Press, 2007.

Larson, Elaine. "The Impact of Physician-Nurse Interaction on Patient Care." *Holistic Nursing Practice* 13, no. 2 (1999): 38–46.

Libster, Martha. *Herbal Diplomats: The Contribution of Early American Nurses (1830–1860) to 19ᵗʰ Century Healthcare Reform and the Botanical Medical Movement.* www.GoldenApplePublications.com: Golden Apple Publications, 2004.

Livermore, Mary Ashton Rice. *My Story of the War: A Woman's Narrative of Four Years Personal Experience as Nurse in the Union Army, and in Relief Work at Home, in Hospitals, Camps, and at the Front During the War of the Rebellion. With Anecdotes, Pathetic Incidents, and Thrilling Reminiscences Portraying the Lights and Shadows of Hospital Life and the Sanitary Service of the War.* Hartford, CT: A. D. Worthington and Company, 1889.

Lomas, Arthur. "As It Was in the Beginning: A History of the University Hospital. Includes Reprints of the 1823 Original Correspondence between Rev. John Dubois on Behalf of the Sisters of Charity and Dr. Granville Pattison." *Bulletin of the School of Medicine University of Maryland* 23, no. 4 (1939): 182–209. University of Maryland Health Sciences and Human Services Library, Baltimore, MD.

MacDougall, Eva. "Review: A Short History of Nursing." *American Journal of Public Health* 22, no. 3 (1932): 342–43.

Maher, Mary Denis. *To Bind Up the Wounds: Catholic Sister Nurses in the U.S. Civil War.* New York: Greenwood Press, 1989.

Manthey, Marie. "The Timeless Values of Nursing." *Creative Nursing* 6, no. 1 (2000): 3–4.

Meehan, Therese. "Careful Nursing: A Model for Contemporary Nursing Practice." *Journal of Advanced Nursing* 44, no. 1 (2003): 99–107.

Melosh, Barbara. *"The Physician's Hand": Work Culture and Conflict in American Nursing.* Philadelphia: Temple University Press, 1982.

Miller, Joan, Timothy McConnell, and Troy Klinger. "Religiosity and Spirituality: Influence on Quality of Life and Perceived Patient Self-Efficacy among Cardiac Patients and Their Spouses." *Journal of Religion and Health* Online, no. September (2006): 1–15.

Nelson, S., and S. Gordon. "The Rhetoric of Rupture: Nursing as a Practice with a History?" *Nursing Outlook* 52, no. 5 (2004): 255–61.

Nightingale, Florence. "Nightingale Papers: Correspondence with Her Parents." British Library 45790, 1850–1869.

———. "Nightingale Papers Vol X Autobiographical and Other Memoranda, 34–196." British Library 43402, 1845–1860.

———. *Notes on Nursing: What It Is and What It Is Not.* Edinburgh, Scotland: Churchill Livingstone, 1980. Originally published 1859.

———. Writings. 1851–1853. British Library #43402, Florence Nightingale Papers, vol. X.

Nightingale, Florence, Michael D. Calabria, and Janet Macrae. *Suggestions for Thought.* Philadelphia: University of Pennsylvania Press, 1994.

Nightingale, Florence, Martha Vicinus, and Bea Nergaard. *Ever Yours, Florence Nightingale Selected Letters.* Cambridge, MA: Harvard University Press, 1990.

Nutting, Mary Adelaide, and Lavinia L. Dock. *A History of Nursing; the Evolution of Nursing Systems from the Earliest Times to the Foundation of the First English and American Training Schools for Nurses.* New York and London: G. P. Putnam's Sons, 1907.

Parse, Rosemarie Rizzo. *Man-Living-Health: A Theory of Nursing.* New York: Wiley, 1981.

Pike, Adele. "Moral Outrage and Moral Discourse in Nurse-Physician Collaboration." *Journal of Professional Nursing* 7, no. 6 (1991): 351–62; discussion 62–63.

Pioneer Healers: The History of Women Religious in American Health Care. Edited by M. Ursula Stepsis and Dolores Ann Liptak. New York: Crossroad, 1989.

Poovey, Mary. *Uneven Developments: The Ideological Work of Gender in Mid-Victorian England, Women in Culture and Society Series.* Chicago: University of Chicago Press, 1988.

Preston, Madge, and Virginia Beauchamp. *A Private War: Letters and Diaries of Madge Preston, 1862–1867.* New Brunswick, NJ: Rutgers University Press, 1987.

Radzyminski, Sharon. "Legal Parameters of Alternative-Complementary Modalities in Nursing Practice." *Nursing Clinics of North America* 42, no. 2 (2007): v–vi, 189–212.

Rafferty, Anne Marie. *The Politics of Nursing Knowledge.* London: Routledge, 1996.

Raines, C. Fay. Correspondence from American Association of Colleges of Nursing to American Medical Association Representatives Dr. David Lichtman and Dr. Craig Anderson, June 11, 2008.

Ramiere, Henri. *The Apostleship of Prayer: A Holy League of Christian Hearts United with the Heart of Jesus.* Baltimore, MD: John Murphy, 1866.

Reverby, Susan. *Ordered to Care: The Dilemma of American Nursing, 1850–1945.* Cambridge, NY: Cambridge University Press, 1987.

Rollins, Gina. "Medical Errors, Poor Communication Undermine Quality of Care, Patient Satisfaction." *Report on Medical Guidelines & Outcomes Research* 13, no. 10 (2002): 5–7.

Rosenberg, Charles E. *The Care of Strangers: The Rise of America's Hospital System.* New York: Basic Books, 1987.

Silvers, Robert B. *Hidden Histories of Science.* 1st ed. New York: New York Review of Books, 1995.

Vogel, Morris J., and Charles E. Rosenberg. *The Therapeutic Revolution: Essays in the Social History of American Medicine.* Philadelphia: University of Pennsylvania Press, 1979.

Wall, Barbra Mann. *Unlikely Entrepreneurs: Catholic Sisters and the Hospital Marketplace, 1865–1925, Women, Gender, and Health.* Columbus: Ohio State University Press, 2005.

Wallace, Meredith, Suzanne Campbell, Sheila Grossman, Joyce Shea, Jean Lange, and Theresa Quell. "Integrating Spirituality into Undergraduate Nursing Curricula." *International Journal of Nursing Scholarship* 5, no. 1 (2008): 1–13.

Watson, Jean. *Caring Science as Sacred Science*. Philadelphia: F. A. Davis Co., 2005.

Zwarenstein, Merrick, and Scott Reeves. "Working Together but Apart: Barriers and Routes to Nurse-Physician Collaboration." *Joint Commission Journal on Quality Improvement* 28, no. 5 (2002): 242–47.

Epilogue – Bibliography

Brown, Esther Lucille. *Newer Dimensions of Patient Care*: Part 1, The Use of the Physical Environment of the General Hospital for Therapeutic Purposes. New York: Russell Sage Foundation, 1961.

Bruté de Remur, Simon Gabriel, and Sister Loyola Law. *Rev. Simon Gabriel Bruté, Bishop of Vincennes in His Connection with the Community, 1812–1839*. Emmitsburg, MD: Daughters of Charity, 1886. Archives of the Daughters of Charity, St. Joseph's Provincial House, Emmitsburg, MD.

Coste, Pierre. *Saint Vincent de Paul: Correspondance, Entretiens, Documents*. Paris: Lecoffre and Gabaldo, 1924.

De Sales, Francis. *Introduction to the Devout Life*. New York: Vintage Books, 2002. Originally published 1609.

DeSisto, Michael, Courtenay Harding, Rodney McCormick, Takamaru Ashikaga, and George Brooks. "The Maine and Vermont Three-Decade Studies of Serious Mental Illness. Ii. Longitudinal Course Comparisons." *British Journal of Psychiatry* 167, no. 3 (1995): 338–42.

Donley, Rosemary. "Nursing at the Crossroads." *Nursing Economics* 14, no. 6 (1996): 325–31.

Emerson, Ralph Waldo. "Circles." In *Selected Essays, Lectures, and Poems*. New York: Bantam Books, 1990.

Peck, M. Scott. *The Different Drum: Community Making and Peace*. New York: Touchstone, 1987.

Ray, Marilyn, Vicki Didominic, Patricia Dittman, Patricia Hurst, Jean Seaver, Barbara Sorbello, and Michele Ross. "The Edge of Chaos: Caring and the Bottom Line." *Nursing Management* 26, no. 9 (1995): 48–50.

Snowdon, David. *Aging with Grace: What the Nun Study Teaches Us About Leading Longer, Healthier, and More Meaningful Lives*. New York: Bantam Books, 2001.

Appendix E – Bibliography

Baer, Ellen. "Nurses." In *Women Health, and Medicine in America*, edited by R. Apple, 451–467. Piscataway, NJ: Rutgers University Press, 1992.

Buhler-Wilkerson, Karen. *No Place Like Home: A History of Nursing and Home Care in the United States*. Baltimore, MD: Johns Hopkins University Press, 2001.

Child, Lydia Maria. *The Family Nurse.* Bedford, MA: Applewood Books, 1997. Originally published 1837.

D'Antonio, Patricia. *Founding Friends: Families, Staff, and Patients at the Friends Asylum in Early Nineteenth-Century Philadelphia.* Bethlehem, PA: Lehigh University Press, 2006.

Fett, Sharla M. *Working Cures: Healing, Health, and Power on Southern Slave Plantations.* Chapel Hill: University of North Carolina Press, 2002.

Fuller, Margaret. *Woman in the Nineteenth Century.* American Transcendentalism, 1843. Full Text on the Web: http://www.vcu.edu/engweb/transcendentalism/authors/fuller/woman (accessed February 2006).

Jameson, Anna. *Sisters of Charity and the Communion of Labour: A Lecture Delivered Privately February 14, 1855 and Printed by Desire.* London: Longman, Brown, Green, Longmans, and Roberts, 1859. Google Books.

Leavitt, Judith., and Numbers, Ronald., eds. *Sickness and Health in America: Readings in the History of Medicine and Public Health.* Madison: University of Wisconsin Press, 1997.

Libster, Martha. (2008). "Elements of Care: Nursing Environmental Theory in Historical Context." *Holistic Nursing Practice* 22, (no. 3) (2008): 160--70.

Libster, Martha. *Herbal Diplomats: The Contribution of Early American Nurses (1830–1860) to Nineteenth-Century Health Care Reform and the Botanical Medical Movement.* www.GoldenApplePublications.com, 2004.

Lynaugh, Joan. "Institutionalizing women's health care in nineteenth- and twentieth-century America." In *Women Health, and Medicine in America,* edited by R. Apple. Piscataway, NJ: Rutgers University Press. 1992.

McBride, Bunny. *Women of the Dawn.* Lincoln: University of Nebraska Press, 1999.

Meehan, Therese. "Careful nursing: a model for contemporary nursing practice." *Journal of Advanced Nursing,* 44 no. 1 (2003): 99–107.

Nelson, Sioban. (1997). "Reading nursing history." *Nursing Inquiry,* 4 (1997): 229--236.

Nelson, Sioban. *Say Little, Do Much: Nursing, Nuns, and Hospitals in the Nineteenth Century.* Philadelphia: University of Pennsylvania Press, 2001.

Nelson, Sioban., and Gordon, Suzanne. "The Rhetoric of Rupture: Nursing as a Practice with a History?" *Nursing Outlook,* 52, no. 5 (2004): 255–261.

Risse, Gunther., ed. *Medicine without Doctors.* New York: Science History Publications, 1977.

Rosenberg, Charles. *Right Living: An Anglo-American Tradition of Self-Help Medicine and Hygiene.* Baltimore, MD: Johns Hopkins University Press, 2003.

Sandelowski, Margarete. *Devices and Desires: Gender Technology and American Nursing.* Chapel Hill: University of North Carolina Press, 2000.

Tannenbaum, Rebecca. *The Healer's Calling: Women and Medicine in Early New England.* Ithaca, NY: Cornell University Press, 2002.

Ulrich, Laurel. *A Midwife's Tale: The Life of Martha Ballard Based on Her Diary, 1785–1812*. New York: Vintage, 1990.

Wall, Barbra M. *Unlikely Entrepreneurs: Catholic Sisters and the Hospital Marketplace, 1865–1925* Columbus: Ohio State University Press, 2005.

For a bibliography of works on historical research in nursing, see the Web site of the American Association for the History of Nursing: http://www.aahn.org/methodology.html.

Additional Readings about Vincent de Paul and Louise de Marillac – Bibliography

Coste, Pierre, *The Life & Works of Saint Vincent de Paul*, translated from the French by Joseph Leonard. Hyde Park, NY: New City Press, 1987.

Dirvin, Joseph, *Louise de Marillac of the Ladies and Daughters of Charity*. New York: Farrar, Straus, and Giroux, 1970.

Flinton, Margaret, *Louise de Marillac Social Aspect of Her Work*. Hyde Park, NY: New City Press, 1992.

Román, José María, *Vincent de Paul*, translated by Sister Joyce Howard. London: Melisende, 1999.

Index

INDEX

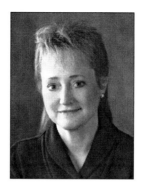

Dr. Martha Mathews Libster, Ph.D., R.N.

Dr. Martha Libster is an educator, clinical nurse specialist, healthcare historian, and "Herbal Diplomat® known internationally for her work on the complementarity of nursing practice, technology, and healing traditions, in particular the use of botanical therapies. She received the American Association for the History of Nursing 2005 Lavinia Dock Award for Outstanding Research and Writing. Dr. Libster is creative director of Golden Apple Healing Arts, LLC, (www.goldenapplehealingarts.com). She is presently the founder of the *Bamboo Bridge*, an international online community, (www.bamboobridge.org).

Dr. Libster is an international speaker on the subjects of integrative care, botanical therapies, self care, healing traditions, and the history of healthcare and health reform. She has over 20 years of clinical experience developing the integration of conventional nursing, technology, and healing traditions. She holds Bachelor degrees in dance education/ movement therapy from New York University and in nursing from Mount St. Mary's College in Los Angeles and a Master's degree in psychiatric nursing with a specialty in infant mental health from the University of Colorado Health Sciences Center. Her doctorate degree is in Humanities – Healthcare History from Oxford Brookes University, Oxford, England. Dr. Libster is presently an Associate Professor of Nursing in the Department of Graduate Nursing Science at East Carolina University in Greenville, North Carolina where she lives in a historic home and herb garden with her husband Harold and her West Highland White Terrier, Sheeva. She is the daughter of a minister, a nurse educated and inspired by the Sisters of St. Joseph of Carondelet, and a student of many religious traditions.

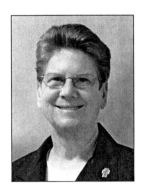

Sister Betty Ann McNeil, D.C., M.S.W.

Sister Betty Ann McNeil, D.C., a native of Virginia Beach, Virginia, entered the Daughters of Charity of Saint Vincent de Paul, Emmitsburg Province, in 1964 and earned a bachelor's degree in social welfare from Saint Joseph College, Emmitsburg, Maryland (1969), a master of social work from Virginia Commonwealth University (1975). As a clinical social worker she has worked in a variety of social ministry roles.

Sister Betty Ann served on the Advisory Committee for the publication of the multi- volume opus *Elizabeth Bayley Seton Collected Writings,* 3 vols. (New York City Press, 2000-2005). Her publications include a monograph, *The Vincentian Family Tree,* a survey of all communities bearing some relationship to Saint Vincent de Paul, Saint Louise de Marillac, and the Vincentian Family, published by the Vincentian Studies Institute (1996). Her most recent work is *15 Days of Prayer with Elizabeth Seton* (Liguori Publications: 2002). She is a contributor to the *New Catholic Encyclopedia* (Catholic University of America Press and The Gale Group: 2002). Numerous articles have been published in *Hospital Progress, Catholic Charities USA, Review for Religious, The Vincentian Heritage, Echoes of the Company of the Daughters of Charity,* and *Vincentiana.*

She has represented the Emmitsburg Province of the Daughters of Charity on the Vincentian Studies Institute of the United States since 1998 and currently serves on the Editorial Board of Vincentian Heritage for the Vincentian Studies Institute of DePaul University, Chicago. Sister Betty Ann has conducted workshops, days of reflection, and retreats internationally on topics related to the history and spirituality of the Vincentian and Setonian tradition. Currently she serves as Provincial Archivist for the Daughters of Charity, Province of Emmitsburg.

Printed in the United States
143588LV00001B/1/P